A Short History of Disease

Other books by Seán Martin

History

The Knights Templar

Alchemy and Alchemists

The Black Death

The Gnostics

The Cathars

Film

Andrei Tarkovsky

New Waves in Cinema

Poetry

The Girl Who Got onto the Ferry in Citizen Kane

A SHORT HISTORY OF DISEASE

SEÁN MARTIN

Oldcastle Books

This edition published in 2022 by
Pocket Essentials, an imprint of
Oldcastle Books Ltd, Harpenden,
Herts, UK
oldcastlebooks.com
@OldcastleBooks

Editor: Nick Rennison

A CIP catalogue record for this book is available from the British Library.

ISBN
978-0-85730-415-5 (Paperback)
978-1-84344-420-6 (eBook)

2 4 6 8 10 9 7 5 3

Typeset by Avocet Typeset, Bideford, Devon, EX39 2BP
in 11.25 on 13pt Perpetua

Printed and bound in Great Britain by Clays Elcograf S.p.A.

FSC
www.fsc.org
MIX
Paper from
responsible sources
FSC® C018072

To the memory of Waldemar Haffkine,
medical visionary and revolutionary

And for all those working in,
and fighting to save, the NHS

Acknowledgements

Thanks are due to the following: Stranger Than Fiction, the Edinburgh non-fiction writers' group; Lois Martin; Dr John Dodgson; Dr David Cavalla; Norma Milne; Ian Dorward; Glenda Martin; Maria McCann; Sarolta Tatár; Ion Mills; and Louise Milne.

Giles Perring and Christine McCourt, in whose house on Jura some of this book was written.

The staff at the National Library of Scotland in Edinburgh, and the staff at the British Library in London.

Thou shalt not be afraid for the terror by night;
nor for the arrow that flieth by day;
Nor for the pestilence that walketh in darkness;
nor for the destruction that wasteth at noonday.

Psalm 91

Contents

Introduction: Definitions, Origins

October is plague season in Madagascar. The humid rainy season begins then, and the warmer temperatures are a breeding ground for the fleas that transmit one of the world's most feared and deadly diseases. Its second pandemic, known to history as the Black Death, hit Europe in 1347 and within two years had killed a third of the population; in some places half. In isolated spots, the mortality rate was one hundred per cent.

So Malagasy authorities were naturally concerned when, in the autumn of 2013, plague began claiming more victims than usual. A rodent disease that remains endemic in many parts of the world, plague finds a conducive home on Madagascar, with the island reporting more plague deaths each year than any other part of the world save the Democratic Republic of Congo. In 2012, Madagascar had 256 plague cases, 60 of them fatal, the highest number recorded anywhere that year.

The International Committee of the Red Cross and the Pasteur Institute were becoming concerned about plague in the island's capital, Antananarivo, in particular the crowded and insanitary conditions of the city's main prison, Antanimora. Its three thousand inmates share their quarters with a thriving population of rats. Hopping from an infected rat – or other rodent – fleas take up residence in bedding, clothing and food, finding human hosts in densely crowded conditions with ease. Staff could be infected just as easily as prisoners, and they had daily contact with the outside world. Unless conditions in

Antanimora improved, the possibility of an epidemic remained.

As it turned out, the epidemic did not happen within the confines of a jail: in December, plague claimed 20 lives in the village of Mandritsara, in the island's northwest. Four other districts reported outbreaks of plague. Of the sixty or so new cases, nineteen proved fatal. Alarmingly, some of these were the more infectious pneumonic form of the disease. Although vaccines against plague have existed since the 1890s, the problem faced by the Red Cross and others in Madagascar is the difficulty in getting the medication to the affected areas – often remote villages in rural areas – in time. 2013 saw the worst outbreaks in years, and the media was soon buzzing with stories about the possible return of the Black Death, or the evolution of forms of the disease resistant to antibiotics.

The Madagascar outbreak was not the only plague outbreak to make the news. A teenage boy had fallen ill that summer, in Ichke-Zhergez, a remote village in the mountainous northeast of Kyrgyzstan, close to Lake Issyk Kul and the Kazakh border. Doctors in the regional hospital at Karakol didn't immediately realise what fifteen-year-old Temirbek Issakunov was suffering from. It was only after he died, on 22 August 2013, that they announced that Temirbek had contracted bubonic plague, probably from the bite of a flea, or eating infected meat.

No one had died from plague in Kyrgyzstan since 1981. Five days later, a young mother and her two children were hospitalised, also showing symptoms of the disease. A press conference was hurriedly called in Bishkek, where government health officials tried to quell fears that an epidemic was upon them. They pointed out that bubonic was not the most deadly form of the disease, and that these were isolated, unusual cases. But they took no chances: a state of emergency was declared, and the doctors who had treated Temirbek were quarantined, along with 105 people who had come into contact with the boy; two teams were dispatched to his home village to round up as many rodents as they could. The authorities in Kazakhstan tightened border controls, and the Chinese withdrew their athletes from the Issyk Kul Sport Games, due to start in early September.

Plague is arguably the most notorious disease in history. That it should still make the news reminds us how much of a threat diseases still represent. The 2014 Ebola outbreak in West Africa took international health authorities by surprise. The outbreak was the first time the disease – first noted in 1976 – had reached epidemic proportions. On 8 August 2014, the World Health Organization declared it a Public Health Emergency of International Concern, and took the unprecedented step of allowing untested vaccines to be used in the field.

Disease has always provoked fear, sometimes worse than the disease itself. In 627, the Chinese emperor T'ai-tsung asked Lu Tsu-shang, 'an official of talent and reputation', to become governor general of Giao province in northern Vietnam. 'You have the ability to pacify this frontier; go and defend it for me, and do not refuse on account of its being far away.' Tsu-shang thanked the emperor, but when the time came to take up the post, refused to go on the grounds that 'In the south there is much malaria; if I go there I shall never return.' Tsu-shang's fear of malaria was greater than his fear of imperial wrath. The emperor was so enraged he had Tsu-shang beheaded.[1]

It is easy to understand the concept of disease in the sense of plague – an epidemic both rapidly fatal and so notorious that it makes its presence felt both in folklore and in metaphor (to 'avoid like the plague') – but what actually *is* disease? Definitions have changed over time.

The Oxford English Dictionary defines 'disease' as:

> A condition of the body, or of some part or organ of the body, in which its functions are disturbed or deranged.
>
> The condition of being (more or less seriously) out of health; illness, sickness.
>
> An individual case or instance of such a condition; an illness, ailment, malady, disorder.[2]

The OED also notes that disease can be used in the substantive sense of an 'absence of ease'; figuratively, as 'A deranged, depraved, or morbid condition (of mind or disposition, of the affairs of a community, etc.); an evil affection or tendency'; and can be combined to form 'disease-germ, -maker; -causing, -producing, -resisting, -spreading, etc.' As a verb it can be to 'bring into a morbid or unhealthy condition; to cause illness, sickness or disease in, to infect with disease.'

As Robert P Hudson notes in *The Cambridge World History of Human Disease*, 'semantic and logical quagmires... await anyone audacious enough to safari through the changing concepts of disease, illness, and health.'[3] Hudson points out that 'Disease has always been what society chooses it to mean – neither more nor less.' Furthermore:

> (1) The definition of disease has varied with time and place in history; (2) the names assigned to diseases are ultimately abstractions, although it is useful at times to act as though they are real; (3) what we mean by diagnostic terms, as with words in general, can be discerned more accurately by what we do with them than by what we say about them.[4]

There have been countless attempts to define illness, disease, and health. (Hudson cites a long list.) The history of disease, however we define it, is undeniably long, far longer than recorded history. This book, short as it is, will – of necessity – be somewhat cursory as a result. It will be largely a social history and, being mindful of semantic quagmires, scientific and medical terms will be kept to a minimum.

We will examine the prehistory of disease, noting its presence in the paleopathological record. Given the limitations of the discipline – as we'll note in the next chapter, only certain diseases leave traces in bones – we will already be in one of Hudson's quagmires. Ancient texts prove to be a veritable semantic minefield, with some ancient diseases remaining unknown. Likewise, ancient epidemics, such as the Plague of Athens, the Antonine Plague and the Plague of Cyprian, all pose epidemiological riddles that have yet to be fully solved. We only get onto scientifically firm ground in the nineteenth century, with the advent of germ theory and crusading figures like Louis Pasteur, Robert

Koch, Rudolf Virchow and Joseph Lister. The twentieth century saw the advent of antibiotics and the development of public health.

It is in these great campaigns, beginning in the Victorian era, that we encounter disease in both the literal sense – people were dying of cholera, typhoid, and the like – and also the figurative: that people were dying was due to their communities being 'deranged, depraved or morbid' due to loose morals, lack of discipline, and poverty.

In the twentieth century, disease appeared in political discourse – Hitler's references to the cancer of Judaism, McCarthy's to communism – while at the same time medicine strode on, confident that all known diseases would be eradicated.

They haven't been, of course. They've outsmarted us, evolving faster than medical research. For the ancients, disease was a punishment from the gods. Gods were replaced with miasmas, miasmas eventually with microbes. Every time human beings have changed their habits or their habitat, they have invited disease to join them.

It is in this sense that disease perhaps has its most useful definition, one we would do well to bear in mind, a definition that behoves us to keep on our toes, to remain ready for disease's next evolution: disease is *dis-ease*, as the OED reminds us, a lack of ease.

1
Prehistory

There was once a time when there was no disease. Life spans were much longer than those we enjoy today, there was no suffering, and people possessed magical powers. They could fly, go to heaven at will, and understood the language of animals.

This is the myth of the golden age, found in cultures the world over. The oldest stories predate Eden: Sumerian cuneiform tablets speak of Dilmun, 'a place where sickness, violence and aging are unknown.'[5] When the sun-god Utu and Enki, lord of soil and earth, brought water, Dilmun flowered and became a beautiful garden. Another pre-Edenic tale is the ancient Persian story of Yima, the first human. During his time, 'there was neither heat nor cold, neither old age nor death, nor disease'.[6] Yima built a beautiful garden, the most widespread image for paradise. This is no coincidence, as Richard Heinberg noted: 'The word paradise itself comes from the Avestan (Old Iranian) word *Pairi-daeza*, meaning a walled or enclosed garden.'[7]

But then disaster struck. Myths of the fall are as widespread as those of the golden age. In Eden, the Serpent tempted Eve to eat the fruit from the Tree of the Knowledge of Good and Evil. In Persia – one of the few stories not to attribute the loss of paradise to the actions of a woman – the Fall was brought about when Yima refused to do the bidding of Ahura Mazda, the Zoroastrian god. Divine displeasure resulted in shorter life spans, pain, toil, conflict, and disease. We have been living in this world ever since.

If paradise in mythology was a garden, in reality, it was probably a beach. Bacteria found at the Strelley Pool Chert in Pilbara, Western Australia, is thought to be around 3.4 billion years old, making it the oldest known form of life yet discovered. At that stage, the Earth was dominated by ceaseless volcanic activity, the continents still in the process of forming, the skies a thick cloud.

We could think of it as an age without disease, but it was also an age without life, or at least life as we know it. We would have found it impossible to breathe, as there was at that stage of Earth's evolution no oxygen: life at Strelley Pool was sulphur-based. The bacteria probably resembled the extremophile bacteria that can be found today in sulphurous caves, acid lakes and in rocks far underground. Rather than being the heavenly arbours of Dilmun, Persia or Eden, the Earth when Strelley Pool Chert was home to the first bacterial life probably more resembled an apocalypse from a painting by John Martin.

Bacteria are not only the original form of life on Earth, but also far and away the most successful and abundant. They had the planet all to themselves for at least a billion years. When the Earth had cooled sufficiently, a type of bacteria known as cyanobacteria began to photosynthesise. That is, they were able to use sunlight to convert carbon dioxide and water into carbohydrates. Oxygen is the byproduct of this process. As Earth's atmosphere began to fill with oxygen, the bacteria slowly began to use it as another energy source.

Around two billion years ago some photosynthetic cyanobacteria invaded other primitive single-celled organisms to form the first plant cells, which were better able to generate energy because they possessed chloroplasts, filaments that were devoted to photosynthesis. Microbial organisms called alpha-proteobacteria amalgamated with other microbes to form mitochondria. These new organisms were eukaryotes, meaning essentially that they were a larger, more advanced form of microbial life. But it is from them that all other life evolved, being powered by chloroplasts and mitochondria.

There were other simple life forms. Single-celled protozoa belong to this category of early life forms. Among their number was thought to be the plasmodium that causes malaria. However, at this very early stage of Earth's history, there were no life forms in which it could cause what we know as malaria; it was simply a microorganism going about its business. Then, as now, that meant finding somewhere to live, generating energy and reproducing. Left to their own devices, most bacteria can reproduce themselves every twenty or so minutes. In one day, a single bacterium can produce a colony of over four sextillion.[8] That stupefyingly large number has twenty-one zeroes after it. Another way of expressing this would be to say that, in a single day, one humble bacterium can produce more of itself than there are vertebrate life forms on the planet.

Bacteria sustain life on Earth. They are in the soil, the air and the water. Each gram of soil contains between one and ten billion bacterial cells, each millilitre of seawater around a million. They are in nature's engine room, constantly transforming matter into energy, constantly purifying, taking in and giving out. In the human body, bacteria outnumber cells by about ten to one (that's roughly 100 quadrillion bacteria to 10 quadrillion cells). Most of them can be found in the gut, and aid the digestion of food, or our immune systems. Others live on our skin, in our mouths, and in places you can't mention in polite conversation.

Another early, very simple and very small life form was the virus. Unlike a bacterium, a virus can't live on its own (it's what's called an obligate parasite). It must of necessity invade a cell and use its host's energy before it can come to life. Once it has done so, a virus will turn the cell it's living in into a production line, spewing out thousands of copies of itself. The virus does not do this out of spite, it's not trying to cause disease, it's simply doing what it's doing. But viral replication nearly always weakens and destroys the cell it's living in, and once the cells start to die off, the organ or organs affected will start to weaken too.

No one knows exactly when viruses first appeared, and to ask why is perhaps to ask the wrong question. It's possible some were the result of imperfect bacterial cell division (although such imperfect offspring usually result in mutated bacteria, rather than viruses). The eminent virologist Dorothy Crawford has dubbed viruses 'rogue pieces of genetic material'[9] which have broken free and found a way to reproduce inside cells. In their natural hosts, viruses can often be benign, only causing disease when they infect a new host. Bats, for example, can carry many viruses that are completely benign to them, but when the viruses make the species jump to humans, they can cause some of the worst diseases currently known, such as Marburg virus disease. We could think of viruses as the microbial equivalent of the Asteroid Belt or Oort Cloud, objects that were too small – or too far away – to become part of larger bodies like planets when the Solar System was forming, and have remained 'free agents' (albeit bound by gravity) ever since. Viruses have always acted to keep life forms in check when any given life form threatens to become overabundant, whether it's human, animal or blooms of algae in the sea.

Out of all the microbes currently known – there are around a million – only 1,415 are known to cause disease in humans.[10] Many are helpful, such as the bacteria that help us digest food, and those that decompose matter and return it to the soil (including human corpses). Some viruses even produce things that we deem beneficial, or pleasing: the bands of colour in variegated tulips, for instance, are caused by a virus. Some bacteria are not naturally harmful to humans, but are only made so by a type of virus called a bacteriophage, or phage for short. The bacteria that cause cholera and diphtheria, for instance (*Vibrio cholerae* and *Corynebacterium diphtheriae*), would be harmless were it not for their resident phages 'switching on' the disease.

And then, around five hundred and fifty million years ago, the so-called Cambrian explosion happened: the first vertebrate life crawled out of the sea and onto dry land.

*

Mediaeval philosophers were fond of referring to the Book of Nature. If you could but read the Book of Nature, they argued, you would attain wisdom. In some senses, they were right: scientists researching the very early history of life on earth have the fossil record to consult. The fossil chapters from the Book of Nature tell us much about the earliest things to have lived on Earth, such as the Strelley Pool bacteria, or the weird and wonderful extinct life forms preserved in the Burgess Shale in the Canadian Rockies.

Human fossils are relative newcomers. Fossils of our ancestor *homo erectus*, from around 1.5 million years ago, show evidence of yaws.[11] This is a tropical disease of the bones and skin that produces unsightly swellings and lesions, and leaves skeletal traces. (Yaws is also related to syphilis, although not transmitted by sexual contact. But more of that later.) Paleopathology can tell us what diseases leave traces in the bone: various forms of dental decay, osteoarthritis, rheumatoid arthritis, osteomyelitis, tuberculosis, leprosy, venereal syphilis, poliomyelitis, fungal bone infections, osteoporosis, rickets, scurvy, thyroid disease, diabetes and anaemia.[12] Tumours can also leave traces, and bones of course will leave clear evidence of trauma (breakages) and disorders of growth and development. Some of these diseases are also found in animal remains. Arthritis, for instance, is found in the remains of cave bears.

Paleopathology has its limitations, however, as Charlotte Roberts and Keith Manchester note. Although a disease may appear to have been present in a body, it is not necessarily the cause of death. Bones can be fragile, and may not survive the process of excavation and examination, so the cause of death is often guesswork. A skeleton may not be representative of the community from which it came – the person could have been a relative newcomer, for instance – and total access to a complete cemetery is the exception, rather than the rule. Furthermore, if a person or community had not developed immunity to a disease due to surviving a previous occurrence, acute infective disease is 'likely to have killed people very quickly in antiquity, especially if the individual had had no previous exposure or experience of the invading organism. Therefore, no evidence of abnormal bone change developed.'[13]

In other words, you die before your bones know what's hit you. Roberts and Manchester point out that 'Many diseases also only affect the soft tissues and therefore would not be visible on the skeleton. It is therefore quite possible that skeletons from the younger (non-adult) members of a cemetery population were victims of an acute, or soft-tissue, disease because frequently they do not have any signs of abnormal bone change. Additionally, their immune systems may not have been fully developed to defend against disease.'[14] Despite these and other limitations, paleopathology can provide vital clues for trying to reconstruct what diseases our ancestors suffered from. 'What can be indicated are the disease processes an individual may have been suffering from in life and whether the disease was active or not at the time of death.'[15]

Human bones aren't the only thing to bear traces of disease. Coprolites, or fossilised faeces, also tell us something about prehistoric disease. From fossilised poo, a general state of health can be deduced. They can tell us whether the person had been infested with parasites such as worms, for instance. As Arno Karlen notes, paleoparasitologists, who study coprolites, prove that 'one man's mess is another's treasure'.[16]

When groups of *homo erectus* moved from Africa to Italy, around half a million years ago, yaws made the trip with them.[17] As to why early humans left Africa, there was probably no one reason. Hunter-gatherer communities could have been following game; they could just have easily been escaping other tropical diseases. Dorothy Crawford notes that sleeping sickness could have been a major problem for early peoples in Africa, as it's endemic to the continent's tsetse fly belt, and is always fatal if not treated.[18] We know that the tsetse fly was active around a million years ago, as fossilised specimens attest. (The fly could also have been responsible for a sizeable extinction of prehistoric horses in North America.[19]) Starting with a headache, sleeping sickness progresses to attack the lymph nodes, produces a rash on the skin and makes the joints ache. When the trypanosome (the protozoan that causes the disease) enters the brain, lethargy, coma and death aren't long in following.

Hunter-gatherer peoples would have been generally healthy, albeit with a fairly short life span of around 30 years. Many of the diseases that affected them would have been 'wear and tear' diseases like arthritis and rheumatism. (Although some of these conditions could have been hereditary, too.) Comprised of several large family groups – perhaps no more than fifty people – hunter-gatherers would have led a life dictated by the seasons and the movements of animals. They hunted, trapped, fished and stalked their prey. This search for food was constant. But there was a balancing act between hunter-gatherer and the environment. As Dorothy Crawford has pointed out, 'On average, hunter-gatherers required around one square mile of foraging area per person, so the number of people in a band was critical: past a certain tipping point further increase would be self-defeating'.[20] It's thought that, if a group got too large, it would practise infanticide, or split into two.

But human populations grew, communities behaving unwittingly like bacteria in ceaselessly splitting into more and more groups, and following more and more big game for food. It did not end well, either for the hunter-gatherers, or the big game. Early humans are thought to have 'exterminate[d] up to 90 per cent of the larger species' between 50,000 years ago in Africa, 20,000 years ago in Europe and Asia and around 11,000 years ago in the Americas.[21] This theory, known as the overkill theory, holds that mastodons, giant sloths and sabre-toothed tigers were all hunted to extinction in order to feed a growing human population. Following them into the cooking pot were gomphotheres, four species of mammoth, ground sloths, glyptodonts, giant armadillos, giant beavers, giant peccaries, the stag moose and the dwarf antelope, brush and woodland musk oxen, the American camel and the American lion, short-faced bears, the dire wolf and the dirk-toothed cat. Australia lost the diprotodon, the 'one-ton wombat', while New Zealand said goodbye to the moa, a flightless bird whose biggest specimen was larger than an ostrich.[22]

The diminishing number of animals to eat, and the threat of diseases like sleeping sickness, would have driven hunter-gatherers further afield. At this point, hunter-gatherers would have increased what is known as the human disease burden. There have been several shifts in this, and they have all caused irrevocable shifts in the pattern of disease.

The earliest human ancestors were apes, who lived largely in the trees. Some diseases would have been either endemic to life in that environment, or at least more common than they would have been on the ground. Certain birds, mammals and insects spend their entire lives in the canopy, and never come down to ground level. Other species, in contrast, require the shade and moisture of life on the ground. All creatures, regardless of what level of the forest they lived in, would have had their own viruses, parasites and diseases. As Arno Karlen notes, 'Changing its niche by only a few meters can radically alter a species' prey, predators and microbes.'[23] Karlen also speculates that it could have been diseases acquired in the trees that may have first forced our ancestors to come down to ground level. Ancestral forms of viral diseases like polio and meningitis could have 'left our arboreal ancestors too crippled to swing through the branches, and enough survivors squeaked out a marginal adaptation to the forest floor to launch a new species.'[24]

When our ancestors shifted their habitat down to the ground, they naturally also made themselves vulnerable to the new diseases that existed there, such as parasitic worms from animal droppings. And the flies that plagued those animals would have given the new ground-based human ancestors sleeping sickness. This was the first shift in disease burden, but over time, our ancestors – and their diseases – adapted to each other. Changes in diet could have led to a second shift: it is probable that our very early ancestors were herbivores, but life on the ground presented them with new opportunities in the shape of animals.

Eating meat, or an increase in the amount of meat in the diet, caused the second shift in the disease burden. Humans were now in more regular contact with animals in order to kill, butcher and eat them. This would have made them susceptible to animal diseases, which were able to make the species jump from animals to humans, known as zoonoses, or zoonotic diseases. This would be particularly true if the animal caught was itself sick; sick animals being slower and easier to catch than healthy ones. However, zoonoses don't enter the human story in quantity at this time, as we'll see.

Arno Karlen speculates that more meat in the diet would have had another lasting effect on human beings: by getting more protein more quickly, early humans would have had more time available for the development of culture. Neanderthals were known to bury their dead, for instance. One grave, from Shanidar cave in northern Iraq, dating from around 60,000 years ago, contains flowers buried alongside the dead man. There is no way the flowers could have got into the grave by accident, as they didn't grow in that locality. Scientists were further astounded to find that the flowers in the grave – hollyhock and yarrow – have medicinal properties.[25]

So, with humans growing in number, they spread out geographically, as we've noted above, causing the third major shift in disease burden. Whether that was due to escaping illness in one area, or chasing animals they wanted to eat, is immaterial for a moment. This new shift in disease burden meant that, as with coming down from the trees, in moving to new lands, humans exposed themselves to new microbes, and new diseases.

This particular shift in disease burden is something most of us are familiar with. When I was growing up, it was a mysterious affliction known as 'holiday tummy'. It happened on holiday, along with traffic jams and bad weather. When at one's chosen destination, one scoured the menu for something sufficiently familiar to eat. Not finding it, one was then forced to sample the local cuisine, usually accompanied by varying degrees of protest or caution. Shortly afterwards, with the strange foreign concoctions safely off the plate and in the tummy, the toilet would need to be visited, usually to more protests, and this time with speed rather than caution. You have eaten new food in a new area, and have exposed yourself to new microbes, and are spending more time than usual in the bathroom. But this, in miniature, is a shift in your disease burden.

Eventually, around 12,000 years ago, humans began to settle, the so-called Neolithic or Agrarian revolution. The hunter-gatherer became a farmer. This caused another shift in disease burden, perhaps the most significant one in history. As soon as people gave up nomadism, they began to attract the attention of microbes in the soil, and also those of animals, which were increasingly being domesticated. It's ironic that doing nothing more than staying put should mark one of the biggest changes in human experience, but that's precisely what it did. As soon as sedentary communities began to appear, people exposed themselves to the billions of bacteria in the soil, and what their gardens and fields didn't give them in the way of disease, their animals did.[26]

This is where zoonoses really began to make their mark. The list of diseases we've caught from our animals is a long one. Tuberculosis from cattle and birds; anthrax from grazing herbivorous mammals; leprosy from mice; rabies from dogs and bats; chicken pox is, unsurprisingly, from chickens; measles probably originated in canine distemper or rinderpest; while the common cold probably comes from horses. There are dozens more examples. The fossilised bones of a mother and child, dating from around 8,000 BC, found in the now-submerged town of Atlit-Yam, off the coast of modern Israel, show that both had suffered from tuberculosis.[27] TB is also thought to have been active in Chile as early as 2,000 BC, which suggests it was brought over the Bering Land Bridge when the Americas were settled some 15,000–20,000 years ago.[28]

Certain roles within communities would have exposed their practitioners to disease: butchers and tanners, for example, would have been coming into contact with animal meat and hides on a regular basis, and would have therefore had a greater exposure to zoonoses. Tilling and ploughing the ground would have exposed the Neolithic farmer to millions of microbes in the soil that could easily enter the human body through cuts or cracks in the skin, or through eating with dirty hands. These were the first 'occupational'-related diseases. Houses that lacked adequate ventilation would have led to respiratory and eye problems.[29]

But it was still a life of hard manual labour: bodies from one of the earliest known settled communities, Aşıklı Höyük in modern-day Anatolian Turkey, occupied between 8,200–7,400 BC, show evidence of joint disease and trauma, and spinal deformities. These suggest rigorous lives of tilling, cutting timber, hauling, and the carrying of heavy loads. (Interestingly, people in Aşıklı Höyük were buried beneath the floors of houses, rather than in a cemeteries.)

After farms, the next stage of the Neolithic revolution was the development of large villages or towns. Bones found at the Neolithic town of Çatalhöyük, close to Aşıklı Höyük, thriving around 7,000 BC, indicate that its inhabitants probably suffered periodic outbreaks of malaria and some form of lung disease, in addition to arthritis, which was common in both young and old alike. Notes made from the 1997 season of excavations at Çatalhöyük suggest that 'Epidemics of infectious disease are a possibility, wiping out whole families or returning year after year. Plague, malaria, enteric dysentery are possibilities. The habitual cleanliness of the house would have controlled infection.'[30]

Given the size of Çatalhöyük – at its largest, it had a population of 10,000 – contagious diseases would have certainly been known. Crowds are good for some pathogens in that they need a certain number of susceptibles in order to remain active. Measles, for instance, as David Quammen notes, 'seems to have a critical community size of roughly 250,000 humans; in an isolated human population smaller than that (on an island, for instance), the virus disappears after everyone has been exposed.'[31] The bigger somewhere like Çatalhöyük and communities close to it got, the more chances diseases had in gaining a foothold. Other diseases couldn't possibly have existed at this time. As Alfred W Crosby notes, 'Because it only persisted by passing from one human to another, smallpox could not have existed with its historical characteristics among the sparse populations of the Paleolithic Age.'[32] When smallpox did finally appear in humans – possibly in late antiquity or the early Middle Ages – it probably came from dogs or cattle (and is related to cowpox, as Edward Jenner would find out many centuries later).

Sheer numbers of people would be aided and abetted by dirt, refuse and sewage. As soon as any of those things contaminated the drinking water and food, diseases would rip through a settlement. This had never been a problem for hunter-gatherers, who would be getting their water from streams or rivers, and probably doing what bears do in the woods, or digging cesspits. Either way, the possibility of contaminating their water and food was minimal.

One burial at Çatalhöyük begs more questions than answers. Like those at Aşıklı Höyük, graves in Çatalhöyük were beneath the floors of the houses. One grave discovered in 1998, known as Space 115 (or Skeleton 3368, Burial 285, cut 3369, Space 115 Midden deposit, to give it a fuller description), however, was not under a house – it would have been out in the open when the body was interred, a space interpreted as a 'courtyard midden', making it 'unique in the records so far'.[33] The body is of a young adult male with seriously diseased bones, which suggests that the man had been an outcast because of his condition.

This midden burial at Çatalhöyük also indicates that disease is not just something that can affect the body and leave traces in the bones, but is also social. The disfigured, disabled or otherwise different were to be regarded as unclean, possessed by bad spirits or perhaps just unlucky, and ostracised (to judge from the uniqueness of the midden grave at Çatalhöyük). People struck low with a disease could have also been subject to early forms of surgery. Again, in the absence of written records, the bone record is our best guide here. Skulls from around the time of Çatalhöyük, perhaps a bit later (maybe 5000 BC), found in locations as diverse as France, Poland, South America and the Pacific, bear the distinctive signs of trepanation. This is the ancient art of drilling a hole in the skull, presumably to let bad spirits out.

As medical historian Roy Porter notes, 'Illness is thus not just biological but social, and concepts of the body and its sicknesses draw upon powerful dichotomies: nature and culture, the sacred and the profane, the raw and the cooked. Body concepts incorporate beliefs about the body politic at large.'[34] If someone within a community is designated sick, Porter argues, it is a reflection of that community's principles of organisation. But the limits of where normal health ends and disease begins are fluid. This is perhaps reflected in modern semantic problems with the word 'disease', that we noted in the introduction. In addition, disease can carry a moral weight. The man seemingly outcast in death at Çatalhöyük could well have been an outcast in life, too.

Some diseases have always been seen as punishment for wrongdoing and sin – leprosy being the prime example, associated in the Middle Ages with lust and improper desire. But as Porter points out, disease could also have a beneficial side: '"Sick roles" may range from utter stigmatisation (common with leprosy, because it is so disfiguring) to the notion that the sick person is special or semi-sacred (the holy fool or the divine epileptic). An ailment can be a *rite de passage*, a childhood illness can be an essential preliminary to entry into adulthood.'[35]

We could almost view the diseases brought about by the Neolithic revolution – the development of agriculture, towns and, in the course of time, cities – as being humanity's own rite of passage, from the 'childhood' of the nomadic hunter-gatherers to the 'adulthood' of settled, 'civilised' life. And we've gained most of our diseases in the process, leaving Dilmun and Yima's garden far behind.[36]

2

Antiquity

The Bible is seething with plagues. In the book of Exodus (Chapters 8 to 12), the Old Testament's infamously wrathful God inflicts ten plagues on Egypt, as a punishment for keeping the Israelites captive. Acting with divine sanction, Moses and Aaron use their staffs, raise their hands and scoop out soot from furnaces to call down afflictions on the land (and, in doing so, become archetypal wizards to rival Pharaoh's own, ancestors to Gandalf and Merlin). The waters in the rivers are turned to blood, killing all the fish; the Nile then teemed with frogs. Lice and flies followed, harming livestock. The Egyptians' animals further suffered in an epidemic, and then – along with their human keepers – developed boils. A storm of hail and fire swept the land, followed by locusts and darkness. Finally, with land and livestock decimated, the firstborn children died.

Such widescreen, epic disasters have turned 'Old Testament' from a noun into an adjective (in the sense of 'Old Testament wrath', and the like). But how many of the ten plagues of Egypt were actual diseases? And could they have actually happened? Was it the hand of the Almighty, or could they have been natural phenomena such as drought. Or a metaphor for a bad harvest, shorthand for hardship? New research suggests that the plagues could have actually happened, but were a series of natural disasters inaugurated by climate change, centred on the ancient city of Pi-Ramesses in the Nile Delta.[37] The reign of pharaoh Ramses II (1279–1213 BC) coincided with a warm, wet period, after which temperatures dropped. This, so the theory goes, caused the Nile to dry up, but not before the warmer temperatures had led the normally fast-flowing Nile to become a semi-stagnant artery of mud. These charming conditions would have been perfect for the formation of a form of freshwater algae known as Burgundy Blood algae (*Oscillatoria rubescens*), which is known to have existed 3,000 years ago and is still with us today. As the algae dies, it stains the water red, hence the water of the Nile becomes 'changed into blood'. (An alternative theory suggests the red colouring could have been caused by *chromatiaceae* bacteria, brought on by a drought.[38])

The algae would also have started a domino effect that produced the second, third and fourth plagues – frogs, lice and flies. The algae would have accelerated the life cycle of frogs, and caused them to leave the river in search of a new habitat. Without frogs, mosquitoes and lice would have flourished in the absence of their main predator, causing insect-borne diseases to flourish; in Old Testament parlance, these were the fifth and sixth plagues – diseased livestock and boils. A volcanic eruption as far away as Crete could have caused a second domino effect, leading to the seventh, eighth and ninth plagues that brought hail, locusts and darkness to Egypt. Volcanic ash could have mingled with thunderstorms to produce hail; it could also have led to higher humidity, leading to a surge in the locust population; and it could also have caused darkness, the clouds of ash creating an eclipse-like gloom.

All of which brings us to the final plague, the deaths of the first-born. One theory suggests that this could have been caused by grain supplies becoming infected by a fungus. Emerging from a period of darkness and disaster, infants would have been the first to be fed, and therefore the first to die.

While this explanation of the ten plagues remains conjecture – indeed, the whole field of Bible-as-history is controversial – such chain reactions are not unknown and, as we will see in Chapter 5, were to cause catastrophe in nineteenth century East Africa.

*

The ten plagues of Egypt are not the only afflictions in the Old Testament: there are over a hundred mentions of disease. The books of Numbers (21:6,8) and Deuteronomy (8:15) both mention a 'fiery serpent', which, it has been suggested,[39] could be a reference to the guinea worm, which causes dracunculiasis, a parasitic infection caused by drinking infected water. Mummies from this period (*c.* 1450–1500 BC) also show evidence of worm infestation. Worms are also mentioned in the Rig Veda, which was probably composed around the same time, offering magical remedies against infestation in both children and cattle.[40]

Elsewhere in Numbers (11:32–35), a plague broke out among the Israelites. Wearying of manna from heaven, they began desiring the varieties of meat they had eaten while enslaved in Egypt. They ate migrating quail, which had been forced to make an emergency landing due to a storm. The Israelites suffer from a 'very great plague' as a result of eating the bird meat. Although Numbers doesn't provide any more information – other than to inform us that the Almighty was not very pleased with the gluttonous Israelites, who suffered many casualties as a result of their impromptu feasting – we could hazard a guess that, if there is any historical basis to the story at all, the Israelites could have contracted avian influenza from the birds. The word 'plague' in the Bible therefore doesn't usually mean plague in the medical sense of bubonic plague. It is a somewhat nebulous term, usually signifying an epidemic, not infrequently mildly catastrophic.

The Bible's relationship to historical fact is equally vague. It is more helpful for our purposes to think of it as containing some truth where diseases and epidemics are concerned, in that the descriptions given by the Biblical writers sometimes – as in the cases discussed – allow us to conjecture what diseases may have been active in that era. The writers themselves certainly saw disease as a divine punishment for the wrongdoings of humanity. This was the mindset of the culture that produced the Bible – and, indeed, of most societies up until the nineteenth and twentieth centuries, when the scientific causes of disease came to be understood. In seeing disease as punishment from the Almighty, the Judeo-Christian tradition is not unique: almost all mythic and religious texts see disease as an affliction sent down from on high for moral transgressions and all manner of wickedness.

However, some religious strictures (such as those from the Book of Leviticus) may have had a more practical origin. As the historian of disease William McNeill noted, the Jewish and Muslim prohibition of pork:

> appears inexplicable until one realizes that hogs were scavengers in Near Eastern villages, quite capable of eating human faeces and other 'unclean' material. If eaten without the most thorough cooking, their flesh was easily capable of transferring a number of parasites to human beings… the ancient prohibition of pork presumably rested rather on an intuitive horror of the hogs' behaviour.[41]

However, in the main, disease was punishment. In Genesis, Eve eats of the fruit of the Tree of Knowledge of Good and Evil: the consequences of this action include pain in childbirth; a multiplication of sorrows; enmity between men and women, between parents and children; patriarchy; and toiling all the days of one's life until humans return to the dust from which they were made (Genesis 3: 15–19). Life spans also shortened, from the 'old as Methuselah' variety – Methuselah himself is said to have lived to the age of 969, Adam to 930 (Genesis 5:27, 5:5) – down to the less mythic 'threescore and ten' (Psalm 90:10).

Expulsion from the Garden saw human beings forced to live short lives of toil and tumult. God tells Adam that a life of toil will bring few rewards:

> …cursed is the ground for thy sake; in sorrow shalt thou eat of it all the days of thy life; Thorns also and thistles shall it bring forth to thee; and thou shalt eat the herb of the field (Genesis 3: 17–18).

God seems to be compelling man to a life of farming, and the Neolithic agricultural revolution, as we've seen, brought forth one of the biggest multiplications of sorrows in human history: the shift to a settled agrarian existence formed another major shift in the human disease burden.

The familial enmity suggested by Genesis took immediate shape in the story of Cain and Abel. The two brothers could be seen as representing the clash between the hunter-gatherer and the settled farmer. After an unspecified argument – possibly over a woman – or because of jealousy when God accepted Abel's offering, but rejected Cain's, Cain kills Abel.[42] God then cursed Cain (Genesis 4:11), afflicting him with the mysterious 'mark of Cain' (Genesis 4:15) and made his farmland barren (Genesis 4:12). Cain became a wanderer, like his murdered brother.

This could explain why Cain then goes on to found the first city, named after his son, Enoch (Genesis 4:17). Cities represent another major change in the human disease burden (as mentioned in Chapter 1). Like farms before them, cities proved to be fertile breeding grounds for disease. Lurking in contaminated drinking water, thriving due to bad or non-existent hygiene, exacerbated by overcrowding, carried from person to person and neighbourhood to neighbourhood by dogs, livestock and insects, diseases flourished in cities. Given the link between the development of urban living and disease, it might be appropriate to suggest that the mark of Cain could be nothing other than disease.

*

Greek myth accounts for the appearance of disease among people with the story of Pandora's Jar which, since a textual corruption in the sixteenth century, has been known as Pandora's Box. Hesiod recounts the story in *Works and Days.* Charged by Zeus with the task of creating humanity, the Titan Prometheus became moved by the lot of (a presumably all-male) humanity, and did all he could to help them. He tricked the gods out of food, donating the fare from a sacrificial feast to humans. Then he really got Zeus's back up: he stole fire. Angered by Prometheus's audacious theft, Zeus ordered the blacksmith Hephaestus to create the first human woman as a means of punishing humanity. Hephaestus set to work, sculpting a figure out of water and earth. Pandora – her name means all-giving, in that all the gods on Olympus gave her a gift – was the result. She was endowed with various divine attributes: Aphrodite gave her beauty, Hermes speech and cunning; Athena clothed her, while the Horae decked her hair with spring flowers. Pandora came to earth as a bride for Epimetheus, Prometheus's brother, and brought with her a wedding present from Zeus: a jar. But upon arriving in Epimetheus's house, Pandora's curiosity got the better of her, and she decided to open the jar, releasing a cloud of spirits that 'scattered pains and evils among men'. As with Eve eating the fruit, this was the moment when humanity became plagued with every known affliction: 'thousands of troubles wander[ed] the earth./The earth was full of evils, and the sea./Diseases c[a]me to visit men by day and, uninvited, c[a]me again at night.'[43] The golden age was over.

From Myth to Medicine: Disease in the Ancient Near East

The Bible is not particularly old: most of the Old Testament was written down between the sixth to first centuries BC; more recent than Hesiod, who wrote in the eighth century BC. The oldest records concerning disease are therefore not Biblical or Classical at all, but are to be found among Egyptian stele and tomb paintings and papyri; Akkadian tablets; and Chinese and Indian medical tracts. According to the historian Manetho of Sebennytos (*fl.* third century BC), Egypt suffered the earliest recorded epidemic, which was said to have occurred in 3180 BC. Writing in his *Aigyptiaka* (*A History of Egypt*), Manetho notes that the reign of the pharaoh Mempses in the First Dynasty was blighted by a terrible epidemic. Unfortunately, he declines to elaborate on what precisely it was, merely recording that '*In his reign many portents and a great pestilence occurred.*'

As in the Bible, ancient Greece and the story of Dilmun, other early cultures such as those of the Babylonians, Hittites and Egyptians, were not without their stories of disease as divine displeasure, or at the very least the work of demons. A gloss in the ancient Egyptian text known as the Edwin Smith Papyrus attributes disease to 'something entering from outside' which is 'the breath of an outside god or death'.[44] Another demon was said to enter the body through the eye, while the Ebers Papyrus refers to the stomach being susceptible to attacks from the *nesiet* demon; elsewhere, deafness is ascribed to inhaling air from the 'beheading demon'.[45] Despite this, it is with writings from ancient Egypt and Mesopotamia that we move from the realms of myth into history for the first time.

An Akkadian tablet from 1770 BC shows that King Zimri-Lim ordered a secretary to write a note for his queen, Shiptu, warning her about a servant woman named Nanna, who was suffering from lesions. The King instructed Shiptu to avoid drinking from shared cups, and not to use a bed or a chair if poor old Nanna had been using it before her. Zimri's note to his queen is possibly the earliest surviving precaution for avoiding contagious disease.

The Babylonians give us the first description of what is probably rabies, as recorded in the Eshnunna Code, a legal document written around 2300 BC. The text describes how the bite of a dog could be fatal, and recommends a fine for the animal's owner.[46]

> If a dog is mad and the authorities have brought the fact to the knowledge of its owner; if he does not keep it in, it bites a man and causes his death, then the owner shall pay two-thirds of a mina (40 shekels) of silver. If it bites a slave and causes his death he shall pay 15 shekels of silver.[47]

However, being of a legal nature, the Eshnunna tablets don't go into detail about precisely *how* a dog bite can be fatal, so we must be cautious with saying that this is definitely rabies. The name of the disease is not mentioned, being of a later coining – rather aptly coming from the Latin, 'to rave', while the name of the virus ('lyssavirus') comes from the Greek *lyssa*, meaning 'to do violence'. As with the Biblical plagues, the Eshnunna Code is another example of how imprecise ancient texts can be when it comes to identifying disease. If a text was to describe some of the symptoms of rabies without mentioning the bite of a dog, then we would be on less certain ground; the disease could be epilepsy or tetanus, for example, which produce similar symptoms. But the presence of a dog (sometimes a bat, fox or jackal), and a bite, followed by madness and death, are strongly suggestive of rabies. (Rabies, or something very much like it, was also known in China, where it is mentioned in a text from the sixth century BC, and it is also described in a first century Indian source.)

Possibly the earliest known mention of epilepsy comes from an Akkadian tablet from *c.* 2000 BC. This text described the symptoms, in which the condition of *antasubbû* as 'a person whose neck turns left, whose hands and feet are tense, and eyes wide open, froth flowing from the mouth and consciousness being lost'.[48] There was a widespread fear that epilepsy might be caused by the 'Star of Marduk' (Jupiter) or demonic possession. Indeed, the name *antasubbû* means 'touched by the hand of a god'.

Disease in Ancient Egypt

The role of demons as disease-causing agencies is attested to by some of the very earliest medical texts that have come down to us – the Egyptian medical papyri. Unlike the Eshnunna Code, Egyptian papyri such as the Ebers Papyrus are actual medical texts, devoting much space to disease, medicine and remedies. Although demonology was present in the Egyptians' medical thinking, it by no means dominates. The papyri are 'by far the most important sources of our knowledge'[49] when it comes to trying to establish what diseases the ancient Egyptians suffered from.

One of the most important papyri – and the longest – was bought by a somewhat shady character called Edwin Smith, an American adventurer and antiquities dealer. On Smith, as the scholar of ancient Egypt John F Nunn comments, 'there are rather diverse views'. He was reputed to 'advise on, and even practise, the forgery of antiquities'.[50] Smith acquired the papyrus at Luxor in 1862, and it has since become known as the Ebers Papyrus, named after the man to whom Smith later sold it. Nothing is known for certain of its provenance, other than that Smith didn't forge it. The papyrus was said to have been found between the legs of a mummy in the Assassif area of the Theban necropolis, but when its importance was realised, the finders were dead – foul play does not seem to have been involved – and the actual location of the tomb was never established. One passage implies that the papyrus dates from around 3000 BC, stating that it was presented to the King of the First Dynasty, the pharaoh Den (whose reign began *c.* 2970 BC). However, such an early dating needs to be taken with a pinch of salt. Assigning a much earlier date to a papyrus – thereby hoping to invest it with the supposed authority that age brings – was common practice. In fact, a passage on the verso dates the papyrus to 1534 BC (in the ninth year of the reign of Amenhotep I).

The Ebers Papyrus is laid out in a somewhat haphazard fashion. Some parts of Ebers seem to assume that 'the diagnosis has already been made and simply lists the recommended treatments.'[51] Other parts are possibly in the wrong order or seem muddled. It starts with three spells designed to be used prior to, or in conjunction with, taking a remedy that the doctor has prescribed.[52] Following this is a section which concentrates mainly on diseases of the belly, worms in particular. From the belly, the papyrus moves down to diseases of the anus. There are various prescriptions 'to relieve a pathological condition of the body', although what this is is impossible to say. Several other diseases are also difficult to identify. Specific terms such as '*wekhedu* of *aaa*' remain obscure.

Although '*wekhedu* of *aaa*' and other terms remain a matter for scholars to puzzle over, we can make a few educated guesses as to what caused the Egyptian gastrointestinal diseases. Parasites like worms (also known as helminths) have been a health hazard in Egypt for millennia, and can infest the human body after infected water is drunk or under-cooked meat consumed, eating food with unwashed hands, or skin contact with larvae in contaminated soil. Worms such as *S. mansoni* and *S. haematobium* are likely to have caused schistosomiasis (bilharziasis), 'still a major cause of chronic ill health in Egypt'.[53] Infection is most likely to have been caused in ancient Egyptians by immersion in river water. The worms lay their eggs in the bladder and the rectum. The eggs are eventually ulcerated through the bladder, and passed in the urine. The main symptom is haematuria (blood in the urine). Centuries later, this disease was still very much in evidence: 'Napoleon's troops reported that Egypt was the land of menstruating men'.[54] Other symptoms can include anaemia, lassitude, loss of appetite, and lessened resistance to other diseases. There may also be interference with liver function, and a possible link to bladder cancer. 'Schistosomiasis of the rectum can be painful and may explain the high percentage of ancient Egyptian remedies for "cooling and refreshing" the anus'.[55] It's also speculated that penile sheaths shown in some murals were worn to prevent infection. It was thought the worm swam up the urethra.

Given the prevalence of such afflictions, Herodotus commented 'that the Egyptians were obsessed with their bowels'.[56] It comes as no surprise to learn that part of the Ebers Papyrus constitutes the 'Book of the Stomach', which concerns itself with various obstructions of the stomach. Various diagnoses have been proposed for the diseases described in this section of the papyrus: obstruction of the lower end of the oesophagus, pyloric stenosis, carcinoma of the stomach, peptic ulceration, even faecal impaction. Even food poisoning is suggested by Ebers paragraph 207, which gives the earliest record of directions for a physician to examine a patient's stools.

After this are remedies 'to cause the heart to receive bread',[57] and remedies for coughs and the *gehew*-disease. Both 'bread' and *gehew* remain unclear. The heart receiving bread could be a reference to a healthy circulation, while *gehew* disease could be in the domain of what modern doctors call ear, nose and throat complaints.

The papyrus continues, discussing treatment of eye diseases, and is 'our main source of information on treatment of eye disease in ancient

Egypt'.[58] This may be the 'book of eyes' referred to by Clement of Alexandria (150–215 AD), who believed that the ancient Egyptians had 42 books of knowledge, six of which were medical. (The other five covered anatomy, diseases, remedies, doctors' instruments and women's diseases.)

Treatment of bites 'both by man and crocodile' is followed by diseases of the head, and what to do with burns, beatings and flesh wounds. But the papyrus returns once more into obscurity with a section dealing with general suffering in relation to 'secretions' (*setja*), and another section dealing with strengthening the *metu*.

Metu is central to ancient Egyptian concepts of life and health. However, we're not sure exactly what *metu* means. It seems to mean different things in different contexts: in some, *metu* seems to mean muscles, in others, the male member or impotence. In another case, 'swelling of the *metu*' sounds as though it could be a post-traumatic aneurysm. Heart disease is also attributed to the *metu*, as are liver diseases and our old friends, diseases of the anus. The Ebers and Berlin papyri (Ebers 856h and Berlin 163h) state that 'all [*metu*] come to his heart... and unite at his anus.'[59] This sounds like the Indian concept of the chakras, or the Chinese meridians, but remains guesswork.

Ebers continues to treat diseases of the tongue; dermatology; teeth; ear, nose and throat; gynaecology.[60] Before we are much the wiser on any of these, 'the content then changes abruptly to a section on household pests.'[61] The *metu* is then discussed again, followed by 'what little is said about the cardiovascular system'. The final part 'is of a more surgical nature' similar to the Edwin Smith Papyrus.[62] (This papyrus, also discovered by Edwin Smith – hence the rather imaginative name – dates from around 1550 BC, and is concerned for much of its length with describing medical procedures, rather than disease.)

Cancer seems to have been relatively rare in ancient Egypt. As John Nunn speculates, this is probably linked with shorter life expectancy, genetic factors and environmental factors.[63] However, 'untreated cancer often produces large tumours before death, and it is therefore surprising that cancers are very rare, as in many ancient populations, in both mummies and skeletal remains.'[64] The Ebers Papyrus contains a reference to 'eating of the uterus', which may refer to a tumour, although there is little scholarly consensus. Nunn does note however that 'one could hardly deny that "eating" is a very graphic description of advanced malignancy.'[65]

The skin diseases mentioned in Ebers could be leprosy. However, as might be expected, the terminology prevents us from making a definite identification. Ebers recommends, 'If you examine a large tumor of *Khonsu* in any part of a man and it is terrible and it has made many swellings.' The physician knew he was powerless to treat it. As the papyrus continues, 'you shall say concerning it: It is a swelling of *Khonsu*. You should not do anything against it.'[66]

As the great historian of medicine, Roy Porter, noted, leprosy 'has a puzzling history. From as early as 2400 BC Egyptian sources contain references to a skin condition interpreted as leprosy, and 900 years later, the Ebers Papyrus mentions a leprous disease seemingly confirmed by Egyptian skeleton evidence.'[67] The Bible appears to mention leprosy as well. Leviticus 13:2 reads, 'When a man shall have in the skin of his flesh a rising, a scab, or bright spot, and it be in the skin of his flesh like the plague of leprosy; then he shall be brought unto Aaron the priest, or unto one of his sons the priests.' In such a situation, the priest would have no option but to cast the person out of the camp, as leprosy was long believed to be highly contagious. (In fact, it isn't, and is actually quite hard to contract. What seems to have inspired terror is the fact that leprosy can disfigure, especially the face.) Leviticus's talk of leprosy – 'living without the camp' – was probably not leprosy in the modern medical sense (Hansen's Disease) but could have been another dermatological complaint such as psoriasis. Nevertheless, the terror the disease inspired was real. Some Egyptian texts refer to the disease as 'the death before death', and lepers were cast out, being exiled to a place called the City of Mud.[68]

Evidence from Mummies

Skeletal evidence, as Roy Porter mentioned, is one of the other main sources for our knowledge of Egyptian disease, although mummies can be just as enigmatic as papyri when it comes to making firm assertions about disease.

The mummy of the pharaoh Ramses V (d. 1145 BC) shows signs of what may be smallpox. Although the surviving medical papyri don't mention anything that sounds like smallpox, Ramses' mummy shows the disease's telltale lesions on its pockmarked face and shoulders. If he did die of smallpox, he would be one of the earliest known victims of the disease. Evidence from other skeletons suggests tuberculosis of the spine, and more obvious deformities such as dwarfism, club foot and hydrocephalus. Guinea worm infestation has also been detected in one mummy, which was known to have caused dracunculiasis. Bones also show evidence of stunted growth, osteoporosis; dietary toxins include lead.[69]

Other diseases have been conjectured, despite a lack of firm evidence from papyri, mummies, potsherds, funerary stelae or other sources. Malnutrition almost certainly afflicted the ancient Egyptians in years of famine. Polio appears to be depicted on some stelae – figures are depicted walking with sticks – and malaria would have certainly been a problem.

There is no firm evidence of plague or tetanus, although both would eventually appear in Egypt.

Disease in Ancient Greece

A thousand years separates the Ebers Papyrus from the next important group of medical writings from western antiquity. In *The History of the Peloponnesian War*, the Greek historian Thucydides gives a graphic account of the epidemic that struck Athens, his home city, in 430 BC:

> The plague first began to show itself among the Athenians. It was said that it had broken out in many places previously in the vicinity of Lemnos and elsewhere; but a pestilence of such extent and mortality was nowhere remembered. Neither were the physicians at first of any use, ignorant as they were of the proper way to treat it, but they died themselves in great numbers, as they visited the sick most often; nor did any human art succeed any better. Supplications in the temples, divinations, and so forth were found equally futile, till the overwhelming nature of the disaster at last put a stop to them altogether.

He describes the symptoms, which included a terrible fever, livid patches on the skin, sore throat, a cough, vomiting, sneezing, fetid breath, convulsions, memory loss, exhaustion and severe diarrhoea. People were afraid to visit the sick, and the dead were buried without proper funeral rites. The death toll was so high – Athens lost a third of its population – that an air of lawlessness began to prevail, with widespread debauchery and crime:

> Fear of the gods or the law of man did not restrain them. As for the first, they judged it to be just the same whether they worshipped them or not, as they saw all alike perishing; and for the last, no one expected to live to be brought to trial for his offences, but each felt that a far severer sentence had been already passed upon them all and hung over their heads, and before this fell it was only reasonable to enjoy life a little.

But what was the Plague of Athens? Thucydides records that there was talk the Spartans – with whom the Athenians were then at war – had poisoned the drinking water, but reserves final judgement. He does observe, however, that surviving the plague made one immune to it for life. Thucydides writes from personal experience: as a general in the war, he contracted the plague himself, but did not make the same mistake certain others did, of thinking they were then immune to all forms of sickness; no doubt they may well have succumbed to other ailments, rendering any celebration short-lived.

Various pathogens have been proposed as the cause of the Plague of Athens, including bubonic plague, influenza, typhoid fever, measles, epidemic typhus, and smallpox, all of which display some of the symptoms described in *The History of the Peloponnesian War*. However, the jury is still out. Paleopathology has so far provided no conclusive answers and scholars are still arguing over the correct interpretation of Thucydides' text. What we do know is that by the time Thucydides was writing, maybe ten to twenty years later, Athens had not only lost the war against the Spartans, but had been forever crippled as a major power. The golden age of Athenian democracy and culture was over, hastened to its grave by the plague – whatever it was.

The Cult of Asclepius

In the wake of the Plague of Athens and the crippling of the city-state's power came the rise of the cult of Asclepius the healer. Its origins are obscure, but it could have been in existence while Thucydides was still writing his history of the war (while the war was still being fought). With the cult of Asclepius, magic maintained its prominence in Greek thinking about disease. The irony was perhaps not lost on Thucydides, who is often regarded as one of the founders of history as a discipline. He downplayed the role of the gods in human affairs, and as such, his work can be seen as a blueprint for later writings about diseases and medicine. But that would have given beleaguered Athenians little succour after losing so many of their kinsfolk to the plague and the lengthy war against Sparta.

Asclepius was the son of Apollo and a mortal woman, reflecting the esteem in which doctors and medical practitioners were held in ancient Greece. Educated by the centaur Chiron, Asclepius used his learning to help humans with his medicinal know-how (plant remedies). So successful was Asclepius at this – indeed, he was said to be able to bring people back from the dead – that Hades, the god of death, complained to Zeus that the underworld was being deprived of its denizens. Zeus agreed that Asclepius had overstepped the mark, and promptly struck him dead with a thunderbolt. (Another version of the story has it that Asclepius was killed because he accepted gold for his services as a resurrectionist.)

Subsequently elevated to the rank of god himself, Asclepius was worshipped as the tutelary deity of medicine, usually depicted as holding a staff around which a snake had coiled itself. This symbol – the caduceus – became synonymous with the healing arts. Asclepius was often shown with his daughters Hygeia (health) and Panacea (cure-all). His sons were known as the Asclepiads, supposedly the first physicians; this title was later bestowed upon all doctors, although it's not certain whether it was a slang term, or one to designate membership of some kind of medical guild.

The Asclepius cult spread during the fourth century BC, and by 200 BC, all towns of significant size in Greece had an Asclepion, or temple to Asclepius. Cos had perhaps the best-known Asclepion, although there were other notable examples at Epidaurus and Pergamon, birthplace of the Roman doctor Galen (for more of whom, see below). Rituals at Asclepia involved incubation, or temple sleep. The patient would sleep before an image of Asclepius, and hope that they would either be made well during the night by the god himself, or be given the cure in a dream (which sometimes required a priest to decipher it the following morning). People came to Asclepia seeking cures from blindness, paralysis, edema, tapeworms, abdominal abscesses, lice, headaches, wounds sustained in battle, infertility, gout, even baldness. If the patient was cured, the event would be commemorated on a plaque placed in the temple precinct: 'Hermodikes of Lampsakos was paralysed in body. In his sleep he was healed by the god.' But how did the gods heal? The experience of Alketas of Halika reveals something of their mysterious ways: 'This blind man saw a vision. He thought that the god came up to him and opened his eyes with his fingers. The first things he saw were the trees of the Temple. At daybreak he left the Temple restored to health.'[70]

The Hippocratic Revolution

However, not all Asclepiads subscribed to the notion that disease had a divine cause. One doctor in particular caused a revolution that affected all subsequent medical practice: Hippocrates of Cos (*c.* 460 BC – *c.* 371 BC). Although Cos had a major Asclepion, Hippocrates, as Roy Porter put it, 'plucked disease from the heavens and brought it down to earth.'[71] Hippocrates was able to do this because of the relative openness of classical Greek culture, 'a quality characteristic of Greek intellectual activity at large, which it owed to political diversity and cultural pluralism.'[72] Unlike ancient Babylon, whose doctors were bound by the Hammurabic code, there was no regulation – to use modern parlance – of the medical profession. Theoretically, anyone could set up shop as a healer, shaman, doctor, exorcist or diviner – all of whose skills were known to have been sought out in ancient Greece to cure sickness.

Little is known for sure of Hippocrates – he exists in the same realm of mythologised history as Homer, Hesiod and Pythagoras. Indeed, a genealogy was drawn up linking Hippocrates to Asclepius, and the famous Hippocratic Oath sworn by doctors begins 'I swear by Apollo the physician, by Asclepius, by health (Hygeia) and all the powers of healing (Panacea), and call to witness all the gods and goddesses...' But Hippocrates needed no dubious links to deities, whether by genealogy or oath, both of which were probably not written down until after his death. He stressed observation and reason over supernatural explanations, and the school he founded was to exert an immense influence. Known as the Hippocratic or Coan School, the collected writings of Hippocrates and his followers were brought together sometime during the third century BC. (Hippocrates was mysteriously able to continue writing books long after his death.)

Although varied in style and substance due to the plethora of authors, the Hippocratic Corpus gives us a much clearer picture of what diseases the ancient Greeks suffered from. Interpretation of the Corpus involves the usual problem with ancient texts, in that definitions are sometimes imprecise, but modern doctors can assert with some confidence that Hippocrates and his followers knew of, amongst others, cholera, pneumonia (described as 'a disease of the ancients'), meningitis, tonsillitis, epilepsy, septicaemia, various gastrointestinal disorders, tuberculosis, brucellosis, tetanus, malaria, and possibly influenza and polio.

The writings on malaria are particularly interesting. Hippocrates was the first to describe the disease's ability to produce fever on alternate days (tertian malaria), or every third day (quartan malaria); its effect on the spleen; its seasonal distribution; and its link to stagnant water. Hippocrates and his school were also aware of the seasonal and environmental risks of infection, as in the case of malaria; the human immune system's tendency to produce fever and swelling as a reaction to infection; and the need to cook meat and fish properly to avoid diarrhoea and food poisoning. Above all, the Hippocratic Corpus attempted to treat every known disease in a systematic and reasoned manner.[73]

Central to Hippocratic thinking was the theory of the four humours, based on the theory of the four elements. Formulated in the fifth century BC by the philosopher Empedocles (*c.* 490–430 BC), the theory held that all things were formed from earth, air, fire and water, and each of these elements had a defining characteristic: wet, dry, hot and cold respectively. From this, Hippocrates developed the idea that the body contained four humours, each comprising a pair of Empedoclean traits: black bile (cold and dry); yellow bile (hot and dry); blood (hot and wet); and phlegm (cold and wet).

As the body was understood to be the microcosm of the great world, so environmental factors also had to be considered. In the tract *On Airs, Waters and Places*, Hippocrates stresses the importance of seasonal influences such as the strength, direction and temperature of winds. What kinds of waters flow? Are they marshy and soft, hard and rocky, or salty and unsuitable for human consumption? And what about the position of the locality itself: is the land high or low, secluded or exposed? What are people's habits like there? Do they eat and drink to excess? Are they idle or industrious?

Health was understood to be a balance of the four humours; this was the natural state of life. Illness only resulted when the humours were out of balance, usually due to a deficiency in one humour, an excess in another, or some unfavourable influence arising from the airs, waters and places. Despite the stress Hippocrates laid on observation and experience, the humoural theory dominated western medical thinking until the Renaissance.

Disease in Ancient China

Records from China about disease are amongst the oldest in the world: the last 3,000 or so years are covered in various forms – historical chronicles, oracle-bones and grave goods. However, like their ancient western counterparts, the Chinese records suffer from the same problems of interpretation, in that the terminology of traditional Chinese medicine is 'based on a system hardly translatable into modern Western terms.'[74] Not only that, but early Chinese script itself poses another problem. As Angela Ki Che Leung notes in the *Cambridge World History of Human Disease*, Chinese writing didn't reach its modern form until around the third century BC, so these early texts on oracle bones and the like are written in pictograms, and an imprecision in the terminology is inevitably present: 'For example, *chi*, which subsequently invariably meant "epidemic disease in general," shows a man alone or lying on a bed with the arrow of the disease shooting into him.'[75] (Disease as an arrow also recurs in Anglo-Saxon ideas about disease – see the next chapter – while the ancient Egyptians also conceptualised disease as being 'something from outside', as we saw earlier in this chapter.)

Furthermore, not only have the concepts of disease changed, but so have the diseases themselves, 'so much so that it is impossible to determine whether an ancient classical term meant the same thing when used in premodern texts, or to find the exact modern counterpart of a disease discussed in old texts.'[76] The term 'fever', for instance, was as vague as it was in western records, where it could stand for any number of conditions.

William McNeill listed 99 epidemics in China between 243 BC and the time of the Black Death in the fourteenth century, based on two earlier compilations, one from the Sung Dynasty (960–1279) and the other put together in the eighteenth century.[77] These are, as we might expect of old sources, rather vague. In 243 BC, for instance, there was 'epidemic throughout the empire', while in 48 BC there was 'Epidemic, flood and famine east of the pass', which O'Neill tentatively identifies as Honan, Shansi and Shantung provinces. Even this scant information is better than that for the late second and early third centuries AD, where a number of epidemics are recorded, but their location and mortality rates seem to have escaped the original compilers completely.

The oldest Chinese records are oracle bones, dating from the Shang Dynasty (*c.* 1600–1046 BC). Written on scapulae and pieces of tortoise shell, they were used for divination. From the oracle bones, we can deduce that the ancient Chinese suffered from diseases of the eyes and ears; had dental problems and speech defects; abdominal diseases; dysuria; beriberi (or something like it); obstetric and paediatric problems; and, in addition, various lethal seasonal epidemics. Scholars are also fairly certain schistosomiasis was known.

Seals from excavated tombs provide another useful source of information about the diseases of the late Chou Dynasty (*c.* 1046–256 BC) and Warring States period (*c.* 475–221 BC). These seals reveal how disease had come to be seen as a field with many different aspects, rather than simply a general notion of ill health. The seal of the physician Wang indicates that he specialised in speech impediments; physician Chang's seal reveals that his speciality was the cure of external lesions; physician Kao treated ulcers; physician Kuo dealt with beriberi and other similar conditions; physician Thu specialised in removing nasal polyps; and physician Chao seems to have been a kind of early psychologist.

Medical texts become an increasingly valuable source of data in the late Chou Dynasty, the so-called Spring and Autumn period (*c.* 771–*c.* 476 BC). The *Yueh Ling* (*Monthly Ordinances*) discusses seasonal diseases. An unseasonally warm or cold spring, autumnal summer or mild winter would spell epidemics. Epidemics in the spring could have been scabies; in summer, bronchitis and pneumonia; in autumn, 'fever' might have meant malaria, and in winter, typhus and tetanus could have developed. Texts written or compiled after the *Yueh Ling* began to differentiate clearly between tertian and quartan malaria. Tuberculosis was also recorded for the first time, as was leprosy.

The *Chou Li* (*Record of Institutions of the Chou Dynasty*, probably compiled in the early Han Dynasty, second century BC) also notes that each of the four seasons has its particular epidemics. Spring has feverish aches and headaches; summer, 'itching scabies-like epidemics'; autumn brings malaria and other fevers; while in winter, respiratory diseases dominate.

A concept of 'airs, waters and places' becomes evident in many of the texts. Another book from the late Warring States period, the *Lu Shih Chun Chiu*, asserts that, in places where there is too much 'light' or clear water, diseases of the scalp (alopecia, ringworm, psoriasis) and goitre will occur. In places where there is an excess of 'heavy' or turbid water, people suffering from swellings and leg ulcers are commonly found, and there will be some who are completely lame (suggestive of beriberi). Acrid water will produce skin lesions, such as abscesses and boils; and where 'bitter' water flows, there will be many people with bent bones (rickets). Only in places where there is 'sweet' water, will people be free of problems. (Indeed, they are said to be 'healthy and handsome'.)

Chinese thinking about disease was not entirely free of superstition. The chronicle known as the *Tso Chuan*, compiled during the Warring States period and covering the years 722 to 468 BC, records some bizarre magical remedies. In the year 638 BC, a deformed witch, probably suffering from rickets, was to be burnt as a remedy for drought until a sceptical official intervened and saved her. The *Shan Hai Ching* records less extreme forms of magic, detailing the medicinal value of certain plants, animals, herbs and minerals.

The *Nei Ching* (also known as *The Yellow Emperor's Inner Canon*), which probably dates from the late Warring States period, was arguably the most important ancient Chinese medical text. It attempted to take the supernatural out of disease, much as Hippocrates did in Greece. No longer were diseases sent by gods, demons or troublemaking ancestors, but were seen to be imbalances of natural processes. Six 'humours' were identified: wind, humid heat, dry heat, damp, cold and aridity. The *Nei Ching* developed an elaborate classificatory system that utilised the concept of Yin and Yang (the two fundamental forces in the universe), the five elements of fire, water, earth, wood and metal, Pa Kang (or the eight diagnostic principles), and the concept of chi, or energy.

Galen & Disease in Rome

The history of disease in ancient Rome is patchy. Livy (59 BC – AD 17) records various epidemics in his *History of Rome*. Between 490 and 292 BC, and especially in the years 212–174 BC, 'a mortality crisis is mentioned on average every 4.3 years'.[78] Rome's health appears to improve after that: from the mid second century BC to the late second century AD, only five epidemics are mentioned (142 BC, 23–22 BC, AD 65, AD 79/80 and 189). However, this could be a result of authorial bias, in that writers often 'paid less attention to inauspicious events'.[79] Epidemics were auspicious, endemic diseases were not, and therefore less liable to be recorded. Late Antiquity is a bit better – that is, worse – with ten epidemics listed between AD 285 and 750. As Walter Scheidel notes, 'This paucity is undoubtedly a function of the nature of the evidence, rather than a reflection of dramatic improvement.'[80]

The most important medical figure in ancient Rome was Galen (129–*c.*216 AD), a polymath – doctor, writer, philosopher, surgeon – who hailed from Pergamon, site of one of the most well-known Asclepions in the ancient world. He is the most important medical figure of the Roman period, and, with Hippocrates, the most important medical authority before the Renaissance. He also wrote voluminously: we have more books by Galen than any other writer from antiquity. He practised in Rome, a city where competition among doctors was far more intense than Athens, and just as deregulated. Rome was a city that, according to the sophist Polemo of Laodicea (*c.*90–144), was the 'epitome of the world'. If so, then it was certainly an unhealthy world: Galen wrote that every day, ten thousand people could be found suffering from jaundice, and an equal number from dropsy.[81]

Despite Polemo's claim, Rome might be atypical of the ancient world. Its huge population of around a million[82] meant that it probably suffered from more diseases than any other city of the time; and cities are fertile breeding grounds for disease, much more so than villages. Some of the city's most persistent health problems were due to a combination of overcrowding, environmental issues and architectural innovation. As Walter Scheidel noted, 'Rome's nodal position encouraged the introduction of new strains of the disease while its exceptionally large population would have made it easier for such arrivals to become endemic and contribute permanently to the metropolitan disease pool.'[83] Susan Mattern sees ancient Rome as rife with disease vectors: 'Rome was, then, an ideal environment for any disease spread by vermin, flies, mosquitoes, feces, dogs, or (because of its densely packed population) through the air, as well as for respiratory illnesses caused by indoor air pollution. One of its most dangerous, pervasive, and characteristic illnesses was malaria.'[84]

The city had always suffered from malaria, due to the proximity of the Pontine Marshes. No one knows the date at which it became endemic in the city, but it was certainly there by the first century BC, when the poet Horace (65 BC – 8 BC) and Livy both made references to it. The disease was worst in late summer, turning all places where stagnant water formed – the *impluvia* or cisterns that caught rainwater, ponds, overflow from fountains and baths – into potential death traps, as this is where the female *anopheles* mosquito would lay her eggs. Susan Mattern notes that 'cases of malaria may have spiked in flood years'.[85] *P. falciparum* is the most lethal form of malaria. This may be the disease that is referred to in ancient writings as the 'semitertian fever'. Writers noted that the fever was periodic, returning every two days. It is this aspect of the fever – the other main one being 'quartan fever', returning every three days – that gives us fairly concrete assurances that the disease in question was indeed malaria. Galen notes that 'we see it every day, especially at Rome.'[86] But one mistake made by Galen, and the Hippocratic writers before him, was thinking fever was the disease, not the symptom. (The Hippocratic Corpus abounds with fevers.) Galen believed that the sickness was created by 'bad air' – which led to the eventual coining of the name 'malaria' (from the Latin, *mal' aria*), in the eighteenth century. Until then, it lurked under a variety of names: semitertian fever, quartan fever, Roman fever, ague.

Since the time of Hippocrates, 'bad air', or miasma, had been commonly thought to either cause or spread disease. While this was incorrect in the case of malaria, it was not too far wide of the mark in others, such as in the case of airborne diseases, like pneumonic plague (see below), which could be transmitted from person to person by coughing – a form of 'bad air', as it were. The miasma theory could also be said to be partially correct in that it intuited the importance of environmental factors in the spread of disease. Dirt, for instance, could spread typhoid (again, this is something we'll come back to later). In the case of ancient Rome, one kind of 'bad air' that led to disease was poor ventilation in the home. The second century AD mummified body of a girl found in Grottarossa on the Cassian Way near Rome showed signs of anthracosis, caused by carbon accumulation in the lungs, a disease more commonly associated with coal miners. But in the case of the girl from Grottarossa, her symptoms were probably caused by smoke from lamps, cooking and fires. She was only around eight years old.[87]

Water supplies in the city also had an unwitting role in the spread of other diseases. The city's aqueducts may have brought fresh water into Rome, but when they overflowed, potentially major health hazards were created. Water from an overflowing fountain would turn the mud of the street into a rich breeding ground for germs. *E. coli* was known to have flourished in such conditions, as did gastrointestinal diseases. Like the ancient Egyptians before them, the citizens of ancient Rome were afflicted by worms; dysentery and diarrhoea could be fatal (especially in children). Animals ran freely: dogs, pigs, goats, even cattle, could be seen in Rome's public thoroughfares on a daily basis. Horace mentions a muddy sow running down the middle of the street in one of his poems, and while the sow herself might have been perfectly happy on her daily round of rooting, animals could act as vectors for rabies, malaria, and also for zoonotic (animal to human) diseases, such as bovine tuberculosis and later, plague. Add muddy feet and unwashed hands to the equation, and you have a direct – and very busy – link between the street and people's homes.

Suetonius (*c.* 69 – after 122) records gruesome confirmation of this. One day 'a stray dog picked up a human hand at the cross-roads, which it brought into the room where [the emperor-to-be] Vespasian was breakfasting and dropped it under the table'.[88] Although the anecdote was no doubt included for its symbolic aspect – the hand was a symbol of power – it illustrates the hazards presented by people dying in the streets and going unburied; unclaimed corpses were usually buried in common pits, or thrown into the Tiber. Suetonius notes that Vespasian, when working as an *aedile*, or public official responsible for the upkeep of public buildings, sewers, and streets, fell foul of the emperor Caligula, who was 'furious because Vespasian had not kept the streets clean, as was his duty, [and] ordered some soldiers to load him with mud; they obeyed by stuffing into the fold of his senatorial gown as much as it could hold'.[89]

Rome's public baths were another hazard. Like the aqueducts and the city's sewers, they were the envy of other cities, and should have gone a fair way to maintaining good standards of hygiene. But in reality they were extremely unhygienic. The Romans had a tradition of 'medicinal bathing' that took place in public baths; both Celsus (*c.* 25 BC – *c.* 50 AD) and Pliny the Elder (23 AD – 79 AD) wrote of its benefits. Bathing was used as a treatment for many diseases, including those known to be infectious, such as leprosy, dysentery and respiratory ailments. However, the potential for spreading disease by way of infected bathwater was high, given that people could be exposing open wounds in the water, while Celsus advised patients suffering from bowel problems 'to bathe their anuses in the hot pools located at these venues but (not unreasonably) warns those with infected wounds not to expose them to the filthy contents of these facilities.'[90] Posterior problems notwithstanding, Galen noted that people urinated in the baths. The hot, smoky atmosphere of the bathhouses likewise could cause people to faint when it wasn't aggravating respiratory problems. The dirty water and humid atmosphere did nothing to keep the cockroaches away. According to Pliny the Elder, they liked the damp warmth (*Natural History*, 11.34).

The combination of dirt, vermin, dead bodies, free range animals, overcrowding – including a permanent influx of population from rural areas, either seeking a livelihood or escaping war – meant that the Eternal City was an eternal crucible of disease. (Despite this, it was, ironically, still one of the more healthy cities of the ancient world; seventeenth century London was dirtier.) Evidence from skeletal remains, and a certain amount of educated guesswork, suggests that Romans also suffered tuberculosis, leprosy, typhoid, all manner of diarrhoeal and gastrointestinal diseases, worms, jaundice, gout, salmonella, anthrax, rabies, epilepsy, hepatitis, elephantiasis and tetanus. Confronted with such a list, it is not surprising to find that most of Galen's patients did not reach old age.

There were other diseases, too. Pliny the Elder devoted the beginning of Book 26 of the *Natural History* to what he termed 'new forms of disease, unknown in ancient times'.[91] One of these was a skin condition Pliny termed *mentagra*, which 'spreads over the interior of the mouth, and takes possession of the whole face, with the sole exception of the eyes; after which, it passes downwards to the neck, breast, and hands, covering them with foul furfuraceous eruptions.' It is 'painless and not life-threatening, but so disgusting that any sort of death is preferable.'[92] Mentagra was transmitted by kissing, and seemed to afflict only upper class males. All of this suggests some sort of sexually transmitted disease, but what it was, we do not know.

The most deadly unknown disease, however, was something Galen himself lived to see. The Antonine Plague – sometimes known as the Plague of Galen's time – broke out during a military campaign in Seleucia in Mesopotamia during the winter of 165–6. By the end of the following year, returning troops had brought it to Rome; it continued to spread throughout the empire and returned regularly until the late 180s or early 190s. Galen's descriptions of the plague are vague, and don't allow us to say with any certainty what it was. He describes it as 'great', and that it lasted a long time; however, Galen did go into some detail about the symptoms. Sufferers developed an eruptive skin rash, sometimes spreading over the whole body, which could become 'rough and scabby' and fall off 'like some husk'.[93] Accompanying this was fever; diarrhoea – including the passing of black and bloody stools; vomiting (in some but not all cases); an upset stomach; fetid breath; and a cough – which sometimes included the regurgitation of blood and scabs. Galen notes 'that the plague was similar to the Thucydidean plague and quotes a passage which includes Thucydides' words about the rash being blistery... in another passage Galen again says the plague was very close in form to the one described by Thucydides.'[94] A rash like the one Galen describes discounts the Antonine Plague being plague in the bubonic sense, where the rashes tend to appear around the buboes in the armpit and groin. Similarly, the rash produced by typhus doesn't behave in quite the same way as the one described by Galen.

The severity of the plague suggests that it was a disease previously unknown in Europe (and therefore probably wasn't the same disease as the Athenian Plague, despite Galen's efforts to compare the two). The historian Cassius Dio claimed there were 2,000 fatalities a day during one of the later outbreaks of the epidemic (in AD 189), 'a figure that has the dubious merit of being at least theoretically possible.'[95] Although numbers cited by ancient writers tend to be more symbolic than literal, we can be certain that a lot of people were dying; it is thought that between a quarter and a third of Rome's population died. The army was also devastated to such an extent that Marcus Aurelius's campaigns against the Marcomanni tribes in the Danube had to be delayed. With Imperial forces seriously weakened, the Marcomanni, and other peoples, were able to slowly encroach on Roman territory. Estimates of fatalities range from between one and five million.

If it wasn't bubonic plague or typhus, what was the Antonine Plague?

Smallpox – 'or something similar or ancestral to it'[96] – has long been thought to be the most likely culprit; or smallpox working alongside another disease new to Europe, measles. A combined attack of two diseases on a virgin population would certainly have been far more deadly than an epidemic of a disease to which people had had time to build up resistance.

A similar mystery surrounds the Plague of Cyprian, which raged across the Roman Empire between 251 and *c.* 270:

> ... there broke out a dreadful plague, and excessive destruction of a hateful disease invaded every house in succession of the trembling populace, carrying off day by day with abrupt attack numberless people, every one from his own house. All were shuddering, fleeing, shunning the contagion, impiously exposing their own friends, as if with the exclusion of the person who was sure to die of the plague, one could exclude death itself also. There lay about the meanwhile, over the whole city, no longer bodies, but the carcases of many...[97]

So wrote Pontius the Deacon, in his hagiography of St Cyprian, Bishop of Carthage, after whom the epidemic was named. Cyprian (*c.* 210–258) described the symptoms in his tract *De Mortalitate*:

> ... that now the bowels, relaxed into a constant flux, discharge the bodily strength; that a fire originated in the marrow ferments into wounds of the fauces; that the intestines are shaken with a continual vomiting; that the eyes are on fire with the injected blood; that in some cases the feet or some parts of the limbs are taken off by the contagion of diseased putrefaction; that from the weakness arising by the maiming and loss of the body, either the gait is enfeebled, or the hearing is obstructed, or the sight darkened... (*De Mortalitate* 14)

These symptoms – diarrhoea, a raging sore throat, vomiting, losing limbs to what sounds like gangrene, general weakness – make it sound as though smallpox was at work, although, as with the Antonine Plague, it could well have been an ancestral variant, or smallpox and measles working together. Bubonic plague has even been conjectured. Whatever it was, it was utterly deadly, with a mortality rate possibly as high as 50 per cent in some areas. Cyprian also noted that 'this Disease attacks our people equally with the heathens' (*De Mortalitate* 8). Historian William McNeill believes this second plague was even more deadly than the Antonine. 'This time reported mortality in the city of Rome was even greater [than the Antonine Plague],' he wrote, 'five thousand a day are said to have died at the height of the epidemic, and there is reason to believe that rural populations were affected even more sharply than in the earlier epidemic'.[98]

The impact of the Plague of Cyprian is difficult to assess with accuracy, but we can certainly count severe population decline as being among its more debilitating legacies. (Whatever the Plague of Cyprian was, outbreaks were said to have recurred, including a severe one in the British Isles in the mid fifth century. The Venerable Bede claimed that, in some places, there were hardly enough people left to bury the dead.) The Cyprian Plague was also a major factor in the so-called 'Crisis of the Third Century', caused by economic depression and what almost constituted open season on the emperor's throne, with over twenty claimants during a fifty-year period (AD 235–85). While the empire was falling apart, Rome remained the hub of the western world, attracting scores of immigrants, pilgrims, mercenaries and merchants, all bringing their diseases with them.

Aside from its depleting of the strength of Rome's armies and weakening her lengthy borders, and thus possibly beginning the decline of Rome, the plague of Cyprian had another lasting consequence. Cyprian's *De Mortalitate* was not a medical tract: it was consolatory. Addressed to fellow Christians, Cyprian reminded his congregation of the tribulations of Job, Abraham and Paul, whose faith was not shaken by adversity:

> … as it is written, "The furnace trieth the vessels of the potter, and the trial of tribulation just men." [Ecclesiasticus 27:6] This, in short,

> is the difference between us and others who know not God, that in misfortune they complain and murmur, while adversity does not call us away from the truth of virtue and faith, but strengthens us by its suffering. (*De Mortalitate* 13)

Cyprian welcomed the plague, telling believers it was a test of their faith. For those yet to be converted, Christianity offered refuge in a world that, as Cyprian admitted, 'is changing and passing away, and witnesses to its ruin not now by its age, but by the end of things' (*DM* 25). With the world changing and passing away, people flocked to the Church for solace. This happened despite renewed persecution of Christians by the emperor Valerian (among whose victims was Cyprian himself).

Not only did the Cyprian Plague swell the Church's rank-and-file, it also helped establish the image of Christ the physician, and with it, Christian influence on medicine and care of the sick. Of the thirty-plus miracles Jesus performs in the New Testament, around two-thirds are healing miracles – curing blindness, leprosy, lameness and cases of possession by demons and evil spirit, which modern medicine would probably classify as psychiatric disorders, although one could be a case of epilepsy.[99]

As Roy Porter reminds us, '"holiness" and "healing" stem from the same root, meaning "wholeness"'.[100] St Luke the Evangelist is traditionally held to be a doctor, 'the beloved physician' (Colossians 4:14). At Pentecost, Christ's disciples are filled with the Holy Spirit and able to heal; Peter cures a lame beggar at the temple gates in the very next chapter (Acts 3:1–10). Thus began a long tradition of healing miracles, often associated with saints, replacing the earlier tradition of incubation, temple sleep and cure by the touch of the (pagan) god. Indeed, so similar was Christianity to paganism in this respect, that EM Forster once remarked it was 'carrying on the work of the earlier firm'.[101] Seeing healing as a religious duty, Christians also established the first western hospitals and hospices in the fourth century, caring for pilgrims and lepers.[102] Hostels and almshouses followed. Despite

Christianity's hostility to all things pagan, Christian doctors happily adopted the theory of the four humours, and continued to regard disease, especially epidemics, as a sign of divine displeasure with a sinful humanity. In this way, the 'work of the earlier firm' was carried on unchallenged in the West until the Renaissance.

The Plague of Justinian

Antiquity is sometimes seen as ending with the closure of the Academy in Athens in the year 529. In his wisdom, the emperor Justinian (527–565) had taken it upon himself to persecute pagan philosophers (amongst others). It was meant to be part of a larger plan to eradicate paganism and heresy from the eastern Roman Empire, which would then be reunited with the western half of the empire, lost to various pagan tribes in the previous century. While Justinian and his general, Belisarius, were busy with this ambitious and ultimately doomed plan, something happened that possibly has a better claim to 'ending antiquity' than the closure of the Academy: the first pandemic of one of the most deadly and feared diseases in history, bubonic plague.

Plague is a rodent disease, most frequently associated (in Europe at least) with the black rat. It is endemic to a number of regions of the world, including parts of Africa, Central Asia, parts of South America and the more temperate regions of the North. It is possibly also endemic in Europe, but on a vastly lesser scale. The plague bacillus, *Yersinia pestis*, lives in the bloodstream of small rodents such as rats, marmots, squirrels or mice. Originally a harmless bacteria in their stomachs, the bacillus evolved over time, enabling it to enter the animals' bloodstream, and becoming lethal in the process.

Rodent fleas are the disease's main vector. When a flea (usually the rodent's familiar, *Xenopsylla cheopis*) feeds on an infected host, the plague bacillus multiplies inside the flea's body, blocking its oesophagus and making it chronically thirsty. Its compulsion then is to bite continually to slake its thirst. When the rodent it has been feeding on dies, it will look for another host to drink from, but, because its foregut is full of undigested, infected blood, it will pass the plague bacillus into the bloodstream of whatever animal it tries to feed on next. The flea becomes, as it were, a highly effective syringe, administering potentially lethal doses of *Y. pestis* to each new host, and with the number of potential hosts diminished due to a plague outbreak, large numbers of fleas would end up living on the same animal; a single rat could have hundreds of plague-infested fleas living on it. With such large numbers of fleas feeding from the same animal, it would hasten the end of the unfortunate host far quicker than if normal numbers of fleas were present, and *X. cheopis* would be forced to go further afield to seek sustenance. That it's also a hardy insect, able to survive for up to six weeks without a host, would help explain why the disease could traverse such huge distances and still remain lethally effective.

X. cheopis does not particularly like human blood but, in the absence of any other host, it will bite. Bubonic plague attacks the lymphatic system, and produces boils or buboes in the groin (the word derives from the Greek word for groin, *boubon*), armpits or neck, usually depending on where the victim was bitten. Bites on the leg would result in buboes in the groin, upper body bites in the armpit or neck, often resulting in the victim developing a limp, a raised arm or a head permanently cocked away from the bubo. Regardless of where they develop, the buboes can vary in size, from that of an almond to that of an orange, are extremely painful and sometimes noisy, being known to make strange gurgling sounds. Most victims will only develop one bubo, appearing between two and six days after the initial infection; if more develop, they will normally be on the same chain of lymph glands. If the buboes suppurate within a week, the victim will usually recover. If not, as happened in the majority of cases, the victim will die. Untreated, bubonic plague has a mortality rate of around 60 per cent.

Although buboes are the most well-known symptom of plague, the victim will likely first become apathetic, quickly developing a high fever, with vomiting, extreme headaches, giddiness, intolerance to light, pains in the abdomen, back and limbs, sleeplessness and acute diarrhoea being not long in following. Contemporary chroniclers also recorded three other symptoms: bruise-like blotches on the skin (possibly caused by subcutaneous haemorrhages) which were termed 'God's Tokens'; severe delirium, which often led to episodes of manic shouting and laughing or, if the victim was still able to stand, dancing or walking aimlessly around in a trance until they collapsed; and, finally, an all-pervasive malodorousness that affected everything the victim's body produced, from breath, sweat and blood to faeces, urine and pus. Plague also has two variants, pneumonic and septicaemic (see the Black Death in Chapter 3), which attack the lungs and bloodstream respectively. These are even more deadly than the bubonic form of the disease.

Why endemic diseases such as plague become epidemics and pandemics is still a matter for research. Usually, a variety of factors will cause the host to leave its native habitat and seek new territories. In the case of the Justinian plague, we can conjecture that rodents in the disease's African reservoir – possibly Ethiopia – were forced out of their natural habitat due to natural factors (drought, for instance), and then travelled north with trade caravans. Trade routes would have continued to play a major part in disseminating the disease once it had gained a foothold in Egypt.

Plague – as an endemic, rather than epidemic, disease – seems to have been known to a number of ancient writers. Aretaeus of Cappadocia (*fl.* 60–80 AD), Rufus of Ephesus (*fl.* 100) and Oribasius (*c.* 325 – *c.* 400) all refer to plague (or something that sounds very much like it), but the major epidemics of their times seem to have been a probable mixture of smallpox, measles, typhus and the ever-present malaria. In the Bible, aside from the ten plagues of Egypt, there was the Plague of Ashdod in the First Book of Samuel. This is more interesting, as it mentions rats.

After capturing the Ark of the Covenant and taking it to the city of Ashdod, the Philistines experienced that old disease chestnut, divine displeasure: 'The Lord's hand was heavy upon the people of Ashdod and its vicinity; he brought devastation upon them and afflicted them with tumours' (1 Samuel 6). The Septuagint and Vulgate versions of the Bible make it clear what this plague is, adding: 'And rats appeared in their land, and death and destruction were throughout the city.' A few verses later, 'the Lord's hand was against that city, throwing it into a great panic. He afflicted the people of the city, both young and old, with an outbreak of tumours.' Once again, the Septuagint is more explicit, by replacing 'tumours' with 'tumours in the groin'. The connection between rats and tumours is reinforced in Chapter 6 where, to placate the wrath of the Almighty, the Philistines have to make gold replicas of five rats and five tumours, as there were five Philistine rulers 'because the same plague has struck both you and your rulers'. Despite these tantalising references to rats and tumours in the groin, the Plague of Ashdod isn't supported by archaeological or paleopathological evidence. The events of 1 Samuel remain in that hinterland between history and myth, like all the other diseases mentioned in the Bible. The same cannot be said, however, for what became known as the Plague of Justinian.

It began in the Egyptian port of Pelusium in the summer of 541, and 'is the first time that we can correctly use the term "plague", for the sickness was undoubtedly bubonic plague.' Prior to DNA analysis confirming *Y. pestis* as the cause of the Plague of Justinian,[103] our chief sources were chroniclers such as the Byzantine historian and lawyer Procopius, whose *History of the Wars* contains an eyewitness account of plague. (As Belisarius's legal adviser, Procopius accompanied the general on many campaigns, where he saw the plague at work.) Procopius describes how the plague started in Egypt, and spread to the rest of the Byzantine Empire, Europe, Persia and the 'barbarian hinterland', by which he probably means the British Isles. Egypt and Asia Minor (modern-day Anatolian Turkey) were particularly badly affected.

Procopius noted that fever was the first sign of plague, with buboes forming after a few days. 'He reports that the mortality rose alarmingly, eventually reaching more than ten thousand each day.'[104] Although we should take ten thousand deaths a day with a pinch of salt, Procopius was voicing the feelings of many when he wrote that Plague of Justinian was 'a pestilence by which the whole human race came near to being annihilated.'[105]

Other chroniclers reported equally grim news. The lengthiest account of the plague is found in the *Ecclesiastical History* of John of Ephesus (*c.* 507–588) who was, even more than Procopius, better placed to witness the annihilation. He was on a diplomatic mission from Constantinople to Alexandria when the plague broke out. Returning home through Palestine, Syria and Asia Minor, he found to his alarm that the plague seemed to be travelling with him:

> During the tumult and intensity of the pestilence we journeyed from Syria to the capital. Day after day we, too, used to knock at the door of the grave along with everyone else. We used to think that if there would be evening, death would come upon us suddenly in the night. Although the next morning would come, we used to face the grave during the whole day as we looked at the devastated and moaning villages in these regions, and at corpses lying on the ground with no one to gather them.[106]

John saw people carrying corpses all day, while others were engaged in the apparently endless task of digging fresh graves. One monastery buried eighty-four of its monks. Houses lay abandoned. Animals wandered untended in streets and on farms.

> Crops of wheat in fertile fields located in all the regions through which we passed from Syria up through Thrace, were white and standing but there was no one to reap them and store the wheat. Vineyards, whose picking season came and went, shed their leaves, since winter was severe, but kept their fruits hanging on their vines, and there was no one to pick them or press them.[107]

The plague seemed to spare no one. John believed that, terrible as it was, it was divinely ordained. As translator Amir Harrak commented, 'John believed that there was a divine plan in the fact that the poor were struck first, so that they might be appropriately buried by the rich, and in the fact that, by the time the rich were struck, there were no survivors to bury them, so that they might rot in the streets, houses and palaces – as in fact happened.'[108]

The emperor Justinian ordered the digging of mass graves, but was then himself stricken; he recovered to rule for another twenty years. Pope Pelagius II was not so fortunate, succumbing to a recurrence of plague in 590. His successor, Gregory the Great, organised public processions 'to demonstrate collective penance'.[109]

Paul the Deacon (*c.* 720–799) wrote a vivid account of plague in Liguria in the 560s. It's one of the best Dark Age accounts of the Plague of Justinian – possibly based on a lost eyewitness account – and is worth quoting at length:

> A very great pestilence broke out particularly in the province of Liguria. For suddenly there appeared certain marks among the dwellings, doors, utensils and clothes, which, if anyone wished to wash away, became more and more apparent. After the lapse of a year indeed there began to appear in the groins of men and in other rather delicate places a swelling of the glands, after the manner of a nut or date, presently followed by an unbearable fever, so that upon the third day the man died. But if anyone should pass over the third day he had a hope of living. Everywhere there was grief and everywhere tears. For as common report had it that those who fled would avoid the plague, the dwellings were left deserted by their inhabitants, and the dogs alone kept house. The flocks remained alone in the pastures with no shepherd at hand. You might see villages or fortified places lately filled with crowds of men, and on the next day all had departed and everything was in utter silence. Some fled, leaving the corpses of their parents unburied; parents forgetful of their duty abandoned their children in raging fever. If by chance long-standing affection constrained anyone to bury his near relative, he remained himself unburied, and while he was performing funeral rites he perished; while he offered obsequies to the dead, his own corpse remained

> without obsequies. You might see the world brought back to its ancient silence; no voice in the field; no whistling of shepherds; no lying in wait of wild beasts among the cattle; no harm to domestic fowls. The crops, outliving the time of the harvest, awaited the reaper untouched; the vineyard with its fallen leaves and its shining grapes remained undisturbed while winter came on; a trumpet as of warriors resounded through the day and night; something like the murmur of an army was heard by many; there were no footsteps of passers by, no murderer was seen, yet the corpses of the dead were more than the eye could discern; pastoral places had been turned into a desert, and human habitations had become places of refuge for wild beasts.[110]

Despite such accounts, scholarly opinion has fluctuated on just how devastating the Plague of Justinian actually was. The French historian Jean Durliat proposed that historians have relied too much on literary sources, which tend to portray the pandemic as a largely urban affair, and almost certainly exaggerated its impact.[111] However, examination of non-literary sources does provide evidence for a dramatic depopulation in the second half of the sixth century. Archaeological evidence from Syria suggests that expansion of both rural and urban settlements abruptly ceased in the second half of the sixth century, which is 'entirely consistent with a pandemic that caused massive loss of life on repeated occasions.'[112]

Other evidence comes from the Byzantine Empire's fiscal records, in that the amount of revenue coming in from taxable land declined dramatically. 'It is thus highly significant that, in spite of Durliat's claims, the advent of the Justinianic Plague and its subsequent recurrences coincided with a period of major instability in the imperial coinage – our best measure of the condition of imperial finances.'[113] There also appears to have been a rise in wages – a development that Justinian himself complained about. But this drop in revenue was real, and would have had an adverse effect on the main recipient of imperial revenue – the army. In 588, army pay was cut by 25 per cent, leading to rebellions on the empire's eastern flank. Things came to a head in 602 with a coup against the Emperor Maurice, followed by a lengthy – and disastrous – war with the Sasanian Empire of Persia. Both the Byzantine and the Persians were weakened by the war, leaving the door open for invasion by the new power in seventh century politics – Islam.

There was trouble elsewhere in the empire. The Balkans and Greece experienced Slavic migrations, the Lombards invaded Italy and the Berbers made inroads into North Africa. While the pandemic's long tail would see the rise of Islam in the seventh century, it would also see the rise of the Vikings in the eighth. Furthermore, as William McNeill has argued (reiterating the view of Belgian historian Henri Pirenne), the power balance of European culture shifted away from the Mediterranean towards the north.[114]

3

The Dark and Middle Ages

The Plague of Justinian had burned itself out by about 550, but the first pandemic – of which it was the first, incendiary, phase – lasted until the mid-eighth century. Among the surviving records for the final stages of the pandemic is *The Chronicle of Zuqnin*, which details the calamities of the years 743–5 in Syria. Even at this late stage, the plague was still capable of burying five hundred people a day.[115] The pestilence started with the poor, and then 'the Destroyer struck those in positions of power'.[116] The Chronicler notes that 'this painful and bitter anguish reigned over the entire world. Just as the rain falls down on the whole earth, or as the rays of the sun spread out over everything equally, so did this plague at this time spread out.'[117]

> ... numerous villages and places suddenly became desolate, without people passing by them or settling in them. The stricken bodies, stretched out on the ground like litter on the surface of the earth, were groaning; and there was no one to bury them since not one of them survived. Thus people were discarded inside those places, swollen, putrid and stinking. Their houses were open like graves, and inside them the owners were rotting from putrefaction. Their furniture, gold and silver were thrown away, and all their goods were discarded in the streets but there was no one to collect them. Vile was gold and silver there! What is more, old men and women with honourable white hair, who had looked forward to being buried in great splendour by their heirs, were discarded in the streets, houses

and palaces, burst open, stinking, with their mouths open. Graceful virgins and beautiful young girls, who looked forward to bridal feasts and elegant and precious garments, were discarded, exposed and rotting together. They became a pitiful lesson for onlookers. If only it had occurred inside graves! Rather, it occurred in houses and market-places! Handsome and cheerful young men turned dark, were discarded and rotted with their fathers.[118]

Loathly Stalkers and Leechbooks, or The Sparrow in Winter

After the mid-eighth century, the plague appears to have disappeared back to its rodent reservoirs in Asia and Africa. Arno Karlen notes that, after the first pandemic finally died down, the Dark Ages were relatively disease-free.[119] This is because the pandemic had wiped out so much of Europe's population – possibly halved it – that there simply weren't enough people left for epidemic and crowd diseases to feed on. It's as though disease, having fed, was sated for a few centuries, and didn't need to gorge again until the High Middle Ages. This could help explain why archaeological finds from this period show mainly bone diseases, breakages and injuries, the kind of evidence paleopathologists have noted in earlier hunter-gatherer societies. Climate change also played a part: from about 800 there were five centuries of warmer weather, until the advent of the so-called Little Ice Age around the year 1300. This meant that the Dark Ages – from the fall of Rome in the fifth century to about the year 1000 – were actually a 'more healthful, less violent era than those before and after.'[120]

It was still an era in which, to judge from evidence from burial sites, there was 'a fairly short life expectancy, a high infant mortality, with women dying young, particularly in childbirth, and a fairly high incidence of bone and joint diseases, such as rheumatism, arthritis and rickets.'[121] Dysentery was common, and the proximity of animals meant the usual susceptibility to zoonoses such as sheep liver fluke.

Another relatively common disease was *lencten adl* ('spring ailment' or 'spring fever') – tertian malaria. Jaundice, pleurisy, pneumonia were also known to have affected the Anglo-Saxons, as well as something called *seo healfdeade adl* (the 'halfdead disease'), which was probably hemiplegia, a form of partial paralysis often caused by a stroke. Housing, for rich and poor alike, was primitive: huts or hovels were heated by a central fire that meant they were smoky – leading to possible eye infections – as well as being dark and damp.

The Venerable Bede (672–735) recounts a story in his *Ecclesiastical History of the English People* that encapsulates both the drafty conditions in such dwellings, and also something of the Anglo-Saxon view of life. At the court of King Edwin of Northumbria (reigned 616–633), when he was considering converting to Christianity in 627, Bede has a noble describe the frailty and brevity of human life:

> The present life of man on earth, O king, in comparison with the time which is unknown to us, seems to me as when you sit at dinner with your commanders and ministers in winter time, with a fire burning on the hearth in the midst in a good warm dining-hall while everywhere outside the rains or snows of winter are raging, a sparrow should come in and fly quickly through the room, who when it has entered by one door soon leaves by another. While it is inside it is not touched by the winter storm, but after a short time of calm gone in a moment, at once it slips from your sight returning from winter to winter.[122]

As the biologist ML Cameron noted in his study of Anglo-Saxon medicine, 'When people lived under such conditions, it is not to be wondered at that their resistance to disease must have been impaired.'[123]

As with the ancient Egyptian belief that disease was 'something entering from outside' which is 'the breath of an outside god or death', and the ancient Chinese pictogram for disease showing a human figure shot with arrows, so the Anglo-Saxons 'had some idea of infective disease; the frequent references to *flying venom*, to *elfshot* and to the *loathly one that roams through the land* can best be explained as showing an understanding of communicable diseases.'[124]

To combat these outside forces, doctors of the time consulted what texts were available. Latin and Greek literature was known to Anglo-Saxon doctors, such as Pliny's *Natural History*, the *De Medicamentis (Book of Medicaments)* of Marcellus Empiricus (*fl.* 400), and Isidore of Seville's *Etymologies* (probably written towards the end of Isidore's life and he died in 636). Very little of Hippocrates' and Galen's work was available to Anglo-Saxons in the original, but much of their teaching was available second (or third) hand, in the paraphrased work of others. Among the most influential of these writers were Oribasius (*c.* 320–400), who hailed, like Galen, from Pergamon; St Augustine of Hippo's personal physician, Vindicianus (*fl.* 364–375); Cassius Felix of Numidia (*fl. c.* 450); and Alexander of Tralles (*c.* 525 – *c.* 605).

Original material was also written, the so-called leechbooks, a mixture of the practical and the magical. (Although, for someone living in the Europe of the eighth or ninth century, the magical frequently was the practical.) The most well-known are *Bald's Leechbook*, possibly written for King Alfred (871–899), and the *Lacnunga*. *Bald's Leechbook* is arranged in the traditional head-to-foot format (a method of organising medical texts that dates back to the Edwin Smith Papyrus, if not earlier) but uniquely, separates the diseases into those whose manifestations are mainly external (Book I), and those whose manifestations are mainly internal (Book II).

Jaundice, chilblains, impotence and even aching feet, amongst others, are to be treated with various plant remedies. Perhaps partly because of the lack of chimneys in houses and halls, as noted above, *Bald's Leechbook* contains nineteen remedies for *eagena miste* ('mistiness of the eyes', 'dimness of vision'). Cameron suggests this 'mistiness' might be due to astigmatism, injuries or infections.[125] One remedy for night-blindness involved eating roast buck's liver, after first anointing the eyes with the meat's juices. Although this might sound like hocus-pocus, it actually worked because the liver would supply vitamin A, 'a deficiency of which is the chief cause of night blindness.'[126] Among the internal diseases in Book II are 'pains in the side', in which 'pleurisy and perhaps pneumonia may be recognized.'[127]

'When all else failed,' Cameron comments, 'the Anglo-Saxon physician could resort to charms, in themselves of no effect, but probably of great psychological benefit to the patient.'[128] The physician could call upon the magical recipes and charms in *Leechbook III*, which appears in the same manuscript as *Bald's Leechbook*, and *Lacnunga*. 'There are conditions which resist treatment even today. It is interesting to find that these are the ailments for which remedies most often have a magical component, as in the one for migraine.'[129]

The *Lacnunga* ('Remedies') is a collection of 200 or so remedies in somewhat haphazard order. It represents the folk magic of the time, including 'two outstanding pagan charms, one for sudden stitch caused by the assaults of witches, elves and Æsir, the other for *dweorh*, a fever with delirium.'[130] Interestingly, as Stephen Pollington notes, amid *Lacnunga*'s magic were some ideas that we would recognise:

> Many *Lacnunga* recipes specify the use of clean materials... which clearly indicates the recognition that tainted or contaminated materials could and would affect the outcome of the treatment. It therefore follows that the importance of cleanliness in medical treatment had at least begun to be recognised. The corollary was also true – that dirty or foul materials had to be avoided to ensure the effectiveness of the treatment. Contagion may also have been recognised, since Bede records the practice of segregating the sick into separate apartments.[131]

Bede also records clear overlaps between Christianity and magic. When Bishop John of Hexham (better known as John of Beverley) was told a young nun in the convent he was visiting had been bled on the fourth day of the moon, he said 'You have acted foolishly and ignorantly to bleed her on the fourth day of the moon; I remember how Archbishop Theodore [Archbishop of Canterbury, 668–690] of blessed memory used to say that it was very dangerous to bleed a patient when the moon is waxing and the ocean tide is flowing.'[132]Bleeding charts have survived, which show the best days of the month for bleeding a patient.

Monks' charts could have done nothing, however, to predict the coming of epidemics. The plague reached England in 664, where it was known as the Plague of Cadwallader's Time (after the King of Gwynedd, who himself died of plague in a recurrence in 682). It's possible that increased contact with Europe after St Augustine's mission to Christianise Britain in 597 led to plague and other diseases reaching England before 664: 'Anglo-Saxon records mention no fewer than forty-nine outbreaks of epidemics between 526 and 1087'[133], although many of these were minor. Irish chronicles record an epidemic in the 540s – probably the Justinian plague – but it's unclear whether it reached Ireland at that time. Given the lack of other evidence, it's probable the first pandemic didn't reach the British Isles at all until the 660s, when various chroniclers described the plague 'in terms that varied from the briefly factual to the nearly apocalyptic.'[134] According to Bede, the plague reached England in the spring of 664, where it first consumed 'the southern regions' before travelling to 'the province of the Northumbrians' where it 'brought low in grievous ruin an infinite number of men.'[135] Recurrences of plague continued on and off, petering out towards the end of the century.

Famines and other maladies

In his classic study *A History of Epidemics in Britain*, Charles Creighton noted that 'The history of English epidemics, previous to the Black Death, is almost wholly a history of famine sicknesses'.[136] Writers were so accustomed to the famine-pestilence cycle that they often assumed outbreaks of the latter to have been caused by the former. Broadly speaking, famines either occur naturally (due to inclement weather – drought, floods, earthquakes, insects) or through human intervention (war, economics). Frederick F Cartwright and Michael Biddiss succinctly summarise the cycle:

> Pestilence, famine and war interact and produce a sequence. War drives the farmer from his fields and destroys his crops; destruction of the crop spells famine; the starved and weakened people fall easy victims to the onslaught of pestilence. All three are diseases. Pestilence is a disorder of the human. Famine results from disorders of plants and cattle, whether caused by inclement weather or more directly by insect or bacterial invasion. And even war may be regarded, though more arguably, as a form of mass psychotic disorder.[137]

Pestilence, famine and war are, of course, three of the Horsemen of the Apocalypse. The fourth, death, follows in their wake. All four were active in northern Europe in these centuries of 'all quiet on the epidemic front', courtesy of the Vikings. That there were Viking raids at all, William H McNeill suggests, is evidence of a 'substantial swarming of population'[138] that had been able to grow due to the European disease pool reaching a state of maturity and balance. In other words, after the plague, people's immune systems and the various diseases doing the rounds of Dark Age Europe were in something like balance. No new epidemiological disasters appeared on the horizon, enabling people to develop resistance to the diseases of the time.

Despite McNeill's proposed stability of the European disease pool, recurrent Viking raids and the warmer climate, the Middle Ages certainly suffered from famines. There was a saying prevalent in the High Middle Ages that England was notorious for famine. Bad harvests could be caused either by too much water (floods, heavy rainfall) or not enough (drought). Late thirteenth and early fourteenth century England, perhaps unsurprisingly, suffered from the former. The Great Famine of 1315 was one of the worst the country ever suffered, being preceded by seemingly endless rain, beginning with a series of unusually wet summers in the mid 1290s. People were reduced to eating grass, dogs, even each other. Death from starvation was accompanied by diseases such as typhus, a disease 'intimately associated with wars, famines and human misfortunes of all kinds.'[139]

Although the name 'typhus' wasn't coined until the eighteenth century (the name deriving from the Greek *typhos*, meaning 'smoky' or 'hazy', a reference to the stupor its victims suffer), historians have long suspected typhus was rife much earlier. It has been proposed as the cause of the Plague of Athens in 430 BC, although this is still debated. Nevertheless, as John C Snyder from the Harvard School of Public Health wrote, 'classic typhus has been one of the major epidemic diseases of all time. It is probable that typhus fever has been exceeded only by malaria as a cause of widespread human suffering.'[140]

Hans Zinsser, in his classic book about typhus, *Rats, Lice and History* (1935), believed that the earliest description of the disease might possibly date from 1083, when an outbreak was recorded by the monks at La Cava Abbey in Salerno, Italy:

> In the year 1083, in the monastery of La Cava in the month of August and September, there spread a severe fever with peticuli and parotid swellings, in which one sees clearly the difference from the Pest, a fever of a different kind – and in this case – accompanied by petechial spots.[141]

The disease is spread by *Pediculus humanus corporis* – the human body louse. The lice live in the warm clothes of humans (wool and cotton in particular) where they lay their eggs. When they feed on an infected person, the louse becomes infected, and spreads the disease via their faeces. If the louse moves to another person and shits, and if that person then scratches where the flea has bitten, the chances are they will get epidemic typhus. Symptoms include fever, headache, delirium (hence 'smoky', 'hazy'), high temperature and, after a few days, a rash (the 'petechial spots' that Zinsser quoted). Fatalities can be around 20 per cent, although they will be higher when other diseases are at work, or the victims are already weak due to malnutrition.

However, there are records of epidemics that do not seem to have been famine-related (although military activity is mentioned in a few cases). Creighton suggests these could have been caused 'probably from a tainted soil'[142], although he doesn't elaborate on this rather vague comment (more suggestive of Victorian moralising or romanticism than actual epidemiological causes). Creighton adds that these references have been found in 'the most unlikely corners of monastic chronicles; but it is just the casual nature of the references that makes them credible, and leads one to suppose that the recorded instances are only samples of epidemics not altogether rare in the medieval life of England.'[143]

In 829, at Christchurch, Canterbury, all but five of the monks died of a pestilence. 897 saw 'a great mortality of man and beast following the Danish invasion which Alfred at length repelled.'[144] In 1010, more invading Danes died of a pestilence in Kent, (according to Ranulph Higden's chronicle), which was described as a *dolor viscerum*, probably dysentery. Miasma theory also made an appearance: 'The stench of their unburied bodies so infected the air as to bring a plague upon those of them who had remained well.' The outbreak was only brought to an end by St Elphege, the Archbishop of Canterbury, who restored people to health by giving out consecrated bread.

Dead bodies spreading illness reappear in a story told late the following century by William of Newburgh (*c.*1136–98), although in this case, the dead body in question is of an altogether more supernatural kind: William noted that a plague broke out in the village of Annan on the Solway Firth, which was thought to have been caused by a revenant.[145] The sickness was only ended when William's informant, who claimed to have been present, organised an exhumation of the revenant's body, which was then summarily cremated.

St Anthony's Fire

St Elphege and his miraculous loaf notwithstanding, bread, consecrated or otherwise, was no guarantee that one would remain disease free in the Middle Ages. If the bread was made from rye contaminated with ergot fungus (*Claviceps purpurea*), the chances are you would develop ergotism, the disease that probably lurks behind a number of evocative mediaeval names: St Anthony's Fire, saint's fire, hidden fire, evil fire, holy fire, devil's fire, and *Ignis sacer* (sacred fire). The St Anthony in question is the desert father and traditional founder of Christian monasticism (*c*.251–356). His relics were returned to France in 1070 by the Count of Dauphiné, and his tomb became a pilgrimage shrine for sufferers of the 'fire' – so-called because one of the visible symptoms was a reddening or blistering of the skin. Indeed, to the shrine was quickly added a hospital for sufferers of the disease, and an order of monks to staff it, the Hospital Brothers of St Anthony.[146]

The disease can take two forms. One, called *convulsive*, afflicts the central nervous system, whereas the second, *gangrenous*, affects the cardiovascular system by constricting the arteries that supply blood to the extremities – hence the reddened and blistered skin, the 'fire'. Which type the sufferer contracted was dependent on the amount of vitamin A in their diet. A diet with sufficient levels of vitamin A – from dairy produce, most likely – would mean the sufferer would probably contract the gangrenous form. Someone living in a village where dairy produce was scarce would be likely to suffer from the convulsive form.

Gangrenous ergotism began with an itching feeling on the feet, the sensation of ants running around them, before the 'fire' became visible. Symptoms of the convulsive form included anxiety, vertigo, noises in the ears, sensations of being bitten or pricked, even stupor. Limbs contracted convulsively, which produced staggering, twitching and other spasmodic movements. Stiffness in the joints would become a lingering symptom. Perhaps most strikingly of all, St Anthony's Fire could produce psychosis, hallucinations,[147] and even serious mental health problems. It's tempting to speculate on the degree to which ergot poisoning, with its visions and terrors, contributed to the demon-populated landscape of the Middle Ages.[148]

Ergotism was a rural disease, flourishing in damp conditions. Areas prone to flooding, such as the Dauphiné, where St Anthony's relics were housed, found themselves plagued by the fire. August Hirsch, the great nineteenth century German epidemiologist, listed 130 epidemics between 591 and 1879, 'acknowledging that these occurrences probably represented the tip of the proverbial iceberg.'[149] In Hirsch's list, most of the epidemics between 591 and the fourteenth century took place in France. An outbreak in 922 of the gangrenous type was said to have killed 40,000 people, while another killed 14,000 in Paris in 1128–9.[150] Indeed, if England was notorious for famine, the same adage held that France was notorious for ergotism, and Normandy for leprosy.

The Disease of the Sinner

Leprosy was the most feared disease of the High Middle Ages. With their decaying flesh, shambling gait, hoarse rasp of a voice and fetid breath, lepers were figures of revulsion, banished from society and regarded with pity and fear. Although most diseases in the pre-modern world were interpreted as punishments from the divine, leprosy developed a special status in this regard: in Christian Europe, it was the disease of the sinner *par excellence*. Even today, leprosy is 'an affliction of almost mythical status'.[151]

The earliest bone evidence of leprosy dates from late Antiquity, when it appeared in Egypt. As Carole Rawcliffe suggests, 'Moving gradually westwards, leprosy appears to have reached Italy with Pompey's victorious legions in 62 BC'.[152] Leprosy made its first appearance in England in the late Roman period. A cemetery in Poundbury, Dorset – dating from the fourth century AD – contains skeletons that bear the telltale lesions of the disease. But paleopathology can tell us only so much. Margaret Cox and Charlotte Roberts remind us that the reality was probably much worse: 'When we look at archaeological bone we may see changes to the normal skeleton but these can never reflect the magnitude of such changes on soft tissue.'[153] One can only wonder what such changes were.

It was possible that the lepers buried in Dorset were not native to the county, or even the country, leaving the possibility that they were Roman soldiers who had contracted the disease somewhere in the Mediterranean basin. That would appear to be the most likely source of leprosy's reaching England. Armies have long been one of the most effective carriers of disease, along with merchants, missionaries, sailors and pilgrims. (But we must also note that armies could often fall victim to disease, and indeed often lost more men to disease than to enemy action – as we will see.)

While the first pandemic of plague was ebbing, leprosy began to spread slowly across Europe. The Anglo-Saxons called it *seo mycle adl*, 'the great disease'.[154] It was always perceived as highly contagious, and prohibitions against lepers were issued in England as early as the seventh century, a century that also saw the building of the first lazar house in Britain. These leper communities were effectively ways of segregating and quarantining sufferers of the disease. By 1300, leprosy had reached epidemic proportions.

Despite its notorious later stages, with its all too visible disfigurements, a person could suffer from leprosy for years and not know it. All they would feel would be a numbness on certain parts of their skin, perhaps some joint pain, but this would be nothing exceptional. Then blotches on the skin would develop that would be impervious to pain. The unfortunate leper-to-be could carry on for years like this, with no symptoms apparently out of the ordinary. Skin complaints were normal and many people were stiff from joint pain caused by arthritis or rheumatism.

Eventually, anyone suspected of having contracted leprosy would be examined by a group of village elders, or in some cases, other lepers. Diagnosis involved various techniques of varying degrees of complexity. At the more 'scientific' end of the scale, the sufferer was subjected to tests such as seeing how long grains of salt took to dissolve in drops of their blood; examining hair or urine; jabbing their extremities with a needle; and, perhaps strangest of all, 'observing facial characteristics through a charcoal flame.'[155] Simpler tests dispensed with the flame and involved deciding whether the suspected leper looked 'loathsome' or 'satyr-like'. Did people 'shudder' at their touch?

Despite the vague air of *Monty Python and the Holy Grail* about these leper tests, they were surprisingly effective. Danish paleopathologist Vilhelm Møller-Christensen (1903–1988) discovered how accurate they had been when he excavated a leper cemetery near Naestved, some forty miles south of Copenhagen. Møller-Christensen found that the cemetery had been linked to a nearby St Jorgen's hospital, which treated lepers between 1250 and 1550. Three quarters of the 650 or so bodies buried there showed signs of leprosy.[156]

As Margaret Cox and Charlotte Roberts noted, skeletal evidence 'can never reflect the magnitude of such changes on soft tissue.'[157] Whatever the bones can tell us, the reality for the person suffering from leprosy would have been much, much worse. Consider the case of this man, whose bones were unearthed in the cemetery of the hospital of St James and St Mary Magdalen, Chichester. He suffered from (according to the skeletal evidence): 'periods of childhood stress, leprosy, degenerative joint disease, non-specific infection and osseous hypertrophy [an enlargement of the bone] in response to his altered posture as a cripple. He also had a nasal fracture, an oblique fracture of the right radius (probably resulting from a fall), a mid-shaft fracture to the left radius, a crush fracture of the left lunate [a bone in the hand], and a compound, oblique, misaligned fracture of the right femur. All of these fractures have associated secondary osteoarthritis and the right femur has corresponding septic arthritis.'[158] It's almost impossible to imagine the daily purgatory of this man's life: the constant crippling pain, the social exclusion, the fear and isolation.

There are two main kinds of leprosy: tuberculoid leprosy (also known as white leprosy), which produces mild joint pains and pale skin, and the far more serious lepromatous leprosy. It is this form of the disease which, in one memorable description, 'erodes noses, swells lips and tongues, erases eyebrows, uproots hair, sculpts facial skin into leonine folds and contorts hands and feet into claws.'[159] Lepromatous leprosy also affects the voice, reducing it to a hoarse whisper, gives the sufferer an unblinking stare, and changes the gait into an ongoing stumble. Over time, lepers will lose all sensation in their skin and muscles; fingers, knuckles and toes can fall off; the nose collapses and the front teeth are lost. The hearing can also possibly be affected (the disease producing a chronic middle ear infection).

In addition to leprosy's horrific litany of afflictions, there was the added isolation and stigma of being a leper. In Europe, lepers were banished from society, being treated as one who had died. (Hence leprosy was dubbed 'the death before death', although white lepers lived in relative freedom in southern France.[160]) This even extended in parts of France, Flanders, and elsewhere, to a mock funeral, the *separatio leprosarum,* which required the leper to wear a black veil and either stand in a freshly-dug grave or kneel before the altar and have the priest tip three spadefuls of earth from the cemetery on their head – a sort of baptism by grave-earth – while a requiem mass was sung.[161] A leper was expected to compose a letter of farewell, known as a *congé*. The most celebrated of these was written by the troubadour Jean Bodel (1165–1210), 'the poet laureate of lepers',[162] who was pronounced leprous in 1202. He wrote that his sadness was without equal; he had initially tried to hide his condition, but now feared the isolation and exclusion he must now face as much as death.[163]

Lepers were forced to dress in a white or grey smock – a forerunner of today's hospital gowns – and were given a bowl in which to collect alms, a stick to point at things they wished to buy, and a clapper or bell to warn people of their approach. They were forbidden to enter churches, or to go to places such as markets, mills, fairs or taverns where there might be crowds. Such was the fear of contagion, lepers weren't allowed to touch anyone except other lepers, were forbidden to eat with anyone except other lepers, and could not wash their hands or clothes in a stream. After 1167, they were forbidden to marry in England, and were not allowed to inherit money or land. They could have sex only with their spouse, assuming said spouse had the stomach for it. If the leper still lived at home, they were not allowed to go outdoors without wearing their smock and carrying their bell or rattle. If funds allowed, lepers could go and live in self-contained communities, known as leprosaria, lazarettos or lazar houses. Bodel, who doesn't seem to have had the financial means to secure a place in the local lazar house, wrote of his attempts to secure a place by appealing to the mayor of Arras. We know Bodel's appeal was successful as, when he died, another poet, Baude Fastoul, asked to be given Bodel's place in the leprosarium.[164]

Lazar houses had originally been part of the Christian concern for charity, which had seen the first western hospitals built in the fourth century AD. By 1300, there were an estimated 19,000 across Europe. The first lazar house in Britain was built in the seventh century, but the majority were founded in the twelfth and thirteenth centuries, just as the epidemic was peaking. They went into decline from the fourteenth century onwards, a possible reflection of leprosy's decline in Europe from that date. (One theory for this is that leprosy was essentially usurped by tuberculosis, a disease that comes from a bacterium of the same genus as *Mycobacterium leprae*, the bacterium which causes leprosy. The theory holds that if pulmonary TB strikes people before leprosy, and they survive, then that would confer immunity against the worst ravages of leprosy.[165] For more on tuberculosis, see Chapter 5.)

Most leper communities were secluded groups of cottages that had their own chapel; some even had their own healing wells or springs nearby.[166] Although some were self-sufficient, or were supported by private donation, many fell under the supervision of monastic institutions. With church influence prevailing, it is not surprising to learn that the 'rules inside leprosy houses emphasised poverty and repentance'.[167] Being built on the edges of towns and villages, and being full of souls who were seen as dead already, 'leper houses were liminal in both essence and in location'.[168] Orders grew up devoted to the care of lepers, such as that of St Lazarus, founded in Jerusalem in 1098 to look after pilgrims and crusaders. (Leprous knights were compelled to join the order, whose first Grand Master, according to legend, was also a leper; Jerusalem even had a leper king, Baldwin IV, who reigned 1174–85.)

'Leprosy,' as Roy Porter noted, 'provided a prism for Christian thinking about disease.'[169]Links were made between lepers and Christ by the likes of Matilda, Henry I of England's first queen (d. 1118), and Hugh of Lincoln, bishop and later saint (d. 1200), who 'prompted a fashion for conspicuous acts of abasement before the most physically repugnant individuals'.[170] One monk, the memorably named Ralph the Ill-tonsured (d. 1062), asked God to give him leprosy 'so that his soul might be cleansed of its foul sins,'[171] of which there were apparently many. If leprosy was good for the soul, it could also be a disease of the soul in others, developing as a result of blasphemy or sacrilege: 'Robert Fitzpernel, Earl of Leicester, was, for instance, allegedly afflicted because he unjustly took possession of an estate lately belonging to Hugh of Avalon, the revered Bishop of Lincoln.'[172]

In tandem with its value as spiritual propaganda, mediaeval physicians argued amongst themselves as to leprosy's cause. Some favoured a corruption of the humours, while others argued for, variously, 'divine will, hostile planetary forces, poor diet, corrupt air, dirt, sexual misconduct, prolonged contact with the leprous and heredity'.[173] The injunctions against leprosy from the Book of Leviticus were still influential, which, coupled with the fear of contagion, did a great deal to help establish the leper houses. But the predominant cause of leprosy to the mediaeval mind was sin, sex in particular; lepers were seen as inherently lusty and lecherous. The fate of Iseult in Beroul's twelfth century *Tristan* – the earliest known version of the story – reflects this. Sentenced to burn for her affair with Tristan, her cuckolded husband, King Mark, is approached by Ivain, a local leper, who has a proposition:

> 'I can tell you quickly what I have in mind. Look, here I have a hundred companions. Give Iseult to us and we will possess her in common. No woman ever had a worse end. Sire, there is such lust in us that no woman on earth could tolerate intercourse with us for a single day. The very clothes stick to our bodies. With you she used to be honoured and happily clad in blue and grey furs. She learned of good wines in your marble halls. If you give her to us lepers, when she sees our low hovels and looks at our dishes and has to sleep with us – in place of your fine meals, sire, she will have the pieces of food and crumbs that are left for us at the gates – then, by the Lord who dwells above, when she sees our court and all its discomforts she would rather be dead than alive. The snake Iseult will know then that she has been wicked! She would rather have been burnt.'

The king listened to him, stood up and said nothing for a long while. He had heard what Ivain had said. He ran to Iseult and took her by the hand.

Iseult cried out: 'Sire, mercy! Burn me here instead of giving me to them!'

The king handed her over to the lepers, and a good hundred crowded around her. Everyone who heard the noise and the shouting took pity on her. But whoever might be sorrowful, Ivain was happy. He led Iseult away along the sandy path.[174]

Beroul not only portrays the fear of leprosy and its perceived link with sexual activity, but also shows how leprosy could be used to dispose of troublesome people. It became, under certain circumstances, a method of social control. The Third Lateran Council (1179) segregated lepers from society, which led to an increase in the building of lazar houses across Europe. Lepers were banned from London in 1346 and 1472, while in France in 1321 lepers were accused of poisoning the wells in an attempt to spread their disease. Many were subject to mob violence, and burnt at the stake. The French king, Philip V, attempted to sequester property and goods belonging to the lepers, finding scapegoats to be a useful source of much-needed revenue. The Jews were also implicated in this apparent plot, although Philip ordered that Jewish communities should not be attacked. Accusations of well poisoning would recur within a generation, and this time the Jews would find themselves bearing the brunt of a Europe-wide paranoia, being accused of spreading the one disease that became feared even more than leprosy: plague.

The Black Death

Plague reached Italy in the autumn of 1347. Ships from the east arrived in Sicily with their crews dead or dying of a strange illness. The sailors had boils in the neck, armpit or groin, suffered from fever, intense pain and delirium, and died within days. The sickness soon spread from the ships into the towns, and people began dying in what seemed like uncontrollable numbers. Relics were brought out of churches, processions held, the intercession of saints sought, but nothing seemed able to stop the progress of the disease. Some ships were repelled, forcing them to put in at other ports, unwittingly spreading the sickness further. The disease quickly reached mainland Italy, and travelled along the Mediterranean coast of France. By the following spring, the whole of Italy, France and the Iberian peninsula were ablaze with plague.

It was like nothing anyone had ever seen before. People could be alive one day, seemingly healthy, only to be found dead in their beds the next morning. So great were the numbers of the dead that the cemeteries were soon full to overflowing. Each city or town hastily dug pits to act as mass graves. When the undertakers died, the dead were left unburied in their houses or in the streets. In Dubrovnik, wolves ran wild in the streets, picking at bodies. (And, in the process, the animals too contracted plague.) To chroniclers and poets, it seemed as if the end of the world was at hand.

The Piacenzan chronicler Gabriel de Mussis, who wrote one of the earliest plague chronicles, echoed the common belief that the plague had been sent as a punishment from God for humanity's sins. God saw 'the entire human race wallowing in the mire of manifold wickedness', and pronounced judgement: 'May your joys be turned to mourning, your prosperity be shaken by adversity, the course of your life be passed in never-ending terror. Behold the image of death. Behold I open the infernal flood-gates... Let the sharp arrows of sudden death have dominion throughout the world. Let no one be spared... Let the innocent perish with the guilty and no one escape.'[175]

The great poet Boccaccio witnessed the ravages of the plague in Florence, where mortality was so high the epidemic was known as the 'Plague of Florence'. In his epic *The Decameron*, Boccaccio has a group of wealthy Florentines fleeing to the hills and entertaining themselves with stories while the plague rages outside their isolated villa. The introduction is perhaps the most celebrated description of the Black Death, and is worth quoting at length as it conveys the sheer scale of the disaster:

In the year 1348, the deadly pestilence appeared in the illustrious city of Florence, the fairest of all Italian cities. Whether it was disseminated by the influence of the planets, or sent by God in His wrath for our iniquities, it had had its origin some years earlier in the East, when, after killing innumerable people, it had spread without mercy from place to place, and, ultimately, to the West.

... in both men and women the pestilence first betrayed itself by the emergence of tumours in the groin or in the armpits, some of which grew as large as an apple, or an egg. From these two parts of the body the tumours soon began to spread themselves in all directions; black or livid spots of varying sizes appeared after this on the arm or the thigh or even around the waist. Like the tumours, these spots were also seen as a sign of approaching death. Doctors could do nothing. Whether they were at fault or whether the disease was untreatable, I do not know. To make things worse, men and women, none of whom were qualified in medicine, tried to treat people as well. Hardly anyone survived. Almost all died within three days from the appearance of the tumours, in most cases without any fever or other symptom.

What's more, the virulence of the disease was increased through merely talking to the sick, just as fire burns things that are brought close to it. And if that wasn't bad enough, it was possible to become infected even by touching the clothes of the sick or anything else that they had touched or used. Once I saw two pigs in the street come up to the clothes of a poor man. He had died of the disease and his things were scattered outside his house. The pigs took the garments between their teeth and chewed them. Almost immediately, they fell down dead, as if poisoned. Had I not seen this with my own eyes, I would have hardly dared believe it, much less set it down in writing.

In these circumstances, people began to shun all contact with the sick, and vowed to stay as healthy as possible. Some thought that to live temperately and avoid all excess would be best. Small groups of people banded together, and lived in isolation. They exercised the utmost care, avoiding every kind of luxury, and ate and drank in moderation. They spoke to no one, in case they should hear about sickness or death, and kept themselves busy with music and discussions and games.

Other people thought that debauchery was the answer, and resorted day and night to taverns, drinking with total disregard for everything, or visiting other people's houses if they saw anything in them that they liked, which wasn't too difficult, as their owners, expecting to die at any moment, had become as reckless as their guests, and threw their houses open to all comers. In this extremity of suffering all laws, both human and divine, were ignored for lack of people to uphold them as they were either dead or sick, and everyone was free to do whatever they wanted.

Some people steered a middle course, neither being wary of their health nor living a life of dissipation. They walked around carrying flowers or fragrant herbs, which they held to their noses, thinking that it would provide some comfort against the air which reeked with the stench of the dead and dying.

Yet others, the most sound of judgement, perhaps, felt that the best medicine was to flee; a multitude of men and women deserted the city, their houses, their estates, their families, their goods, and went into voluntary exile, fled to the country, hoping that God would not pursue them with His wrath, but would only destroy those who stayed behind.

Whatever course of action people took, many died. Citizen avoided citizen, neighbours lost all feeling for each other, families met only rarely; so afraid were people of this disease, that brother forsook brother, nephew uncle, brother sister, and often husbands their wives; what's more, scarcely believable, is that parents abandoned their children, and left them to their fate, as if they had belonged to strangers. The huge numbers of sick had no choice but to rely on the charity of what few friends they had left, or servants, who demanded high wages for their care, (despite not being qualified) and who merely looked after the immediate wants of the sick, and watched them die; they very often died too. There were so few people left to care for the sick that no woman, however fair or well-born she might be, shrank, when stricken with the disease, from the ministrations of a man, and willingly exposed to him every part of her body; some received the man's physical attention rather than medical aid. Possibly, with better care, some may have survived, but the combination of so virulent a plague and such poor medical aid resulted in huge mortality, with deaths taking place day and night; those who witnessed it – or even heard about it second hand – were struck dumb with amazement.

Traditionally, during a funeral, the women would gather inside the house and wail their laments, while the men would gather outside with the priest to carry the body to the church requested by the deceased in their will. However, with the pestilence raging so furiously, these arrangements were soon dropped. Most died without a crowd of mourning women; most would-be mourners were either dead or out getting drunk, which was good for the health of the women, who did not have to go near a corpse or mix with others. Most biers were not carried by friends and neighbours, but by the desperate *becchini*, who hired themselves out for such awful tasks, and would carry the body, not to the church of the deceased's choice, but to whichever one was nearest to hand, with four or six priests in front carrying possibly a candle or two; nor did the priests bother to conduct too long and solemn a funeral service, and with the help of the *becchini* hastily dumped the body in the first open grave they could find. It was worse for the poor. They stayed in their homes, where they sickened by the thousand each day, and, being without help of any kind, could not hope to escape death. They died at all hours in the streets; those who died at home were not missed by their neighbours, until they noticed the stench of their putrefying bodies; the whole city was a sepulchre.

It was common practice for people, moved more by fear of contamination than by charity towards the deceased, to drag the corpses out of the houses with their own hands, aided, perhaps, by a porter (if there was a porter to be had), and to lay the bodies in front of the houses, where any funeral cart that made the rounds might have seen them. Sometimes, in the morning, there would be more dead piled up in the streets than the cart driver could count; often, whole families were loaded onto the biers. Priests arrived to find that they were burying not one, but six or eight, sometimes more. People had become indifferent to the suffering all round them, and the dead were disposed of as if they were goats.

There was not enough consecrated ground for the vast number of corpses which day and night – almost every hour – were brought to the churches for burial. When the cemeteries were full, they dug a huge trench which they put the new corpses in as they arrived by the hundred, piling them up like goods in the hold of a ship, tier upon tier, each layer of bodies covered with a little earth, until the trench could hold no more.

The surrounding countryside suffered as harshly as the city. There, in villages, or in open fields, by the roadside, on the farm, in the home, the unfortunate husbandmen and their families, bereft of doctors' or servants' care, died day and night, not as men, but rather as beasts. They too, like the Florentines, abandoned normality, believing each day to be their last, and stopped working in the fields and tending their animals, and instead drank and ate all they had stored. They denied shelter to their cattle, sheep, goats, pigs, fowl, even to their dogs, and drove them out into the fields to roam in the unreaped corn.

Boccaccio believed that, between March and July 1348, one hundred thousand people in Florence and the surrounding countryside fell victim to the plague. Mediaeval figures are notoriously unreliable; 'one hundred thousand' should be taken to mean probably half that figure. Still, it was an appalling mortality rate, and it was happening right across Europe.

Boccaccio's belief that the pestilence originated somewhere in the interior of Asia was widely shared and, unlike the numbers mentioned in contemporaneous death tolls, is almost certainly correct. The Arab historian Ibn al-Wardi, who witnessed the Black Death at Aleppo and died of it himself in 1349, believed that the pestilence had originated some fifteen years earlier in the 'land of darkness', by which he probably meant Mongolia. If this were the case, then it would mean that plague was raging in Central Asia in the early-to-mid 1330s.

Chinese records note that the Great Mongol Khan Jijaghatu Toq-Temür died on 2 October 1332, aged 28, and his sons followed him in rapid succession. The chronicles are peppered with stories of natural disasters and cataclysms that were afflicting China at the time with alarming – one might be tempted to say almost Old Testament – severity. In 1333, famine followed a drought; following the famine, there was a deluge; 400,000 are said to have died. An earthquake caused Mount Tsincheou to partially collapse, and huge faults appeared in the landscape. The following year, 1334, was no better: Houkouang and Honan provinces experienced drought, followed by a famine attended by clouds of locusts; an earthquake in the Ki-Ming-Chan Mountains brought floods that were so bad they created a new lake; in Tche the dead were said to amount to more than five million. If this wasn't bad enough, the earthquakes that had caused Mount Tsincheou to cave in continued up until 1345, along with further floods and crop-destroying locusts.

Amidst all this chaos, humans would not have been the only occupants of China and Mongolia to have become virtual refugees in their own land: the lives of the rodent population would have been equally disrupted. It is probably this series of disasters that forced them to migrate, taking with them the plague bacillus. They must have headed south, taking the plague to India, and west, where they would have infected traders on the Silk Road. The plague-carrying fleas easily made the jump from rats and marmots to establish a new home in the cloths, rugs and furs bound for Europe and the markets of the Middle East. By 1346, the plague had reached the Crimea, where the ships that brought the Black Death to Sicily in October of the following year are thought to have originated.

The Black Death transformed Europe into a giant theatre of mortality, the kind of nightmare landscape imagined by Pieter Bruegel in his painting *The Triumph of Death*, in which armies of the dead relentlessly round up and mow down the living. Arriving in mainland Italy in January 1348, it immediately began to capitalise on the work already started by poor harvests and famine; 600 a day were said to have died in Venice. Genoa, Pisa, Rome and Florence soon fell. Riven by political infighting, Italian city states were forced by the plague to put their differences aside, or perish.

The town of Pistoia provides a good example of how the city fathers coped with the crisis, as here the civil ordinances published during the Black Death have survived. On 2 May 1348, when the first reports of cases were coming in, the council drew up its first set of preventative measures. No one was to visit any area where plague was already raging, such as Pisa; if anyone was already there, they were forbidden to come back. No goods were to be imported into the town, including corpses. Markets were monitored closely, with only local produce being allowed to be offered for sale. Funerals were to be family-only affairs, and bells were not to be rung. Town criers and trumpeters were likewise silenced. Three weeks later, on 23 May, the travel restrictions were lifted, as, by now, regardless of whether one went to Pisa or not, one was just as likely to catch the plague in Pistoia. Food regulations, on the other hand, were tightened up. On 4 June, a team of town gravediggers was appointed; no one else was to bury bodies but these 16 men. On 13 June, the rules for the defence of the town were redrafted, to allow the rich to choose a proxy to serve in the ranks for them if they so desired. This is unusual, as despite their obvious advantages of wealth, Church and State did their inadequate best to protect all members of society during the Black Death.

Although in Pistoia, the council did as much as they could to limit the damage, in Orvieto the council performed less conscientiously. The town had around 12,000 inhabitants and had been prosperous, despite heavy losses incurred during the ceaseless struggles between the Guelphs and the Ghibellines. The political uncertainty and instability this produced, in addition to the famines of 1346 and 1347, had crippled Orvieto's economy and, by the time the Black Death struck in the spring of 1348, the average Orvietan was in no mood for yet more disaster. The town council met on 12 March, and all mention of disaster was studiously avoided. The plague was raging 80 miles away in Florence, and perhaps they felt that there was nothing they could do to avoid it. The town had one doctor and one surgeon, who both worked full time. There were also a good half dozen citizens who were qualified in medicine and could be prevailed upon to offer their services as and when the need arose. For a town of Orvieto's size, this was not bad going. There was only one properly equipped hospital, however, with several other institutions managing as best they could on private donations and worse facilities. Public hygiene, as in most mediaeval cities, was virtually non-existent. In repeated – and seemingly ineffectual – ordinances, the council forbade such traditional street activities as the rearing of animals, the tanning of skins and the disposal of waste from windows.

The Black Death hit Orvieto particularly hard: around 50 per cent of the population were dead within three months of its arrival in April 1348. Unlike Pistoia, no ordinances were published with preventative measures. In fact, the plague does not appear in city records until June, when a new council was elected. But it was too late: the plague was raging at near to full strength, and of the seven councillors elected, two were dead by 23 July and three more were in their graves by 7 August. Any pretence of trying to hold council meetings was scrapped; even the city's most important religious ceremony, the procession of the Assumption, had to be abandoned.

In Siena, work had to be halted on the new cathedral. The Black Death struck just as the transept had been built and the foundations of the choir and the nave had been laid; the masons died and no one was left to continue their work. The wool industry effectively ceased to exist, and the import of oil was halted. On 2 June, all Siena's courthouses were closed down for three months and gambling was banned for all time. (The loss of revenue was so great, however, that this prohibition had to be repealed six months later when the worst of the epidemic was past.) So much money was bequeathed to the church in inheritances and donations (made no doubt with the salvation of at least the donor in mind) that all the regular taxes the Church collected were suspended until 1350.

One of the best-known of Sienese plague chronicles was written by Agnolo di Tura. 'Father abandoned child,' he writes, 'wife, husband; one brother, another, for this illness seemed to strike through the breath and the sight. And so they died. And no one could be found to bury the dead for money or for friendship... And in many places in Siena great pits were dug and piled deep with huge heaps of the dead... And I, Agnolo di Tura, called the Fat, buried my five children with my own hands, and so did many others likewise. And there were also so many dead throughout the city who were so sparsely covered with earth that the dogs dragged them out and devoured their bodies.'

Some merchants, fleeing across the Alps, tried to find safe haven in the Lombard town of Bobbio. They sold what goods they had, but either they themselves were carrying plague, or their merchandise was flea-infested, for the man who purchased their goods suddenly died, along with his entire family and several neighbours. One can only assume that the merchants must also have died and been buried together in the common pit. More woes from the same town are noted by de Mussis: 'one man, wanting to make his will, died along with the notary, the priest who heard his confession, and the people summoned to witness the will, and they were all buried together on the following day'. In Piacenza, de Mussis' hometown, 'Cries and laments arise on all sides. Day after day one sees the Cross and the Host being carried about the city, and countless dead being buried... pits had to be dug in colonnades and piazzas, where nobody had ever been buried before.' Another chronicle notes 'the physician would not visit; the priest, panic-stricken, administered the sacraments with fear and trembling... no prayer, trumpet or bell summoned friends and neighbours to the funeral, nor was mass performed.' In Padua 'the bodies even of noblemen lay unburied and many, at a price, were buried by poor wretches, without priests or candles.'

The *Chronicle* of William of Nangis, perhaps the best contemporary account of what happened in Paris, records that, 'There was so great a mortality among people of both sexes… that it was hardly possible to bury them. In the Hôtel-Dieu de Paris… for a long time more than 500 corpses were carted daily to the churchyard of St Innocent to be buried. And those holy sisters, having no fear of death, tended the sick with all sweetness and humility, putting all fear behind their back. The greater number of these sisters, many times renewed by death, now rest in peace with Christ.'

Although 500 deaths a day in one parish alone seems like a typically inflated mediaeval figure (it has been suggested that this is a misprint of 50), the death toll in Paris was severe, with perhaps as many as 50,000 people dying during the second half of 1348. The rich fled, leaving the poor to face the brunt of the plague as it stalked the narrow streets. William of Nangis records that priests fled, too, making his 'holy sisters', who no doubt went to the grave in their droves while attempting to alleviate the suffering that raged around them, all the more remarkable.

Some people reacted with less than Christian actions. Knowing they were almost certainly going to die, they spent what little time remained to them in drinking and dancing. Looting and licentious living were commonplace, even more so than in Florence. To a casual observer, there can have seemed little difference between plague victims experiencing the feverish convulsions known as the dance of death, the *Danse Macabre* that inspired countless paintings, and those who staggered out into the street too drunk to walk in a straight line. When even Pope Clement had agreed that the plague had been sent by God as a punishment for their collective sins, what use was it in trying to remain alive? Eat, drink and be merry, for tomorrow we die.

Extreme forms of behaviour got worse as the plague progressed through Europe. In Germany, a group known as the Flagellants began holding public penances, at which group members would whip themselves in an attempt to appease the Almighty. Onlookers were encouraged to confess their sins. At first welcomed even by the Pope, the Flagellants' processions became ever more extreme. They began to see themselves in an increasingly messianic light: not only did they need to rid the world of plague, but Christendom itself needed to be saved. When they announced that they could absolve sins, the Pope withdrew his blessing, and the movement faded into obscurity.

The Flagellants were responding to one of the main theories about the cause of the Black Death, namely that it had been caused by the sins of humanity. Such had been the thinking behind the causes of the Plague of Justinian eight hundred years earlier. Penance and prayer were encouraged across Europe. In Hungary, pillars were erected as a sign of collective repentance. The pillars often depicted figures whose intervention was sought to lift the pestilence: the Virgin Mary, Saint Sebastian (a patron saint of pestilence victims), Saint Roch (a patron saint of epidemics, depicted on later pillars), Saint Joseph, Saint Augustine of Hippo, Saint John the Baptist, and Saint Christopher.

For the Viennese, the Black Death was thought to be spread by the Pest Jungfrau, a beautiful maiden who flew through the air in the form of a blue flame and killed people by simply raising her hand. When her victims expired, they were seen to exhale a blue flame, which was taken to be the Jungfrau's departure as she sought her next victim. In Lithuania, there was a similar legend: that the plague was a woman who killed her victims by waving a red scarf at their windows or doors.

But the main theory was that a miasma was responsible. Miasma theory – the belief that foul air could disseminate disease – was as old as Hippocrates. When the Pope sat beside a fire in his palace in Avignon, he believed he was keeping the miasma at bay. His ploy was successful, and he survived the plague, but not for the reasons he assumed. There was no miasma for the fire to dispel: the fire saved the Pope's life by keeping the rats away.

Philip VI of France commissioned the hallowed Medical Faculty at the University of Paris to find out exactly what had caused the unparallelled calamity of the Black Death, and they quickly reported back to him with their findings. The cause, it seemed, was astrological in nature, not medical: an unfavourable conjunction of Saturn, Jupiter and Mars that took place in Aquarius at 1pm on 20 March 1345 seemed to be at the root of all their suffering. Conjunctions of Jupiter and Saturn were regarded as bringers of death, and the added presence of the fiery Mars would indicate that, had they but known it three years earlier, disaster was bearing down upon them. (Planetary movements would also be implicated when syphilis first reached Europe in the late fifteenth century, as immortalised in a print by Albrecht Dürer. See Chapter 4.)

The general feeling was that the epidemic had struck because the atmosphere had become corrupted, and the plague had spread from place to place like a cloud of poison gas. One theory held that this miasma was caused by the sea becoming choked with dead fish. Another believed that the noxious atmosphere was caused by corpses that had lain too long unburied after a war that had no doubt been raging recently somewhere in the East.

Others believed earthquakes were responsible, pointing out that the plague had arrived in mainland Italy the same month that an earthquake hit the Friuli region (it struck on 25 January 1348). As with the fire/miasma theory, this was correct, but not for the reasons that contemporary chroniclers believed. They held, once again, that the earthquake had released foul airs from the bowels of the earth. In reality, the earthquakes that may have played a part in the pandemic were those that struck China in the early 1330s, displacing the rodent populations, who carried the plague bacillus with them to new lands.

Another theory held that the Jews were responsible, causing plague by poisoning the wells. Such an accusation had been made against lepers in the Languedoc in 1321, who had, so the rumour went, been acting on instructions given to them by the Jews. On that occasion, the lepers had come off worse, and many were burned at the stake. Now the Jews bore the brunt of rumour. At Chillon in Switzerland in the autumn of 1348, a number of Jews admitted to poisoning the wells, their confessions extracted under torture. The Pope tried to intervene, pointing out that Jews were dying of the pestilence as well as

Christians, but his entreaties fell on deaf ears. The Chillon Jews went to the stake. Worse was to come. In Basle the Jews were herded into a specially constructed building and burned to death. Mass burnings occurred across Germany. At Esslingen in December 1348, the Jewish community committed mass suicide rather than go to the stake.

Ruprecht von der Pfalz took the Jews living on his lands under his personal protection and nearly provoked a revolution, earning himself the nickname 'Jew Master' in the process. Only Casimir, King of Poland, seems to have been almost entirely successful in preventing slaughter in his lands. (Detractors claimed he had been under the thumb of Esther, his Jewish mistress.) Despite the efforts of figures such as Casimir and Ruprecht, many Jewish communities were wiped out altogether, or permanently displaced. Europe would not see anti-Semitism on this scale again until the rise of Hitler.

There was little people could do except flee the plague, as Boccaccio's characters did. In the Moroccan town of Salé, a certain Ibn Abu Madyan gave the idea of isolation an unusual twist: he walled himself up alive in his own home. He had enough food and drink laid in to last, he reasoned, and decided to sit out the plague. His gambit worked: he survived, emerging into a world very different from the one he had left.

One isolation tactic has survived to the present day. During a later outbreak of plague in 1377, the city of Ragusa (modern Dubrovnik) insisted that ships coming in from Venice and elsewhere be kept in the harbour for 30 days. This was later extended to 40, from which we get the modern word quarantine (from the Italian *quaranta giorni*, meaning 40 days).

Miasma theory prevailed, as did the teachings of Hippocrates and Galen but, as neither had had experience of a plague epidemic, their works weren't much use. Indeed, the first person to call was the priest so that the last rites could be administered. With such daily contact with the stricken, it is not surprising that the death rate among the clergy was particularly high.

The Arab doctor Ibn al-Khatib (1313–1374) was almost alone in believing that the plague was contagious.[176] He noted how waves of infection always seemed to coincide with 'the arrival of contaminated merchants and goods from foreign lands where plague was raging'.[177] In contrast, Ibn al-Khatib pointed out that the tent-dwelling nomads of the desert remained healthy during the pandemic.[178]

Ibn Khâtimah, who disputed with Ibn al-Khatib over the contagion theory, witnessed the effects of the plague at first hand in his home town of Almeria, where he noted something that inadvertently supported the theory of contagion: in Suq-al-Khalq, a market area with lively trade in blankets, clothes and bedding, the mortality rate was almost 100 per cent. It was, in other words, a place with a very active flea population. The Byzantine historian Nicephorus Gregoras was one of the few contemporary writers to mention rats, noting that they too were dying in the houses they frequented.

Estimates of mortality by modern scholars put the death rate at approximately 30 per cent. In some places, such as Florence, it was higher – probably 50 to 60 per cent. Some smaller communities were wiped out altogether. In England, the country with the best records, we read of higher mortality in certain areas. At Carlisle, the castle lands were left untenanted for 18 months, due to all previous tenants dying, while at West Thickley, Co. Durham, the ecclesiastical roll read simply 'they are all dead'.

The Effects of the Black Death

One immediate effect of the pandemic was the invention of quarantine. Wages rose across Europe, due to the lack of a full workforce. People travelled in search of work, weakening feudal ties. Such was the movement of labour that the manorial system never recovered. Needing the workers, but fearing the power shift that higher pay might bring about, Europe's monarchs and nobles capped wages in an effort to maintain the status quo. Unrest began to simmer, finally coming to the boil in England in 1381 with the Peasants' Revolt. Similar popular uprisings occurred in France and Low Countries. Although the revolts were quelled, the damage was done: the Black Death had helped the feudal system to its grave.

The church also suffered. The huge numbers of clergy who perished tending their flocks were hurriedly replaced, but often the incoming incumbents were not as well trained. Some were less than eloquent in Latin, leading to a rise in the vernacular. It is not a coincidence that groups like the Lollards came to prominence in the years after the Black Death, advocating worship in the common tongue of the people, rather than the Latin of the elites. It was a mere half a dozen generations from John Wycliffe and his (illegal) Bible translated into Middle English to Martin Luther.

One of the puzzles about the pandemic is its virulence. What made it the worst pandemic in history, if judged in terms of proportion of population killed? The natural disasters that had afflicted China in the 1330s helped make the population more vulnerable to disease. Much of Europe had been similarly stricken in the first decades of the fourteenth century. There had been no major earthquakes, granted, but repeated crop failures, heavy rains and famine, saw Europeans weakened by malnutrition, starvation and poverty. In a sense, Europe was the victim of its own success: the High Middle Ages had seen the general standard of living improve; the economy grew, wages rose. And so did the population. By 1300, Europe's population was outstripping its resources. Intensive farming was weakening the soil.

That being said, the Black Death was much more virulent than the Plague of Justinian. Plague chronicles recount that the plague was just as active in the winter months, suggesting that pneumonic plague was raging alongside its bubonic form, which usually does most of its work in warmer months. Pneumonic plague, like TB, can be spread from person to person through coughing and expectorating. It's also possible that the third form of plague, septicaemic, was also at work. This form of the disease goes straight into the blood, where it causes septic shock. No buboes form. Death can come within twenty-four hours. This might account for the stories of people going to bed healthy and being found dead the next day.

Yet none of these three main forms of plague can explain why the Black Death spread quickly in sparsely populated countries, such as Norway. Theories have since been put forward to try and explain this, claiming that another disease such as anthrax must have been working alongside plague.[179] Anthrax spores have been found in plague pits but to date there is not enough conclusive evidence.

Historian GM Trevelyan argued that the Black Death was at least as important as the industrial revolution, while David Herlihy argued that the Black Death was 'the great watershed', without which there were would have been no Renaissance, and with no Renaissance, no industrial revolution.[180] The prevailing view now is that the pandemic accelerated changes that would have happened anyway, such as the end the feudal system, while at the same time delaying other transformations, such as the Renaissance, which had already started in Italy by 1347, but then went into enforced hiatus for around a century while the pandemic did its work.

As the Plague of Justinian can be seen to close Antiquity, so the Black Death brought the Middle Ages to an end. The plague would continue to recur in Europe into the Renaissance, a world haunted by its danse macabre.

4

The New World

When Christopher Columbus reached the New World on 12 October 1492, he noted in his journal that the native people – the Arawaks – were friendly and peaceful. 'With fifty men we could subjugate them all and make them do whatever we wish.'[181] He was so impressed by their gold jewellery that he took a number of them prisoner, insisting they take him to the source of the gold. Columbus began to make plans to sell them as slaves, and to make good Christians out of them. (He wasn't averse to his crew raping the women, either, nor was that seen as incompatible with Christianity.[182]) And so began one of the most disastrous episodes in history: the arrival of the Old World in the New.

The disaster was not just cultural and political: Columbus's belief that he could 'subjugate them all' with fifty men proved to be an uncannily accurate prediction of what actually happened. The Spanish conquistador Hernando Cortes landed in Mexico in 1518 with only a few hundred men. The Aztecs, like the Arawaks before them, were peaceful and offered the Spanish gifts of gold; Cortes himself was regarded as a minor deity. (Or at least, that's what he told the King of Spain in a letter home.) His forces bolstered by other indigenous peoples who effectively acted as Spanish mercenaries, Cortes managed to conquer the Aztec empire (modern-day Mexico) in just a few short years following his arrival. He was greatly aided by smallpox. In fact, the disease did most of the work for him.

Smallpox had in fact been present in the New World for around a dozen years by that time. It was introduced into Newfoundland by

Portuguese explorers in 1506 (who also brought tuberculosis with them). The following year, an outbreak occurred on Hispaniola – probably courtesy of the Spanish – where 'whole tribes were exterminated',[183] as the German medical historian August Hirsch matter-of-factly put it. In 1515, it appeared in Puerto Rico, introduced by African slaves; the native Arawak and Calusa population was reduced from 50,000 to 600 within 25 years.[184] When considering such a catastrophic fatality rate, it comes as no surprise to learn that smallpox was nicknamed the 'cruel disease,' the 'Angel of Death', and the 'Destroying Angel'.

Smallpox's early history is a matter of conjecture. Because it's a crowd disease, and can only be passed from person to person, it couldn't have survived among the scattered populations of the Americas; even if it had been present prior to the arrival of Europeans, its critical community size would never have been reached, and it would have died out. However, there's no evidence for New World smallpox prior to Cortes. As we saw in Chapter 2, the Egyptian pharaoh Ramses V may have been a victim of smallpox. The Bible and the Greeks are also silent on the subject of smallpox, which leads us to the tentative conclusion that it may not have reached the Mediterranean by the time of Hippocrates (fifth and fourth centuries BC). It is possible that the disease was active in ancient China: a manuscript from 1112 BC refers to a disease which may have been smallpox, where it was referred to as 'venom from the mother's breast'[185] but there is little firm evidence until we get to the fourth century AD. In the West, smallpox was once considered the disease behind the Plagues of Athens (430 BC), Antoninus (second century AD) and Cyprian (third century AD), but these epidemics are now generally thought to have been caused by something else (see Chapter 2). St Nicaise, Bishop of Rheims, is traditionally said to have suffered from smallpox – indeed, he was later made into the patron saint of those afflicted by the disease – although his death in 452 was not a result of his illness: the Huns beheaded him on the steps of his church. Marius, Bishop of Avenches in Switzerland, mentioned an outbreak of a disease he called *variola* in 570 AD, as did

Gregory of Tours a decade later, and this is the name that medicine was to adopt for the virus.

Two strains were eventually identified in the twentieth century, *Variola major* and *Variola minor*.[186] Both seem to be descendants of an earlier virus, the prehistoric taterapox. Of the two, *V. major* is by far the more lethal, with a 25 to 30 per cent mortality rate if untreated. But *V. minor* seems to have been the first to develop, possibly between 1,400 and 6,300 years ago in West Africa. The Yoruba, who came to live in the lands where *V. minor* originated, made supplications to a god of smallpox, Shapona, suggesting that the disease had been endemic there longer than anyone could remember. Some time between 400 and 1,600 years ago, *V. major* evolved, probably in Asia.[187] This conjecture might help explain why 'There is some indication of smallpox in China by the fourth century, and stronger evidence for its arrival in Japan in the 730s.'[188] If this is correct, we could conjecture that the eighth-century Japanese outbreak was the newly-evolved *Variola major*, and that the smallpox from which Ramses V suffered, and that noted by Marius and Gregory of Tours, was *Variola minor*.

From Japan in the 730s, smallpox began slowly creeping westwards. By the turn of the ninth century, it had reached Baghdad. The great Arab doctor Rhazes (Muhammad ibn Zakariyā al-Rāzī, 854–932) knew of both strains of the disease, described in his *Treatise on Smallpox and Measles*. Rhazes described smallpox as a prevalent childhood disease. It seems, by this time, smallpox existed in most of Asia, parts of northern Europe, sub-Saharan Africa and Indonesia.[189] Towns, cities and trade routes, spreading across Asia from the Pacific to the Atlantic, were well enough established – and large enough – to give the disease a substantial reservoir. By the turn of the first Christian millennium, then, smallpox was a threat, but did not loom so large in mediaeval consciousness as leprosy, famine and the ever present 'fevers'.

All this changed, however, by the time Cortes invaded Mexico. What happened remains a mystery: either there was a further mutation of the *V. major* virus; perhaps it did not appear in late antiquity or the Dark Ages at all, but was only now, in the early years of the sixteenth century, making its murderous appearance. Whatever viral changes were afoot, the result was catastrophic. The virus was possibly introduced into Mexico by an African slave in the spring of 1520, a few months after Cortes had entered the Aztec capital Tenochtitlán for the first time.[190] What happened next is recorded by the Spanish friar, Fray Toribio Motolinía, in his *History of the Indians of New Spain* (1541):

> ... when the smallpox began to attack the Indians it became so great a pestilence among them throughout the land that in most provinces more than half the population died; in others the proportion was a little less. For as the Indians did not know the remedy for the disease and were very much in the habit of bathing frequently, whether well or ill, and continued to do so even when suffering from smallpox, they died in heaps, like bedbugs. Many others died of starvation, because, as they were all taken sick at once, they could not care for each other, nor was there anyone to give them bread or anything else. In many places it happened that everyone in a house died, and, as it was impossible to bury the great number of dead they pulled down the houses over them in order to check the stench that rose from the dead bodies so that their homes became their tombs. This disease was called by the Indians "the great leprosy" because the victims were so covered with pustules that they looked like lepers. Even today one can see obvious evidences of it in some individuals who escaped death, for they were left covered with pockmarks.[191]
>
> ... it extended over all parts of their bodies. Over the forehead, head, chest. It was very destructive. Many died of it. They could no longer walk, they could do no more than lie down, stretched out on their beds. They couldn't bestir their bodies, neither to lie face down, nor on their backs, nor to turn from one side to the other. And when they did move, they cried out. In death, many [bodies] were like sticky, compacted, hard grain... many [of the survivors] were pockmarked... some were blind... this pestilence lasted sixty days, sixty lamentable days.[192]

Nearly half the population of Mexico died of smallpox in six months. 'Whatever the number of dead, this outbreak was a catastrophe, and of a scale far exceeding its earlier rampages on Hispaniola, Puerto Rico and Cuba.'[193] The Aztec Empire could not withstand such an onslaught. Their gods had abandoned them, it seemed.

While it was doing its work in Mexico, the disease cut swathes of people down in Colombia, Cuba, Peru, Puerto Rico, Venezuela and Yucatan. By the time Francisco Pizarro arrived to conquer South America for the Spanish crown in 1532, he was effectively leading a rearguard force, mopping up what the Destroying Angel had started. The Incas, like the Aztecs before them, saw their world collapse around them. In the 1550s, Chile and Brazil fell to smallpox, with conquistadors and missionaries following in its wake. The Jesuits, keen to convert local populations, held mass baptisms. Like the Aztec practice of communal bathing, this only served to spread smallpox further.

North America survived relatively intact until the seventeenth century. This was due in large part to the fact that colonial attentions prior to this period had been directed elsewhere: at navigation, exploration, mapping and surviving the apocalyptic convulsions that Europe was going through, the crucible of Renaissance and Reformation. But almost as soon as colonists began to set foot in North America in earnest, the death toll began to mount exponentially. A smallpox epidemic began in New England in 1614, killing large numbers of Massachusett, Micmac, Pawtucket and Wampanoag. So drastically were Native American numbers cut, that when the *Mayflower* landed in 1620, the tide was already turning in favour of the white settlers (even if they didn't know it at the time). Other tribes, such as the Algonquin and Abenaki, fell victim before the decade was out. As happened in Mexico, the indigenous populations believed their own gods had let them down, and the Europeans had little, if any, sympathy. Between the arrival of the Pilgrim Fathers and the end of the seventeenth century, it is thought that up to 90 per cent of North American native peoples were wiped out – millions died – a catastrophe on a par with the Black Death or both world wars. It was another triumph for Civilisation, and Christianity.

Why did it happen? The short answer is that, from 1492 onwards, explorers, conquistadors, missionaries, mercenaries, merchants and settlers carried their diseases across the ocean, taking the Old World disease pool with them. The native peoples of the Americas were a virgin population, ripe for infecting.

The Americas are thought to have been settled in prehistory by peoples crossing the Bering Land Bridge (*c.* 30,000 BC or later). Whatever viruses and bacteria that came over with them from Palaeolithic Asia were probably weakened by the cold of Siberia, Kamchatka and Chukotka and effectively finished off by the Alaskan climate. Only the hardiest could have survived – whether human, animal or bacteria. As a result of this isolation from the Eurasian landmass, the disease pool of the New World evolved along very different lines to that of the Old. There was no smallpox, as we've already noted. Tertian malaria, yellow fever, dengue, measles, diphtheria, typhoid, scarlet fever and influenza were also unknown. These would all be imported by the white man and his African slave; the Native Americans stood little chance of resisting infection.

Prior to Columbus, there seem to have been few epidemiological disasters. It's possible that the main disease-related crisis was the collapse of the Mayan empire in the eighth and ninth centuries AD. This has been attributed to, variously, drought, famine, war, poor trade and unsustainable population growth. All of them may have played their part. We should also consider the role of Mayan farming practices. Maize and beans were Mayan dietary staples for centuries, so much so that it seems to have led to iron deficiency anaemia. Skeletal evidence from Mayan children shows that they had been suffering from an acute form of iron-deficient anaemia.[194] In addition, the soil was poor in iron, leading to less iron in crops and mothers' milk. The Mayan diet was also low in vitamin C, which the body needs to absorb iron. Further vitamins were lost through the Mayan custom of soaking maize in water, which created a deficiency in folic acid and vitamin B12. Factor in further iron loss through sweating, suffering from hookworm, tapeworm and other parasites that were an unavoidable hazard of Mayan farming. Mayan diet also lacked zinc, which stunted growth and the ability to resist infection. The combined effects of poor diet, anaemia, vitamin deficiency and parasite infestation produced a weakened people, much less able to withstand disasters both natural and man-made. When adverse circumstances began to pile up during the eighth and ninth centuries, it spelled the end of the great period of Mayan civilisation.

The dwindling of the Mayans notwithstanding, Aztec codices contain references to disease, but these could be famine- and crop-failure related, 'and may not have been the result of the sort of human-to-human infectious chain that existed in the Old World.'[195] Three disasters are mentioned by the codices, dated to the years 780, 1320 and 1454, 'but the decipherment of Aztec codices is an inexact science at best.'[196] In general, native Americans, regardless of where they lived, enjoyed good health in comparison with Europeans and also a longer life expectancy – some even reached the grand old age of fifty.

However, the 'good health' seen by the first explorers was relative. Arno Karlen notes that 'when native peoples first met Europeans, their societies ranged from hunter-gathering to advanced Neolithic, their health from good to adequate to wretched.' Evidence from bones, mummies and coprolites shows high rates of dysentery, intestinal parasitic diseases, infections from wounds, non-pulmonary tuberculosis (probably caught from birds, cattle or horses), and pinta, a non-venereal skin disease linked to syphilis. They possibly had syphilis as well – see below – pneumonia (in bacterial and viral forms), and hepatitis A. The jury still appears to be out on malaria.[197]

Advocates of pre-Columbian malaria point to the fact that the Aztecs gave quinine to malarial Jesuits in the 1620s. This drug, still used today, is derived from the bark of the cinchona tree. But at what stage did the Aztecs acquire this knowledge? Some suggest malaria was either brought over the Bering Land Bridge with the first settlers, or, in a more controversial theory, was imported by Japanese explorers to Ecuador when they are thought to have made contact with the Valdivian culture at some point between 3500 BC and 1800 BC. What we can say for certain is that, when Europeans arrived in the New World at the end of the fifteenth century, malaria travelled with them, largely carried by African slaves.

Two diseases were totally unknown in the Old World: Chagas' disease and Carrión's disease, or Oroya fever (bartonellosis). Chagas' disease, while similar to African trypanosomiasis (sleeping sickness), seems to have originated in northeastern Brazil and evolved independently. It is at least two thousand years old: mummies from the Tarapaca Valley in northern Chile have revealed Chagas' signature digestive tract problems, and it remains endemic in that part of Chile to this day.[198] Carrión's disease is similarly old; indeed it seems to have been represented on pieces of pre-Columbian Peruvian pottery known as *huacos*. Originating in the Andes, it is a parasitic condition that can cause fever and anaemia and can lead to unsightly boils known as 'Peruvian warts'.

The Great Pox

One disease that quite possibly travelled back to Europe on Columbus's ships made an appearance after the Battle of Fornovo on 6 July 1495. Charles VIII of France, fighting to claim the throne of Naples, inflicted a decisive defeat on the forces of the Holy League, a group of powers including the Papal States, the Duchy of Milan and Venice. Following the battle, Marcello Cumano, a military physician serving with Venetian forces, noted that:

> Several men-at-arms or foot soldiers, owing to the ferment of humours, had pustules on their faces and all over their bodies. These looked rather like grains of millet and usually appeared on the outer surface of the foreskin or on the glans, accompanied by a mild pruritis [a desire to scratch]. Sometimes the first sign would be a single pustule looking like a painless cyst, but the scratching provoked by the pruritis subsequently produced a gnawing ulceration. Some days later, the sufferers were driven to distraction

> by the pains they experienced in their arms, legs and feet, and by an eruption of enormous pustules which lasted… for a year and more if left untreated.[199]

Another doctor, Alessandro Benedetti, noted how the new disease was spread:

> Through sexual contact, an ailment which is new, or at least unknown to previous doctors, the French sickness, has worked its way in from the West to this spot as I write. The entire body is so repulsive to look at and the suffering so great, especially at night, that this sickness is even more horrifying than incurable leprosy or elephantiasis, and it can be fatal.[200]

It was called the great pox to differentiate it from smallpox, although it is better known as syphilis.

It seems to have first reached Europe two years before the siege of Naples. The Spanish physician Ruy Diaz de Isla attended Columbus and his crew in Barcelona in March 1493, shortly after their return from the New World. Some of the crew were clearly ill with something, although the sailors themselves attributed it to the rigours of the voyage. It soon began to spread in Barcelona, and was to follow in the wake of Columbus and his men as they made their triumphant progress. Diaz de Isla dubbed the disease the Serpent, equating syphilis with the serpent in the Garden of Eden, and the pox with the Edenic island of Hispaniola. This intuition proved to be accurate, as syphilis was eventually found to be caused by a snake-shaped bacterium, *Treponema pallidum*. Diaz de Isla would go on to treat 20,000 syphilis victims, during which time he identified the three stages of syphilis, primary, secondary and tertiary (see below).

Some of Columbus's sailors – either from the historic 1492–3 voyage, or more likely the second voyage of 1493–4, which saw the Admiral take many more slaves – were thought to have fought in Charles's army at Naples, and they then infected prostitutes after the city was taken in

February 1495. By the time of the engagement at Fornovo, syphilis had passed into the ranks of Holy League troops, possibly due to the same prostitutes maximising their business opportunities by servicing both sides in the conflict.

This first European syphilis was much worse than its modern descendant. In other words, it behaved like any new disease hitting a virgin population (a rather unfortunate phrase in this context) for the first time. Smallpox, making its first American landfall at the same time as syphilis began to rampage through Europe, behaved with equal ferocity for exactly the same reasons. (No prior experience of a disease meant there was no immunity in the host population.)

Because of its perceived origin within the ranks of Charles's army, syphilis was dubbed 'the French disease', or, as Alessandro Benedetti put it, 'the French sickness'. The name 'syphilis' was coined by the Italian humanist-physician Girolamo Fracastoro (also known by the Latinised form of his name, Fracastorius), in his poem *Syphilis, sive morbus gallicus* (1530), although the name didn't start to gain wide usage until the late eighteenth century.[201] Fracastoro describes how the shepherd Syphilus falls foul of the gods by cursing them for sending a heat wave that kills his cattle. The gods respond by striking Syphilus down with the 'unspeakable disease', giving the shepherd the unfortunate distinction of becoming the first human to suffer from syphilis.

Syphilis is caused by a spirochetal bacterium, *Treponema pallidum.* (A spirochete simply means a bacterium that is spiral-shaped. Yaws, Lyme disease and relapsing fever are also caused by spirochetes. They are most often found in mud or water, or, within the body, in blood, lymph or sweat.)[202] It is transmitted mainly by sexual contact, although it can be passed by a mother to her foetus; this hereditary form is known as congenital syphilis.

When Europeans reached the Americas, syphilis seems to have adapted especially for them. As Andrew Nikiforuk noted, 'for the Arawaks the disease was probably a mild yet common skin infection that was no more irritating than a case of scabies.'[203] They could pass it by skin-to-skin contact or by sharing eating utensils. (This endemic form of syphilis is sometimes known as bejel.) But in Europeans, who not only generally wore more clothes but lived in a colder climate, the bacteria made their home in 'the most hospitable environment they could find: European genitals.'[204]

It was on the genitals, or the mouth, where chancres – the first signs of the disease – appeared. This is the first sign of syphilis's three stages, the primary, which usually appears two to four weeks after the initial infection. The chancre will usually disappear after a couple of weeks, perhaps leading the sufferer into a false sense of security that the disease has left them. During primary syphilis, buboes can also appear, which no doubt would have led the afflicted into believing that they had contracted the plague. As a result of this, syphilis came to be dubbed 'the great imitator' by the eminent Canadian doctor William Osler (1849–1919), as it produced symptoms that appeared to be those of other diseases (plague, meningitis and heart disease in particular). Syphilis is at its most infectious during the primary stage.

Secondary syphilis sees painless skin rashes appear all over the body. The sufferer will get headaches, fever, a feeling of exhaustion. They might lose some hair, 'resulting in an almost moth-eaten appearance to the scalp'.[205] And they will feel an ache in their bones. This is the sign that the spirochete is spreading throughout the body, burrowing its way into the unfortunate person's bones. Alessandro Benedetti once performed an autopsy on a woman who had suffered from syphilis and noted that her bones 'were tumorous and suppurated to the very marrow'.[206] After a few weeks, the secondary symptoms disappear. Again, the person with syphilis would be forgiven for thinking that they were clear of the disease.

But then comes the tertiary phase. This will only develop in around one third of untreated cases, but when it does develop, the results can be horrific. Taking between one and twenty years to develop, the symptoms of tertiary syphilis can include further tumours and suppurating abscesses, 'from which issued a villainous and infected mud which almost made the heart stop beating.'[207] Inside the body, the bones are further destroyed, 'producing especially horrific mutilations when the nasal and palate bones have been destroyed.'[208] The cardiovascular system is attacked, causing aneurysms, while in the central nervous system, meningeal syphilis can develop, which will eventually shut the body down altogether. During this time, the syphilitic will develop the stumbling gait of a leper, and is quite likely to become blind, insane and violent.

After the campaigns of 1495, Charles's army disbanded; the soldiers, mercenaries and camp followers dispersed through Europe, taking syphilis with them. By 1496, it was in France, Switzerland, Germany and Holland; by 1497, England and Scotland; by 1499 it had reached Hungary, Poland and Russia. When Vasco da Gama set out for India in July 1498, a number of his crew were syphilitic, and would live to introduce the disease to the subcontinent.[209]

As the disease spread, so did the horror stories. Diarist Bernardino Zambotti, writing in late 1496 of syphilis's effects in Ferrara, noted that the disease was incurable, 'following excruciating pains in the bones and nerves, accompanied by massive pustules all over the body.'[210] The stricken 'screamed day and night without respite, envying the very dead.'[211] One merchant in Perugia was 'so consumed by the disease between the thigh and the torso that it was possible to see everything that he had inside his body.'[212]

Doctors were powerless to stop the disease. They tried bloodletting. Ruy Diaz de Isla prescribed sexual abstinence, good hygiene, and eating well. The prescription in Fracastoro's poem was quicksilver. None of it did any good, although quicksilver – mercury – became a popular method for treating syphilitics in the sixteenth century. Quite why is a mystery: it frequently did more harm than good. Doctors, it seemed, wanted to be seen to be doing something to justify their fees.

A link with sexual activity was soon established, and syphilis, like leprosy before it, became the disease of the sinner. The radical Florentine preacher Savonarola saw it as divine punishment for the excesses of the age; the French invasion of Italy and the advent of the pox were seen as signs of the imminent end of the world.[213] Humanist scholar Joseph Grünpeck saw signs of a different kind: he attributed the advent of the pox to the 'Great Conjunction' of Jupiter and Saturn that occurred on 25 November 1484.[214]

This date appears on one of the earliest known depictions of the disease, a woodcut of a syphilitic man by Albrecht Dürer. The man stands beneath an astrological emblem representing the conjunction, displaying ulcers on his legs, arms and face. That he is dressed in the garb of a *landsknecht*, or mercenary, suggests Dürer was well aware that the disease was being spread by returning soldiers. (It is one of the artist's earliest woodcuts, dating from 1496.) The image illustrates a poem about epidemics by the humanist scholar Theodericus Ulsenius, and carries the title *Der Syphilitische oder Die Franzosenkrankheit* 'The Syphilitic, or the French Disease'), although this was probably added later, after the publication of Fracastoro's poem in 1530.[215] Swiss artist Niklaus Manuel Deutsch created a more chilling image around 1517. *Death as a Soldier Embraces a Young Woman* shows death in the tattered rags of a *transi* soldier, embracing a girl, one hand thrust between her legs. The anonymous *St Anthony and the Syphilitics* of 1520, (now in Lübeck) is a gentler depiction. A man and a woman, their faces bearing the signs of advanced stages of the disease, are brought before the saint in a woodland scene. They are introduced to Anthony by none other than Mary Magdalene, herself long associated with repentance for sins of the flesh;[216] here those sins are embodied by a small group of naked girls just inside the treeline behind the saint.

Everyone blamed everyone else for the pox. The Italians referred to it as 'the Spanish disease' or 'the French disease'. (The Germans and the English preferred the latter.) The French, for their part, dubbed it the 'Pox of Naples'. The Japanese, who had suffered their first outbreak in 1569, called it the 'Portuguese Sickness' after the sailors who had introduced it. The Portuguese called it the 'Castilian Disease'. For the Chinese, it was the 'Ulcer of Canton', a reference to the city where the first outbreaks had been recorded (introduced by the Portuguese, again). Tahitians, in the eighteenth century, called it the 'British Disease'. (Captain Cook thought it was the fault of the French.) The Persians called it the 'Disease of the Turks', while the Turks called it the 'Christian disease'.[217] As one historian of epidemics remarked, 'In this way syphilis announced the birth of nationalism.'[218] The Spanish writer Oviedo, who spent ten years as an administrator on Hispaniola, was in no doubt as to where the disease came from. Writing to the King of Spain in 1526, he advised, 'Your majesty may take it as certain that this malady comes from the Indies, where it is very common amongst the Indians, but not so dangerous in those lands as it is in our own.'[219]

By the time Fracastoro published his poem, syphilis had spread very rapidly across the Old World. No one was exempt (except the celibate, of course). In particular, the rich and powerful could be as susceptible as the poor. Ivan the Terrible (1530–1584), Tsar of Russia, suffered from it, leading to madness and cruelty. In one insane rage, he attacked his pregnant daughter-in-law, causing her to have a miscarriage; and in 1581, he notoriously murdered his own son. Another son, Feodor, was thought to suffer from congenital syphilis and in a moment of madness – one of many, it seems – proposed marriage to Elizabeth I. Robert Desowitz notes that the Cardinal Bishop of Segovia and Pope Alexander VI (Alexander Borgia) were also thought to be syphilitics.[220] Another Borgia, Cesare (1475–1507), was syphilitic and had to wear a mask over his face to cover the disease's ravages. So too was another Pope, Julius II (1503–13), who is remembered for commissioning Michelangelo to paint the Sistine Chapel's ceiling. Julius is thought to have contracted the 'French disease' from Rome's male prostitutes. On Good Friday 1508, he was unable to bare his foot to be kissed by worshippers as it was completely covered with syphilitic sores.

Less certain is the case of Henry VIII of England. Like Ivan, he became a tyrant, and was prone to fits of violence. He also suffered from a possibly telltale ulcer on his leg. He is said to have undergone a personality change in the late 1520s, around the time he was starting to push for divorce from his first wife, Catherine of Aragon. From then on, Henry became ever more the tyrant, breaking with Rome, proclaiming himself head of the Church of England and, in a massive larceny operation, stole vast amounts of land and wealth when he dissolved the monasteries. After changing the landscape of faith in England forever, he then began to backtrack in the early 1540s, allegedly showing signs of remorse for his actions. Could the English Reformation have been driven by a syphilitic tyrant and his henchmen?

*

There is ongoing debate about the origins of syphilis. One argument holds that it started in the Americas, as de Isla and Oviedo believed, mutating in the 1490s when it came into contact with Europeans. Objections to an American origin were raised even while the disease was causing terror and shame across sixteenth century Europe. Scholars pointed to the Bible, and the illnesses Job suffers: 'the days of affliction have taken hold upon me. My bones are pierced in me in the night season: and my sinews take no rest.' (Job 30.16–17) The references to pains in the bones were seen as proof that syphilis had been part of God's plan since time immemorial. Not content with the word of God, humanist doctors scoured the works of Hippocrates, Celsus and Galen.

Later participants in the debate 'claimed to have identified the pox in the Babylonian poem of Gilgamesh, in the Ebers Papyrus, and in the ulceration of the genitals described by Paul of Aegina, Pliny the Younger, and so many others. What is the "country sickness" Horace refers to? What is the ficus which, according to Juvenal and Martial, makes doctors smile and results from debauchery, particularly pederasty? And don't the Arab doctors also describe a plethora of lesions on the genitals and anus – ulcers, chancres, warts, verrucae and rhagades?'[221]

Modern objections to the American or Columbian theory of origin revolve around the disease's links to other ailments of the same genus – pinta, bejel and yaws. This theory holds that a form of syphilis was long endemic in Africa and in Europe but went unrecognised until the 'French' or 'Neapolitan' disease appeared after the Battle of Fornovo. This theory maintains that what had often been taken for leprosy in the Middle Ages could well have been syphilis.

Another theory – that of the 'dual origin' – is a variation on these themes, maintaining that there were two forms of the disease, one from Africa spread by social contact, and the other strain that developed in the Americas, that was also spread by social contact until it became a sexually transmitted disease once it encountered Europeans.[222] The African strain eventually spread north into Europe, where it was taken for leprosy ('pre-Columbian' syphilis), while the American strain came back with Columbus.

Of the theories, the Columbian is best backed up by paleopathological evidence,[223] although the cause of the pre-Columbian camp has been bolstered by a number of archaeological discoveries in Britain. Bodies from Hull Priory, Blackfriars in Gloucester and Whithorn in Galloway – all of people who had died before Columbus's return to Europe in 1493 – showed evidence of the bone damage characteristic of syphilis.[224] How syphilis – if that is indeed what it is – reached late mediaeval Britain remains unknown. Similarly, in 2010, the body of a young man from an Anglo-Saxon cemetery at Apple Down in Sussex was also found to show evidence of syphilis.[225] He had died in the sixth century AD. This discovery would appear to support a 'dual origin' theory for the beginnings of syphilis, although it remains controversial.

*

Europe's aggressive drive outwards in the sixteenth century was marked by disease. As the *Cambridge World History of Human Disease* notes, 'In the sixteenth and seventeenth centuries, dozens of "new" diseases seemed to demand or defy medical explanation.' Many of these diseases were the result of Europe's 'outward urge' (to borrow a phrase from John Wyndham). This onslaught of new diseases, combined with the invention of the printing press and Renaissance humanism's desire to debate and explain the world in new terms, produced some of the earliest medical descriptions we have of diseases like typhus, scarlet fever, rickets, 'the "English sweate" (whatever that was), and even anorexia nervosa.'[226]

The 'English Sweate' is the odd one out in this group, as it remains one of the great unknowns of Renaissance epidemiology. It first appeared in London in September 1485, shortly after the new Tudor king, Henry VII, had been victorious at Bosworth Field. As the humanist scholar – and sometime courtier – Polydore Vergil commented, it 'was taken by many as a bad omen'.[227]

The sickness struck quickly, its victims succumbing to acute feverish sweating, becoming comatose and dying within 48 hours. It seemed to strike men more than women, and, unlike so many diseases we've looked at, affected the rich more than the poor. It also seemed to home in on Englishmen – the Scots, Welsh and Irish being largely immune. There were recurrences in 1508, 1517, 1528, and 1551, each time affecting a comparatively small number of people. The *Chronicle* of Edward Hall (1497–1547) reports that the 1517 outbreak 'was so cruel that it killed some within three houres, some within two houres, some merry at dinner and dedde [dead] at supper. Many died in the Kynges court, the lord Clinton, the lorde Gray of Wilton, and many Knightes, gentlemen and officers.'[228]

Justus Hecker (1795–1850), the German physician and writer who arguably did more than anyone else to start the study of the history of disease,

> blamed the English climate and the habits of the English nobility. [T]he English sweating sickness was a spirit of the mist, which hovered amid the dark clouds. Even in ordinary years the atmosphere of England is loaded with these clouds during considerable periods, and in damp seasons they would prove the more injurious, as the English of these times were not accustomed to cleanliness, moderation in their diet, or even comfortable refinements. Gluttony was common among the nobility as well as among the lower classes; all were immoderately addicted to drinking.[229]

Modern theories have tended to steer clear of the weather and drink as causes: it was quite possibly a virus (or a new arbovirus) brought to England by Henry VII's Flemish mercenaries, who were immune to the 'sweate' themselves. But it disappeared in 1551, and has not reappeared since.

Hecker was also fascinated by another mystery disease that was contemporaneous with the English Sweate: the dancing mania. The most celebrated case occurred in Strasbourg in the summer of 1518, when a woman started to dance in the street. Bystanders began to join in. Soon hundreds were dancing, and wouldn't – or couldn't – stop. At the peak of the phenomenon, about 400 people were dancing. The authorities decided to let them carry on, in the hope that they would exhaust themselves. They didn't. Some danced themselves to death. Eventually, the remaining dancers were bundled into wagons and taken to the shrine of St Vitus at Saverne, thirty or so miles away, which seems to have had the desired effect.

The Strasbourg outbreak had not been the first. The earliest recorded spate of mass dancing occurred in Flanders in the seventh century.[230] In the thirteenth century in Germany, a group of children danced from Erfurt to Arnstadt, which may have inspired the legend of the Pied Piper of Hamelin. In 1278, around 200 people were stricken with the mania on a bridge across the Meuse. The bridge collapsed. In 1374, there was a major outbreak in Aachen, which spread to a number of cities in western Germany and the Low Countries.

There were further outbreaks after 1518, too. In 1564, on St John's Day, there was an outbreak in Flanders, said to have been witnessed by Pieter Bruegel, who made an engraving of the dancers. (The image remains in a copy by Hendrik Hondius.)

What could have caused this bizarre behaviour? Hecker believed the dancing was an attempt to ward off disease, plague in particular, stoked by religious fervour.[231] More recent scholarship argues that, in each case, the communities affected were recovering from trauma and hardship, such as floods, famine, plague.[232] An additional factor may have been the cult of St Vitus, who was thought to be able to curse people by making them dance. Weakened by famine and its resultant illness, the people of Strasbourg may have begun to dance to appease the saint, and then entered a trance state. The more people who joined in, the harder it was to stop. It's significant that the epidemic seems to have stopped after the dancers were taken to the shrine of St Vitus to pray.

Modern medicine explains St Vitus Dance in terms of Sydenham's chorea, a streptococcal infection that causes involuntary jerking movements. (Another chorea, Huntington's, causes similar movements, but is the result of a genetic abnormality.) The condition takes its name from Thomas Sydenham (1624–89), the doctor and medical reformer who was dubbed 'the English Hippocrates'. Sydenham's work helped move the study of disease and the practice of medicine away from the classical model of the humours, and into the modern era. Humoural theory wasn't quite dead in Sydenham's time, but was starting to look unwell.

Concepts of disease – and the medicine required to treat them – had been changing for a century or more by Sydenham's time. The iconoclastic Swiss doctor Philippus Aureolus Theophrastus Bombastus von Hohenheim (*c.*1493–1541) adopted the alias Paracelsus – 'greater than Celsus', a reference to the first century Roman doctor – and publicly burned the works of Galen and Avicenna at Basel in 1526. Paracelsus questioned unthinking acceptance of tradition and authority, and stressed the importance of observation and experiment.

Such observation and experiment saw Renaissance scholars looking both outwards to the world around them, and inwards, into the workings of the human body. In the same year that Nicolaus Copernicus published *De revolutionibus orbium coelestium* (*On the Revolutions of the Celestial Spheres*, 1543), which overturned the geocentric model of the heavens, Andreas Vesalius's *De humani corporis fabrica* (*On the Fabric of the Human Body*) represented a huge advance in the fledgling science of human anatomy.

The work of Vesalius began hammering nails into the coffin of humoural theory (although it took a very long time to die, and was still widespread in the eighteenth century). Surgical and medical schools such as the Royal College of Surgeons in Edinburgh and the Royal College of Physicians in London were founded. William Harvey (1578–1657) discovered the circulation of the blood in 1628, which contributed more nails to the coffin, as did the discovery of the lymphatic system a few years later by Olaus Rudbeck (1630–1702) and Thomas Bartholin (1616–1680). Developments in the manufacture and use of microscopes by Robert Hooke (1635–1703) and Antonie van Leeuwenhoek (1632–1723) effectively invented the science of microbiology. For the first time, human beings were able to see cells and bacteria, which were dubbed *animalcules*. The founding of the Royal Society in London in 1660 encouraged Hooke, Leeuwenhoek and others to present their findings, and The Society dedicated itself to the furtherance of knowledge.

Among those invited to present work to the Society was London haberdasher John Graunt (1620–1674). In *Natural and Political Observations Made upon the Bills of Mortality* (1662), Graunt published his findings on the bills of mortality, which had been published every week in London since 1592. The bills listed the mortality numbers in each parish, and were later modified to include causes of death as well.

Some need no explanation: Aged, Stillborn, Worms, Cancer, Gangrene and Fistula, Childbed (probably puerperal fever or other complications of birth), Consumption and Tissick (both tuberculosis), Falling Sickness (epilepsy), French Pox (syphilis), Frighted (heart attack?), Grief, King's Evil (scrofula), Bit with a Mad Dog (rabies), Bloody Flux (dysentery), meagrom (migraine), Made away with themselves, Leprosy, Measles, Palsy and Plague.

Other people left this world in a slightly more memorable manner: Fainted in Bath, Excessive Drinking, Suddenly (heart attack or perhaps what is now known as Sudden Adult Death Syndrome) or Found Dead in the Streets. And then there are still other causes that are perhaps most memorable of all: Teeth (possibly dental abscesses or oral gangrene), wen (a tumour, so presumably cancer), Rising of the Lights (probably obstructions of the windpipe), Blasted, or Planet Struck (sudden paralysis, or becoming 'confounded').

Writing in his Preface, Graunt said he had 'found some Truths, and not commonly believed Opinions, to arise from my Meditations upon these neglected Papers.' In finding truths and not commonly believed opinions, Graunt became one of the first demographers. For the first time, relatively accurate data was available on the prevalence of disease. Gone were the wild estimates, guesswork and exaggerations of mediaeval accounts. Modern public health initiatives all begin with Graunt.

*

In the Americas, so many Indians died from smallpox and other Old World diseases that the Spanish and Portuguese were forced to import slaves from Africa in order to run their plantations and colonies. Black Africans were naturally immune to smallpox, as many had suffered from sickle cell disease (also known as sickle cell anaemia), which was endemic in many parts of Africa. That sickle cell disease gave immunity to smallpox was a biological fluke which condemned millions of Africans to lives of servitude in the New World. In a further horrible irony, freed slaves returning to Africa found themselves susceptible to diseases that they had been immune to – or that did not exist at all – in the New World.

The East Indies, too, quickly fell within the compass of European imperial ambition. The Portuguese explorer Vasco da Gama sailed for India in 1498, taking syphilis with him. But at sea, another disease manifested itself. Some of da Gama's crew became lethargic, with their skin drying and tightening, hair knotting into clumps; fresh wounds no longer healed. Then their gums became swollen and purple, and they began to lose their teeth. This latter stage is the classic symptom of scurvy, caused by a deficiency of vitamin C in the diet. In this case, it would have been occasioned by a lack of fresh fruit and vegetables. At its worst, the disease would have caused old fractures to break again, accompanied by tubercular lesions and cardiac haemorrhage.[233] Scurvy would blight sailors of all nations for more than two hundred years.

The English and Dutch conducted experiments into the problem. It was noted that sailors recovered quickly when reaching port and eating fresh fruit and vegetables. However, it was not possible to keep these fresh on long voyages. The Dutch tried planting orchards in their territories on Mauritius and St Helena, and even created gardens on some of their ships. This appears to have had some success in reducing the mortality rate while at sea.[234] An English doctor, Edward Ives, who served as ship's surgeon in the 1740s, tried an alternative idea. Ives persuaded his admiral to carry supplies of the best Devon cider. While these lasted, none of the five hundred men aboard died.[235] After numerous such trials and experiments, the English began to provision their sailors with lime juice at the end of the eighteenth century, earning the nickname 'limeys'.

Scurvy was not just restricted to the sea. 'Land scurvy', or pellagra, afflicted primarily poor city dwellers. The disease was first recorded in the eighteenth century among impoverished farmers of northern Italy and Spain, who had become dependent on maize brought back from the New World. Maize was easy to cultivate, and provided substantial yields. It began to replace barley, wheat and millet. Its economic potential was not lost on Europe's elites. The Austro-Hungarian royal family, the Habsburgs, 'actively fostered its production not only because maize provided a staple food for the peasants, but because its greater yields meant larger tithes for the royal coffers.'[236] And when said peasants developed pellagra, 'members of the upper classes... tended either to deny the existence of the disease or to blame its appearance on the inherent moral weaknesses of its victims.'[237] Thus, the rich blamed the poor for something the rich themselves were responsible for. But as cities grew in the nineteenth century, pellagra would become one of the least worries of Europe's poor.

*

The poor were also more likely than the rich to be on the receiving end of harsh treatment if they found themselves detained in an asylum for the mad. The poor would have heavy fetters and chains put on them, as they were 'fit only for the pauper lunatics: if a gentleman was put in irons he would not like it,' or so said Thomas Monro (1759–1833),[238] head physician at London's notorious mental asylum, Bethlem Royal Hospital, better known as Bedlam. Indeed, the Board of Governors at Bedlam referred to the patients as 'prisoners' and 'the poor'.

Conditions had long been harsh: records survive of a sixteenth century patient whose leg was 'so ulcerated that it is thought it must be cut off', while another patient complained that 'her foote was rotten'.[239] In 1631, an inquiry found that Bedlam was so underfunded that its patients were close to starvation. By the time Samuel Pepys was writing his celebrated diary, the 'poor' were better fed, but had become a tourist attraction: he noted in his Diary for 19 February 1669, 'All the afternoon I at the office, while the young people went to see Bedlam.' An entry fee of one penny would admit the curious, where they could wander at will, looking at the patients as if they were specimens in a zoo.

In 1699, the writer Ned Ward (1667–1731) published his account of just such a day out:

> We heard such a rattling of chains, drumming of doors, ranting, hollering, singing and rattling, that I could think of nothing but Don Quevedo's *Visions* [possibly a reference to Francisco de Quevedo's 1608 satire *The Dream of Hell*] where the damn'd broke loose, and put Hell in an uproar.[240]

Ward witnessed one of the 'shatter-brained fraternity' expose herself to a young girl, shouting, 'I've got hair where you've got none', and narrowly escaped being soaked in urine by one patient, the 'bread and cheese' man, who took great delight in hurling the contents of his chamber-pot at visitors. Another inmate didn't seem to use a chamber pot at all, as he 'smelled of urine and ran round his cells clapping his hands and shouting "halloo, halloo, halloo..."'[241] In art, Hogarth's *A Rake's Progress* No 8: *In the Madhouse* (1732–3) and Goya's *Yard with Lunatics* (1793–4) and *The Madhouse* (1812–19) captured the desperate condition of the 'distracted'.

Such treatment reflected the fact that the mad were down in the sewers of public opinion, along with lepers, prostitutes and the disabled. No one knew what caused madness. For centuries it had been on the borderlands of the demonic, with exorcism being the principal remedy. If demons weren't responsible, then an imbalance of the humours was to blame, or the influence of the moon. By the nineteenth century, the etiology had shifted away from supernatural causes to the relatively bland, not to say downright eccentric: domestic disturbances and disappointed love – the latter affecting women in particular – were thought to have made more people 'nervous' 'than the sword has slain'. Other potential causes of madness were thought to include 'mistaken perceptions of real religion', 'hard, intense and long-continued studies', 'the fearful associations of being awoke from sound sleep while the house is on fire', 'blows on the head' and onanism.[242] The French doctor Philippe Pinel (1745–1826) believed that physical factors – such as 'an organic lesion of the brain' – caused insanity, or that emotional disorders might play a part.[243]

There was no agreement on treatment. The practice of trepanation – drilling a hole in the skull – is thought to be one of the oldest methods of controlling mental illness; skulls from the Bronze Age have been found bearing the telltale holes and cracks of the trepanner's art. This rather extreme method was still being practised during the Renaissance, as evidenced by Hieronymus Bosch's painting, *The Extraction of the Stone of Madness* (*c.* 1494). From the seventeenth century onwards, institutionalisation was generally seen as the way to proceed. The prominent London physician Thomas Willis (1621–75) advocated administering regular thrashings to patients, while Thomas Monro admitted before a government enquiry in 1815 that at Bedlam, 'We apply generally bleeding, purging and vomit'.[244] Others advised drugs such as opium, concoctions of agrimony, ivy and vinegar, or shock treatments such as throwing the lunatic into a river. A cold bath would suffice if there was no river nearby.

This was all far behind what was going on in the Ottoman Empire. In the hospital founded in Edirne by Sultan Bayezid II (1481–1512), fragrant scents were employed to calm patients. Flowers were thought to affect the humours. Violets, for instance, were said to have a cool and moist temperament, and therefore were good for treating the opposite qualities of yellow bile. This didn't always work: the flowers used 'as a type of olfactory therapy' were sometimes trampled on by the patients, or simply eaten.[245] Other forms of quite humane-seeming therapy were tried, including the use of theatrical performances. The Ottoman Turk writer and traveller Evliya Chelebi visited Edirne in 1651, where he noted music was also being used, 'and many of the insane were reported to have been relieved by this "nourishment of the soul"'.[246]

Things had not always been so progressive in the Muslim world. The hospital in Damascus that was treating insane patients by 1185, where, according to the Muslim traveller Ibn Jubayr, there was 'a system of treatment for confined lunatics, and they are bound in chains.'[247] The Berber writer and diplomat Leo Africanus (*c.* 1494 – *c.* 1554) visited the hospital in Fez and noted conditions as bad as those at Bedlam: 'The walls of their rooms were strengthened with heavy beams of wood and iron. The person who was in charge of feeding them constantly carried a whip, and when he saw an agitated patient, he administered a good thrashing.'[248] The tradition of going to look at the mad also existed. In 'The Three Madmen's Tale' from *The Book of the Thousand Nights and One Night*, we read of this:

> 'What do you say to a visit to the maristan [asylum], my lord? We have often spoken of exploring a house of fools together, but we have never done so yet. To my way of thinking, the mad have a more subtle understanding than the sane. They behold differences and affinities which are hidden from common men, and are often visited by strange visions.'[249]

The 'differences and affinities which are hidden from common men' that some asylum patients were privy to was not necessarily madness. In the early sixteenth century, Sir Thomas More described one patient who was in Bedlam because he had 'fallen in to ye frantike heresyes'[250] while Ned Ward met a man on his 1699 visit who spouted anti-monarchist views from the confines of his cell. When Ward informed the man he was committing treason by saying such things, the man surprised Ward by agreeing with him, and offered a lucid defence of his position:

> 'Truth is persecuted everywhere abroad, and flies hither for sanctuary, where she sits as safe as a knave in a church, or a whore in a nunnery. I can use her as I please and that's more than you dare do. I can tell great men such bold truths as they don't love to hear, without the danger of a whipping-post.'[251]

As Bedlam historian Paul Chambers notes, 'The man was quite correct. So long as he was classified as mad, he was free to express his anti-establishment views without fear of repercussion. Should he ever be declared sane and released then these same views would more than likely land him in prison or the pillory.'[252] Chambers speculates that the anti-monarchist might have been Richard Stafford, a fervent Jacobite who was admitted to Bedlam in 1689. This was a quicker way of getting him off the streets, where he had been 'dispersing books and pamphlets full of Enthusiasm and Sedition',[253] than taking him to court. As the French philosopher Michel Foucault argued, the growth in asylum building from the seventeenth century onwards in Europe was a symptom of the ruling elites' need to control their populations, freethinking in particular.

Epileptics could also find themselves in Bedlam and similar institutions if there was no one to look after them in the outside world. As with the 'distracted', early mental asylums didn't really know what to do with epileptics, given that no one really knew what caused the disease. It was generally best to lock them up out of sight, as some thought epilepsy might be psychologically contagious: merely seeing someone have a fit might bring one on in the observer.[254]

Epilepsy was long associated with ideas about demonic possession and malign astrological influences. The Arabs referred to it as the 'Divine Disease', echoing the ancient Babylonian belief that epilepsy was caused by the 'touch of a god'. From the early Middle Ages epilepsy had been associated with madness. Isidore of Seville, writing in the seventh century, referred to epileptics as *lunaticus*. Sometimes these 'lunatics' were thought to have prophetic visions, and enjoyed the status of a holy fool.

Despite the longstanding supernatural associations, some medical authorities had surmised quite early on that epilepsy was a 'disease of the brain'. Despite its title, the Hippocratic text *On the Sacred Disease* argues that epilepsy had natural causes and should be treated accordingly, with a regimen based on diet and exercise. There is some evidence that, when trying to ascertain the causes of epilepsy, certain later Greek physicians – Herophilus (335–280 BC), Erasistratus (304–250 BC) and Asclepiades of Bithynia (*c.*124–40 BC) – 'tended to think in terms of the brain and nervous system'.[255] These early intimations of epilepsy as a neurological condition were finally confirmed in the nineteenth century. But after Soranus of Ephesus (*fl.* second century AD), who was 'perhaps the last for some time to think about epilepsy in this way', came Galen and humoural theory, which influenced nearly all subsequent writers and physicians until the nineteenth century.

However, epilepsy retained its stigma. *On the Sacred Disease* is critical of the superstitions surrounding epilepsy, such as the efficacy of avoiding baths, eating goat meat or wearing black in curing the disease. Those who advocated such things were, according to Hippocrates, no better than 'conjurors, purificators, mountebanks, and charlatans'. Another widely held belief was that epilepsy could be cured by drinking fresh human blood. In Roman times, epileptics were known to enter the arena to drink blood from gladiators' wounds. The historian of epilepsy, Owsei Temkin, might have been thinking of this practice when he wrote, 'To the ancients, the epileptic was an object of horror and disgust and not a saint or prophet as has sometimes been contended.'[256] Epilepsy – like madness – was seen as making a person unclean, and Romans had the custom of spitting whenever they saw an epileptic, which was thought to keep the demon that caused the disease at bay. They also avoided drinking from the same cups as epileptics, and eating from the same platters. Like leprosy, epilepsy was the disease of the sinner.

5

Early Modern to 1900

> Returning one evening, somewhat later than usual, to my own house, my attention was attracted, just as I entered the porch, by the figure of a man reclining against the wall at a few paces distant. My sight was imperfectly assisted by a far-off lamp; but the posture in which he sat, the hour, and the place, immediately suggested the idea of one disabled by sickness. It was obvious to conclude that his disease was pestilential.

So begins *Arthur Mervyn,* the novel by Charles Brockden Brown, first published in 1799–1800. The pestilential disease which the man on the porch – the hero, Arthur Mervyn – is suffering from is yellow fever. A major epidemic decimated Philadelphia in 1793, which forms a major part of the plot. (Indeed, the novel's subtitle is *Memoirs of the Year 1793.*) Arthur describes the scene in the Welbeck mansion:

> I wandered over this deserted mansion, in a considerable degree, at random. Effluvia of a pestilential nature assailed me from every corner. In the front room of the second story, I imagined that I discovered vestiges of that catastrophe which the past night had produced. The bed appeared as if some one had recently been dragged from it. The sheets were tinged with yellow, and with that substance which is said to be characteristic of this disease, the gangrenous or black vomit. The floor exhibited similar stains...
>
> The door opened, and a figure glided in. The portmanteau dropped

> from my arms, and my heart's blood was chilled. If an apparition of the dead were possible, (and that possibility I could not deny,) this was such an apparition. A hue, yellowish and livid; bones, uncovered with flesh; eyes, ghastly, hollow, woe-begone, and fixed in an agony of wonder upon me; and locks, matted and negligent, constituted the image which I now beheld. My belief of somewhat preternatural in this appearance was confirmed by recollection of resemblances between these features and those of one who was dead.[257]

Yellow fever is first definitively recorded in 1648, when it broke out in Campeche, a Spanish outpost on Mexico's Yucatan peninsula. The first omen was a thick fog, which appeared in March, according to Diego López de Cogolludo in his *Historia de Yucathan*. The fog was so dense there was an eclipse-like darkness for several days. The indigenous Mayans took the fog as 'a sign of great mortality of people in this land, and for our sins'.[258] Great mortality did indeed follow. The first cases were reported in June. Cogolludo lamented that Campeche was 'totally laid waste'.[259] He referred to the disease as the *peste*, noting that victims were 'taken with a very severe and intense pain in the head and of all the bones in the body, so violent that it appeared to dislocate them or to squeeze them as a press.' The pains were frequently followed by a 'vehement fever', in which they could become delirious. If the disease worsened after that, the victim would vomit 'putrefied blood and of these very few remained alive.'[260]

What was this mysterious new disease that was bringing Spanish possessions in Latin America to their knees, and how did it get there? Yellow fever is an acute viral haemorrhagic disease, thought to be native to Africa. It's what is called an arboviral disease – that is, transmitted by an arthropod vector. In the case of yellow fever, the vector is the female *Aedes aegypti* mosquito, affecting humans and monkeys with her bite. Aside from the 'severe and intense pains' and 'vehement fever' recorded by Cogolludo, the symptoms of yellow fever include a slowing of the heart rate – unusual for fevers, which usually cause the opposite. Worsening kidney function causes jaundice, and bleeding can occur from eyes, mouth, nose and rectum. The 'putrefied blood' Cogolludo mentions earned the disease the nickname *el vomito negro* (black vomit).

From its probable home in Africa, yellow fever was almost certainly exported to the New World on slave ships, the mosquitoes laying their eggs in the vessels' freshwater barrels. In addition, the slave trade was undergoing changes in the seventeenth century. Originally the province of the Spanish and the Portuguese, by the time yellow fever broke out on Yucatan in 1648, the Iberian powers were facing competition from the Dutch, British and French. With more slaves being taken to the Americas, plantations were getting larger, and needed more slaves. To cite the example of Barbados, by mid-century, the number of property holders had fallen from 11,000 to less than 800. This also resulted in plantations amalgamating and with the larger plantations, there came the demand for more labour. When English colonists arrived in 1627, the island had virtually no slaves at all. In 1645 – just three years before the first confirmed case of yellow fever – there were 5,600. By 1667, there were 82,000.[261] In addition to the massive increase in slaves, sugar came increasingly to replace – or at least complement – tobacco and cotton.

Not all the ships on the seas in the summer of 1648 were European colonists. Some were probably pirates. But it mattered little: mosquitoes were not fussy travellers, and could hitch a ride on any ship with a fresh water supply. From Yucatan, yellow fever spread to the French colonies of St Kitts and Guadeloupe in the summer of 1648. One-third of St Kitts's population perished within eighteen months. It then struck Cuba; a third of Havana's residents died between May and October 1649.[262] The disease also seems to have been active on Barbados, where yellow fever (or something very much like it – it was described as a 'nova pestis' or a 'new distemper'), may have broken out in September 1647.[263] It remained such a potent threat that it even appears to have slowed down – hindered, certainly – European exploitation of the Caribbean. In 1665, 1,500 British troops seized the French-held island of St Lucia. Within two years, the number of British soldiers on the island had fallen to a rump force of 89. The French were not responsible: yellow fever did most of the work.[264]

With the increased sea traffic – slavers, imperialists, colonists, traders and pirates – it was only a matter of time before yellow fever reached mainland North America. A British fleet is thought to have introduced the disease into Boston, Massachusetts, in 1693, the first continental North American city to be infected. Charleston, North Carolina, Philadelphia, and New York City were all affected within a decade, losing between seven and ten per cent of their populations. But it proved to be a difficult disease to predict. From 1737 to 1743, yellow fever was an annual visitor to the eastern seaboard of America. It then disappeared until 1762, when it flared up again until 1765. Another long silence ensued, until the 1793 epidemic in Philadelphia.

Yellow fever then began to dog the newly-independent United States, becoming perhaps the most significant disease in the country's early history, just as it had done in the Caribbean in the seventeenth and early eighteenth centuries. There was so much yellow fever in Louisiana that Napoleon decided to abandon his plan to pursue a North American empire. The disease had already claimed the lives of thousands of French soldiers on Haiti (then fighting for independence), and further losses could not be sustained. Napoleon ordered his foreign minister, Talleyrand, to sell Louisiana to the American government in 1803. (That was certainly not the end of yellow fever in the state: in the 1840s, Irish immigrants, fleeing the great famine at home, are thought to have been responsible for the huge rise in the number of yellow fever cases in New Orleans.) Florida lost so much of its population to yellow fever in the 1820s and 1830s that statehood was delayed, while Memphis, Tennessee, was nearly abandoned as uninhabitable after epidemics in 1878 and 1879. Such continuing disasters would have shocked the Gothic imagination of Brockden Brown and his hero, Arthur Mervyn.

There was very little health officials could do to stop the successive epidemics, which usually struck in the summer. Ships arriving from affected areas were forced to fly a yellow flag – the Yellow Jack – and then had to undergo a period of quarantine. Established to combat the plague (the first quarantine was introduced in fifteenth century Dubrovnik), quarantine was used in the US from the 1793 Philadelphia outbreak onwards. Although one of the few relatively effective tools the urban health boards had at their disposal, it was not always popular. Commercial interests frequently opposed quarantine, as cargoes – such as bananas – wouldn't keep for 40 days. Opponents pointed out that, of the eight American epidemics following 1793, quarantine had stopped none of them. The problem was simple: although the disease could burn itself out on a ship held for thirty or forty days, nothing prevented the disease-carrying mosquitoes from alighting.

There were those who thought yellow fever was contagious. These 'contagionists' were usually to be found supporting quarantine. An opposing camp – unwittingly echoing the miasma theorists of the Black Death – declared the main cause to be dirt and squalor causing 'bad air'. This 'explained' why victims who did not know each other could be affected. However, sometimes all these factors were present, but there was no yellow fever. One doctor in New Orleans noted however, that sometimes all the ingredients for a supposed miasma might be present, but without yellow fever occurring: 'What a quandary the yellow fever wizards must be in!... We have heat and moisture, dead dogs, cats, chickens, etc, all over the streets, and plenty of hungry doctors; yet Yellow Jack will not come.'[265]

The American army doctor Walter Reed tried to make Yellow Jack appear in a potentially fatal experiment that took place in Havana in 1900/01. While the US had been the victor in the Spanish-American War of 1898, she had lost more men to yellow fever than to enemy action, and Reed had been appointed by the Surgeon General to look into the matter. Reed and his colleagues, Jesse Lazear, James Carroll and Aristides Agramonte, wanted to test the theory that yellow fever was caused by mosquitoes. The theory had been first put forward by the Cuban doctor, Carlos Finlay (1833–1915), but Finlay never made the decisive discovery that the vector is the female *Aedes aegypti* mosquito. Another possible source of inspiration was the British army doctor, Ronald Ross, who, in 1897, discovered that malaria was transmitted by mosquitoes (see below). Carroll allowed himself to be bitten by mosquitoes that had fed on yellow fever patients. Despite becoming very ill, he survived. Lazear was not so lucky. He died from yellow fever on 26 September 1900, two weeks after being bitten and so delirious in the final stages that it took five men to hold him down.[266]

Undeterred, Reed set up another experiment, which took place in wooden huts dubbed 'Camp Lazear' in honour of his fallen comrade. Reed had one group of volunteer soldiers placed in a hut full of filthy blankets and clothing covered with blood and vomit from yellow fever victims. But, crucially, there were no mosquitoes. In another hut, conditions were pristine, but Reed introduced mosquitoes. The volunteers in this hut contracted yellow fever; those in the blood-and-vomit-infested hovel emerged merely in need of a bath and some fresh air.

Subsequently, a sanitation campaign took place, spearheaded by another army doctor, William Crawford Gorgas, whose previous attempt to clean up Havana in 1898 had failed due to the campaign's focussing on classic 'miasma-producing' areas such as dirty streets and piles of refuse. When Reed told Gorgas about the results at Camp Lazear, Gorgas went on the offensive, draining mosquito breeding grounds – especially any standing fresh water near houses – spraying with insecticide, and introducing screens and insecticides into sick rooms. As a result of Gorgas's improved methods, Havana was free of yellow fever by 1901, and Gorgas went on to tackle the situation in the Panama Canal (see below), which was decades behind schedule due to yellow fever and malaria. A yellow fever vaccine was finally developed in 1937 by the South African virologist Max Theiler (1899–1972).

Despite these major advances, questions about yellow fever remain. Why has it never invaded Asia, despite the continent's abundant population of mosquitoes and tropical environments? Do Asians have innate immunity? Or is it because encephalitis occupies the same ecological niche? A further puzzle is that the mosquito *aedes albopictus* spreads yellow fever and dengue fever in America, but not in Asia. No one knows why it should be a vector on one continent, but not another.

The disease has clear links with emergent capitalism, militarism, and imperialism. Indeed, each of these three inter-related things could be said to have caused yellow fever to become an epidemic disease. As Margaret Humphreys writes,

> Yellow fever serves as an early example of an 'emerging disease' and as a warning against the disruption of tropical habitats. In its jungle form the disease is not particularly threatening, and where it exists in equilibrium with a stable society, it causes only a minor childhood disease. Developed countries that disrupt such a balance do so at their peril. In many ways it is fair to say that yellow fever is the price that Europeans and their progeny paid for the sin of slavery.[267]

*

While yellow fever was doing its work in the newly-independent United States, and people were lamenting the lack of a health company to deal with the problem – 'We have fire companies, we have insurance companies, and we have banking companies; but no company could equal the extensive or essential benefits desirable from a health company'[268] – a doctor in Berkeley, Gloucestershire, made a momentous discovery. Edward Jenner (1749–1823) noticed that milk maids who had contracted cowpox did not catch smallpox. 'What renders the Cow-Pox virus so extremely singular… is that the person who has been affected is for ever after secure from infection of the Small-pox,' he wrote.[269]

In May 1796, Jenner decided an experiment was in order. He chose James Phipps, the eight-year-old son of his gardener, and a young dairymaid, Sarah Nelmes, who had contracted cowpox. Jenner took a scraping of material from a cowpox pustule on Sarah's hand and scratched it into the boy's skin. Six weeks later, Jenner inoculated James Phipps with the smallpox virus taken from the pustule of a smallpox patient. The disease didn't 'take'. Jenner then vaccinated his own son with cowpox with equal success. Jenner's process became known as 'vaccination' from *vacca*, Latin for 'cow'.

Jenner did not invent the process of vaccination. A semi-legendary account places its origins in eleventh century China.[270] However, we're on firmer ground with evidence from sixteenth century China. Inoculation for smallpox is mentioned in a book of 1549, but not described until the reign of the Longqing emperor, (1567–72).[271]

The process spread slowly along the Silk Road from China. In 1717, Lady Mary Wortley Montagu (1689–1762), wife of the British ambassador in Istanbul, caused a minor stir in London society circles by having her four-year-old son inoculated against smallpox. This method of 'engrafting', as Lady Mary called it, involved rubbing smallpox scabs – 'as much venom as can lie upon the head of her needle'[272] – into open wounds. (It was also known as 'variolation'.) The method had long been practised by the Turks, who possibly learned it from the people of Circassia in the northwestern Caucasus.

Lady Mary had herself been a victim of smallpox, losing her famous looks (including her eyelashes)[273] at the age of 26 (in December 1715). Fascinated by Ottoman culture, Lady Mary resolved to save her son from the possibility of contracting the disease when she heard about the 'engrafting' procedure, writing in her *Turkish Embassy Letters* of how a woman appeared with 'a nutshell full of matter of the best sort of smallpox'[274] when she arranged for her son to be inoculated. (She also had her three-year-old daughter inoculated in 1721.)

Lady Mary's pioneering efforts started an interest in inoculation in England, although it was not entirely trusted, by dint of its origins in darkest Asia, by way of the Turk. As a safety precaution, engrafting was first tried out on six Newgate convicts who had been condemned to hang – three men and three women – who were offered the choice of being 'engrafted' in return for freedom. Although condemned to hang, the six could quite likely have been taken by typhus, or one of the other diseases that were so frequently to be found in the prison that they were virtually members of staff. Conditions in Newgate were so bad – it was little better than an open sewer – that many inmates died before reaching the gallows. King George I allowed the experiment to go ahead on the grounds that 'carrying on this practice to perfection may tend to the general benefit of mankind'. The engrafting was a success:

none of the six became seriously ill, and in September 1721, all six were released from Newgate Prison, free from smallpox.

The need for inoculation was rather more pressing in the Colonies. A smallpox epidemic gripped Boston that same year. The Puritan minister Cotton Mather encouraged inoculation after being told about the process by his African slave. Mather then told Zabdiel Boylston, a physician practising in Brookline (then a village outside the city). Boylston began inoculating patients, but made himself and Mather very unpopular in the process. Despite the epidemic raging around them, many Bostonians – including other doctors – were suspicious of the process of inoculation, and underlined their hostility by firebombing Mather's house and forcing Boylston into hiding 'with curses, assault, and threats of hanging.'[275] However, it became clear that inoculation worked, when it was found that, out of the 248 people Boylston had treated, only six had died. Both he and Mather were made members of the Royal Society.

Both the Newgate experiment and the experiences of Mather and Boylston made the notion of public health, if not immediately possible, then at least notional. There had been early incarnations of what we would now call public health policy during plague epidemics, but these usually amounted to little more than monarchs or city fathers ordering more plague pits to be dug for the dead, or suggesting measures that we now know to be largely useless, such as hanging heavy curtains in windows to ensure plague-producing miasmas didn't seep into people's homes. 1721 marked a turning point, as inoculation showed that procedures could be carried out that actually worked, 'for the general benefit of mankind'. In Russia the great reforming tsar, Peter the Great, was an advocate and ordered his doctors to begin using inoculation. Spain, on the other hand, was bound by a church every bit as suspicious as New England Puritans, and inoculation didn't catch on there for nearly a century. Despite these attempts to introduce inoculation, smallpox remained a major killer in eighteenth century Europe.

In Britain, Edward Jenner played a key role in early public health, and the eradication of smallpox in particular. Although initially ridiculed by some, who feared that being inoculated with bovine material would make them develop cow's heads from various parts of their anatomies, Jenner's work soon found acceptance from the medical establishment, and he was amply rewarded financially by the government. Safer and more reliable than variolation, vaccination spread to other countries, including Spain. The 1804 expedition to the Americas and China led by Dr Francisco Javier de Balmis (1753–1819) was possibly the first international healthcare undertaking. Balmis set out not to conquer new lands, but to conquer smallpox in Spanish America. Jenner's work marked a turning point in the struggle against disease, a struggle that, as the new century progressed, gave many indications of being successful.

*

While the likes of Jenner and Balmis were trying to rid the world of smallpox, another disease became quite fashionable in polite society. It was known as the White Death because it gave the sufferer a wan appearance that was immortalised in paintings and literature. Such paleness conveyed good breeding, intelligence and sensitivity. It was also called consumption, because it caused weight loss, as if the person were being visibly consumed by the sickness. For some artists and writers, getting it was almost a career move. Lord Byron is said to have remarked 'I should like to die of a consumption, because the ladies would all say "Look at poor Byron! How interesting he looks dying."'[276]

The White Death was, of course, tuberculosis. The poet – and medical student – John Keats wrote of 'the weariness, the fever, and the fret' in 'Ode to a Nightingale'. It was a reference that was at once both autobiographical and prophetic: his mother and brother died of tuberculosis (in 1810 and 1818), and Keats himself died of TB in Rome in 1821, at the age of 25. The disease was a death sentence at that time. When Keats coughed up blood in February 1820 – the first sign that he was ill – he knew immediately what it meant. 'I know the colour of that blood,' he told his friend and roommate Charles Brown. 'It is arterial blood; – I cannot be deceived in that colour; – that drop of blood is my death-warrant; – I must die.'

Tuberculosis is one of the oldest diseases known to humanity. As we saw in Chapter 1, paleopathological remains from the submerged Neolithic village of Atlit Yam off the coast of Israel suggest the disease has been plaguing humans for at least the last 9,000 years. TB has left a long trail across many medical texts from antiquity, too. Babylonian, Assyrian, Chinese, Hindu, Greek, and Roman sources all describe the disease. The earliest description of tuberculosis may be Chinese from as early as 2700 BC, while in the West, the Hippocratic writings refer to it as phthisis, which they believe to have been caused by 'evil air'. Hindu texts from around 1200 BC describe treatment for pulmonary TB, as do Mesopotamian writings from the seventh century BC.[277] And in that time, TB has been known by more names than just the White Death, phthisis and consumption. Depending on what part of the body it attacks, it has also been known as scrofula, *Lupus vulgaris* (the common wolf) and Pott's Disease.

Behind these names is a chronic bacterial infection, caused by the bacillus *Mycobacterium tuberculosis*. It can affect cattle as well as humans (*Mycobacterium bovis*), and it was long thought to be a zoonosis. Now research suggests that either humans gave TB to cattle – a process known as anthroponosis or reverse zoonosis – or that the human strain emerged before the bovine.[278] TB can affect almost any organ of the human body, as well as the central nervous, circulatory and lymphatic systems, and can also attack the bones and joints, the spine (when it is known as Pott's Disease) and the skin (cutaneous TB, one of whose forms is *lupus vulgaris*). Its most common form is pulmonary tuberculosis, when the bacillus attacks the lungs and is spread from person to person through airborne droplets. (Keats is thought to have contracted the disease from nursing his brother Tom, who died just over a year before Keats himself became ill. Such a relatively long incubation period is not uncommon with TB; some can be much longer.) Symptoms include coughing, bloody sputum, night sweats, weight loss and difficulty breathing. In this incarnation, the disease was known as the White Death, consumption and the graveyard cough.

If the bacillus settled in the lymph glands, however, tuberculosis would manifest as glandular swellings around the neck. This form of TB was often the result of drinking milk from infected cows. (Louis Pasteur would change all that, as we will see.) It was simply a case of the bacilli, once inside the body, taking the shortest route to the closest lymph nodes. 'Thus, bacilli ingested in contaminated milk would tend to manifest their presence in the neck and intestinal regions, whereas those inhaled would concentrate in the lungs.'[279]

In this form, tuberculosis was thought to be a separate disease known as scrofula, the King's Evil or the Royal Disease, and had a longstanding association with royalty in England and France. It was not that monarchs of either country were thought to be particularly susceptible to the disease; on the contrary, they were thought to be able to cure it by the laying on of the Royal Hands. This appeared to work, as the swellings would often go down after being touched by the King or Queen, which might account for the longevity of the practice.

The Royal Touch, as it was known, is thought to have begun in France after Louis IX returned from crusade in 1254 (although it may also have had something to do with the French king's saintly reputation: he was canonised in 1297). There is a further link between Louis, disease and crusade: that he went on crusade at all was said to be due to his recovering from a serious illness, an apparently miraculous cure. Disease, royalty and cure were therefore linked in the popular imagination. Henry III of England, keen to keep up with the man idealised as the most Christian of monarchs, began his own practice of 'Royal Touch' in the following decade. This was, significantly, the time of the Second Barons' War (1264–67), in which Henry needed all the signs of royal authority he could get. The Royal Touch was one way of asserting the House of Plantagenet's divine right to rule.

Indeed, England had its own saintly king, Edward the Confessor (1042–66), who was said to have had healing powers, and was proclaimed a saint in 1161. (The only English monarch to be canonised, as Louis was in France.) As Kenneth Kiple noted, 'by taking up Edward the Confessor's healing tradition, the Plantagenets were, in effect, linking themselves with saintliness... The political benefits from such efforts could be enormous.'[280]

Henry's successor, Edward I, continued the practice and is known to have touched thousands of his subjects. Again, with Edward's campaigns in Wales (the office of Prince of Wales as heir apparent to the English throne begins with Edward), involvement in the Scottish Wars of Independence, and expulsion of England's Jews in 1290, the Royal Touch reminded the royal subjects that the King's actions had divine sanction and could not be questioned. Christ had been a miracle worker and healer, so now was the king.

The Royal Touch continued to have political significance. It helped bolster dubious claims to the throne, or weak monarchs. Charles I (1625–49) made a return to touching his subjects after losing the civil war to the parliamentary forces of Oliver Cromwell, and was still performing the Royal Touch as late as October 1648, just three months before his execution.[281] When the monarchy was restored in 1660, Charles II (1660–85) was urged by his physician Richard Wiseman to resume the practice of touching. It proved to be a popular move: the largest number of people touched was in 1684; so many, in fact, that a stampede ensued.

The touch continued in France, too, where the reigning Bourbons were becoming even more unpopular than Charles I and James II (1685–8) of England. The boy king Louis XV touched more than 2,000 people at his coronation in 1722. Louis XVI – the last French monarch before the 1789 Revolution – was perhaps the most avid dispenser of the Royal Touch of all the later Bourbons. (Not that it did him much good in the long run.) Interestingly, in territories where there was no concept of the divine right of kings – such as the German and Italian states – scrofula was hardly ever seen as a disease in its own right.

Queen Anne (1702–14) was the last British monarch to touch, despite being Protestant. Old habits were clearly dying hard. She touched the young Samuel Johnson in 1712, although he wasn't cured. Nonetheless, Johnson kept his 'touch piece', a gold coin minted for the occasion and threaded on a white ribbon that the Queen hung round the necks of all 300 people touched that day. Johnson wore his for the rest of his life.[282]

By the time Keats died from pulmonary tuberculosis, scrofula was a political antique, and would soon become a 'nosological antique' too. August Hirsch still used the term (he was writing in the 1860s),[283] although it was becoming increasingly apparent scrofula was a form of tuberculosis, not a separate disease. A new vocabulary was needed 'because of increasingly strident demands for a new precision from physicians determined to transform medicine from an art to a science.'[284]

*

Medicine's transition from an art to a science had been going on in fits and starts since the time of Paracelsus and Vesalius. The word 'tubercle' was first used in 1689 by the English physician Richard Morton (1637–98), in his treatise *Phthisiologia*. He used it to describe the small nodules of inflamed tissue that were found in the lungs of people who had died of what, in Morton's time, was still being referred to by the Greek word phthisis.

Hippocrates believed phthisis was caused by 'evil airs'. In the sense that pulmonary TB is spread by droplets, coughed, sneezed or otherwise expectorated from person to person – it can even be transmitted when speaking – Hippocrates was quite right. But as cities grew in the nineteenth century as a direct result of the industrial revolution, 'evil airs' began to spread. For the better off, tuberculosis in its pulmonary form was often seen as the result of a sensitive disposition, or heredity. For the less well off, no such niceties could be entertained. Pulmonary TB afflicted 'hardworking people' (to borrow a phrase from our hardworking politicians), and hit them hard.

If Hippocrates had come back in the nineteenth century, he would have been horrified by the 'airs, waters and places' he would have seen. As little towns darkened into big cities, the airs were choked up by smog from Blake's dark satanic mills, the waters fouled by inadequate sewerage and faulty drainage, and places for living and working reduced to little better than Newgate Prison had been at the time of the smallpox experiments, rendered almost uninhabitable by overcrowding, dirt, damp, dust, poor or non-existent ventilation, and cold. But of course, such buildings were far from uninhabited: despite the conditions, the poor did not have the luxury of leaving. Under these conditions, pulmonary tuberculosis became one of the great endemic diseases of the nineteenth century, and the crowded, dirty city became its favoured breeding ground.

Getting away from the city for cleaner air was one of the recommended treatments. In *Nicholas Nickleby*, when Smike contracts tuberculosis, Nicholas is advised 'that the last chance and hope of his life depended on his being instantly removed from London.' Nicholas takes his friend to 'that part of Devonshire in which Nicholas had been himself bred' on the grounds that it was 'the most favourable spot'.[285] Becoming more wracked by the disease each day, Smike has a vision of conditions which were the very opposite of the great urban breeding grounds of tuberculosis:

> He fell into a light slumber, and waking smiled as before; then, spoke of beautiful gardens, which he said stretched out before him, and were filled with figures of men, women, and many children, all with light upon their faces; then, whispered that it was Eden – and so died.[286]

Such beautiful gardens were beyond the reach of most TB sufferers in the nineteenth century; Smike was lucky in that at least he got to spend his final weeks away from London and its fatal filth. For the urban poor who were not blessed with friends like Dickens's hero, there was little they could do.

Various treatments had been tried over the centuries. The Greeks and Romans favoured balancing the humours through diet, drugs, changes in lifestyle, and surgery.[287] A wholesome diet was thought to be beneficial, as nourishment was thought to combat the 'consumption' of the body. Freshness was encouraged in food, especially milk (from any source, animal or human). In her history of tuberculosis, Helen Bynum recorded some of the further dietary treatments, including hyssop and fleawort boiled in sour wine; horehound, pine nuts, parsley and pepper with honey; and inhaling 'the fumes of ivy'. Galen had a potion that was comprised of a pound of mountain squill plant, soaked for a month in vinegar, and then administered each morning 'when patients had to be brought back from the edge of despair.'[288] Fasting was recommended sometimes, but had to be practised cautiously in case it encouraged further consumptive wasting. Unlike in ancient remedies for epilepsy, bathing was encouraged. Myrrh oil with lupines could be applied to the feet, and then replaced with butter. Gentle exercise was also encouraged, provided the patient didn't overdo it. Surgical procedures mainly involved bloodletting, especially if the patient was spitting blood. Humoural theory dictated that spitting blood was due to a build-up of blood, therefore bleeding was the logical remedy.

Further aid could come in the form of a change of air: 'This was no two-week pick me up in the sun, but the sombre search for a dryer, lighter climate with gentle, favourable winds.'[289] It would be beneficial if the journey involved travel by boat. 'Sea voyages were considered intrinsically healing because of the motion of the boat, including nausea (purging) and exposure to sea air, particularly when patients were spitting up blood. If this was beyond the patient's strength (or purse), a sojourn to the nearest coast should be attempted.'[290] Failing that, fresh air must be got into the patient's room. So if the patient couldn't afford a trip to Egypt or Libya, the doctor would have no option but to simply leave the door to their room open.

After the end of classical antiquity, methods did not change very much. The Arabs recycled and adapted Hippocrates and Galen in their own way, as they had with other diseases. Isaac Judaeus (*c.* 840–932) and Avicenna (980–1037) both wrote on tuberculosis, although some of their treatments were specific to their countries and climates.

We are unsure of rates of infection in the Middle Ages. As Helen Bynum noted, a French archaeological dig exhumed 2,498 skeletons from seventeen burial sites dating from the fourth to the eleventh centuries, revealing an inferred rate of infection of 1.2 per cent (29 of 2,498).[291] 'This figure is thought to be low in comparison with modern rates.'[292] Such a low rate of infection indicates both the rural nature of life in the early Middle Ages, tuberculosis's difficulty in spreading in such small communities, where the chain of infection was likely to die out, and also the disastrous effect urbanisation had on human health in the eighteenth and nineteenth centuries, when it is thought that virtually all city dwellers were infected with the TB bacillus.[293] One development in the natural history of disease that may have helped TB in the Middle Ages was its dominance over leprosy, as noted in Chapter 3. A theory emerged in the 1940s proposing that TB gave immunity from leprosy, but new evidence from DNA studies of human bones from the first to sixteenth centuries might offer an alternative explanation. The study showed that leprosy sufferers were often co-infected with tuberculosis as well, and it has been suggested that TB, being faster-acting, killed the sufferers before leprosy was able to.[294]

Regardless of precisely how tuberculosis gained its foothold, it had become widespread by the early nineteenth century, as revealed by advances in medicine. The French doctor René-Théophile-Hyacinthe Laennec (1781–1826), the inventor of the stethoscope, observed the damage wrought by the disease during post mortems. He found tubercles in patients' intestines, livers, spleens, kidneys, glands, on the skin and in the membranes around the brain and spinal cord. It became clear that phthisis, consumption, *lupus vulgaris*, scrofula and Pott's were different manifestations of the same disease. In the 1830s, the word 'tuberculosis' was introduced into medical usage by Johann Lukas Schoenlein (1793–1864), a professor of medicine at Zurich, an acknowledgement that these various tubercle-producing afflictions were all part of the same condition. But the precise nature of the disease still drew no clear consensus from the medical profession. As the composer Frédéric Chopin wrote,

> I have been sick as a dog these last two weeks; I caught cold in spite of 18 degrees of heat, roses, oranges, palms, figs and three most famous doctors of the island [he had gone to Palma in Majorca for health reasons]. One sniffed at what I spat up, the second tapped where I spat it from, the third poked about and listened how I spat

it. One said I had died, the second that I am dying, the third that I shall die.[295]

Typhus

Tuberculosis was just one of a group of diseases that flourished in the squalid conditions of the nineteenth century city. Typhus, for instance, was ever present. The link between squalor and typhus was not lost on the German epidemiologist August Hirsch, who wrote that 'The history of typhus... is the history of human misery.'[296] The disease thrived anywhere dirty or crowded, as its nicknames testify: jail fever, ship's fever, camp fever.

London, like all cities, had suffered repeated typhus epidemics. At the Old Bailey in 1750, the passageway connecting Newgate Prison with the courtroom was so overcrowded with lousy prisoners waiting to be tried it had caused an outbreak. Typhus did the hangman's work for him, killing one third of Newgate's inmates in the outbreak. But it was no respecter of class: two judges, the lord mayor, aldermen and other court officials were also taken. A report blamed the outbreak on overcrowding and filthy conditions caused by the 'horrid neglect of gaolers, and even of the sheriffs and magistrates, whose office it is to compel the gaolers, to the most rigorous repeated orders and attention to their duty'.[297]

These courtroom flare-ups were known as 'Black Assizes' and had been a feature of law and order since the sixteenth century. In 1577 the trial at Oxford of a Catholic bookbinder, Rowland Jenks, had been afflicted. He had been accused of disseminating 'Popish' books, and the ensuing scandal had resulted in far too many people attending the trial to see the bookbinder receive his just desserts. Typhus took advantage of the crowded courtroom, and around 400 people are thought to have died as a result of attending the trial. Jenks got off lightly by comparison: he only had his ears cut off.

One solution to the Black Assizes would have been to install more windows, not only at Newgate and the Old Bailey, but in other court rooms and prisons across the country, and in any building likely to be crowded, such as tenements. However, due to the 1696 window tax, this was beyond the financial reach of many; even the better off were forced in some cases to brick windows up. (The tax remained in place until 1851.)

The German doctor Rudolf Virchow (1821–1902) found similar problems when he visited Upper Silesia in 1848. Virchow studied an epidemic of typhus in the region, and found that peasants were living in squalid conditions, and were infected with body lice but refused to bathe. They subsisted on a meagre diet of potatoes and vodka, which did nothing to strengthen their immune systems.

Port cities could also be particularly susceptible. New diseases could be frequently brought in by ship – crew, passengers, cargo or the ubiquitous ship's rats could all act as vectors. The Black Death might be the most significant occurrence of infestation through ports, but it was certainly not the last. Both Liverpool and New York were hit by a typhus epidemic in 1847. Despite the fact that the Atlantic Ocean separated the two cities, both epidemics had the same cause: immigrants fleeing the great famine in Ireland.

The Irish potato crop in 1845 was infected by the fungus *Phytophthora infestans*. The 1846 crop was wiped out, the 1847 was meagre, and the year following was another wipe-out. As Ireland was heavily dependent on its potato crop for its main source of food, this was catastrophic. The 'famine fevers', typhus and relapsing fever, soon began their work, aided by dysentery, diarrhoea and scurvy. The British government's response was inadequate, probably more by accident than design. The 1846 Fever Act was intended to combat the crisis, but seems to have been ineffectual due to a lack of government spending: there simply weren't enough doctors or other health workers to deal with the situation. Government intervention in Ireland was further weakened by the need to deal with the outbreaks of typhus in Liverpool and elsewhere. In the eyes of those in Westminster, Ireland was always a dirty, troublesome and insignificant backwater; its problems were always 'beyond the pale'. Disaster in England always took priority over those in Cork, Clare, Kilkenny and Galway.

The combination of famine, fevers, and an incompetent public health response was a catastrophe that had an incalculable impact on Irish history. Between 1845 and 1851, the population of Ireland dropped from around 8.5 million to 6.5 million. One million died, and another million emigrated, mainly to the US and Canada. It was 'one of the most dramatic demographic collapses in Western history.'[298] It left a lingering collective memory, both among the remaining population, and the diaspora. Many 'held the British government responsible for the human disaster, perhaps through the inefficiency of its actions to relieve suffering, perhaps (in the minds of angrier Irish memories) through a policy of genocide that deliberately allowed the Irish to starve... [although] few historians would [now] accept the latter version.'[299] Anglo-Irish relations would never recover.

The situation in Ireland in 1846 was beyond anything anybody – in government or out – could imagine. The common perception that typhus was contagious – miasma theory was still alive and well – caused many to flee, leaving their dead unburied and unshriven. Many took to the roads, taking their diseases – and their body lice – with them. Food distribution centres and soup kitchens became rife with disease. If the soup kitchens ran dry, some committed crimes so that they would be jailed, knowing they would get a meal in prison. (They would probably also get typhus.) There seemed to be no escape. Even emigration didn't solve the problem: thousands died in transit to North America; the vessels that bore them became known as 'coffin ships'.

Many also fled across the Irish Sea to England, Wales and Scotland. So many starving and ill Irish immigrants arrived in Liverpool in the spring of 1847 that it caused an immediate crisis. The need for extra hospital beds was so acute that feverish Irish were given beds in temporary hospital wards set up in dockside warehouses known as fever sheds. Four old prison ships were requisitioned and hastily put to use as hospital ships. At all costs, the ailing immigrants had to be kept out of the city's wealthier areas, and contained in the 'fever districts', which were, in all cases, the poorer parts of the city, with the worst housing and sanitation, among them the wards of Vauxhall, Exchange,

Great George, Scotland, Lime Street, Abercromby, St Anne's and St Peter's.[300] Those who didn't end up in fever sheds found cheap lodgings in the cellars of the fever districts, but the filthy conditions only served to exacerbate the conditions that typhus, dysentery and diarrhoea thrived in. (Many wanted to avoid 'capture' by the hospital authorities in case they were sent back to Ireland after treatment.)

There was little the overworked doctors and hospital staff could do: nearly 60,000 people contracted typhus in Liverpool; at one point, 88 per cent of them were Irish.[301] The epidemic became known very quickly as 'Irish Fever'. Liverpool's city fathers did not look too kindly on them, as might be expected. The prejudices of the time dictated that the Irish only had themselves to blame: typhus was seen to be the result of 'over-crowding, drunkenness, and every other kind of vice'.[302]

Once the epidemic had burned itself out by early 1848, the city fathers, rather than tackle the acute problems of the slums, 'paid scant attention to sanitary reform: instead, they sought to rectify Liverpool's "black spot" image through lavish schemes of civic ornament and grandeur, urban "boosterism" befitting the "second metropolis."'[303] The result was, as might be expected, similar troubles when typhus returned, as it did in 1865–6, when it was accompanied by cattle plague (rinderpest) and cholera. The Irish were once again blamed for the epidemic (Irish drovers being apparently responsible for the cattle plague); and the Irish once again suffered the most.

Despite the severity of the 1865–6 epidemic, it didn't equal 'Black '47', as it quickly became known. 1847 saw 30,000 deaths in total across England and Wales. 60,000 contracted typhus in Liverpool alone. In the view of the city's Medical Officer for Health, Dr William Duncan, Liverpool became a 'city of plague', the year being 'calamitous'. Historian Frank Neal has calculated that, in Liverpool, 7475 died of typhus in 1847, 70 per cent of whom – around 5,500 – were Irish immigrants.[304] This figure, he feels, justifies the Registrar General's comment from his third quarterly report for 1847, that Liverpool in that year became 'the hospital and cemetery of Ireland'.[305]

*

Irish immigrants to North America had plenty of experience of poverty and disease well before Black '47 and the famine years. Typhoid was thought to be 'like typhus' since the French doctor Pierre Louis (1787–1872) coined the name in 1829. It was identified as a separate disease by the American doctor William Wood Gerhard (1809–72), who was studying an outbreak affecting mainly Irish immigrants living in Philadelphia in the winter of 1835–36, and even contracted the disease himself. In Britain, William Jenner (1815–98) announced independently of Gerhard in 1850 that typhus and typhoid were distinct diseases; Jenner went one better than Gerhard by managing to contract both diseases in the course of his researches. It still took another ten years or so, and several epidemics, before the theories of Gerhard and Jenner were widely accepted, and the efforts of a third doctor, William Budd (1811–80), before public health policy in Britain was changed.

Typhoid is one of the great diseases of urban filth. Caused by the bacterium *Salmonella typhi*, it thrives in areas with poor sanitation and infects humans via faecal-oral transmission. In layperson's terms, if particles of human shit containing the bacteria get into the drinking water, you are likely to get typhoid. Its symptoms include abdominal pain, intense headache, high fever and a distinctive 'rose rash' on the chest and abdomen. Untreated it can be fatal in 10–20 per cent of cases. Typhoid is thought to have become a problem whenever there was a need in human settlements to dispose of sewage. Prehistoric facilities were of the 'bear in the woods' variety, of course. But as soon as humans invented the cesspit, they were in trouble. Or rather, they were if the cesspool could in any way leak into the drinking water supply. You don't need a huge city for typhoid to become a problem, as was shown by what happened in the early attempts to establish a colony at Jamestown, Virginia. 105 settlers arrived in April 1607 with the intention of starting a new colony in the name of King James I. When fresh supplies and colonists arrived the following year, only 35 of the original settlers were still alive. Over the next two decades, it is thought that 6,500 out of 7,500 colonists died from typhoid.[306] However, at the time Gerhard and Jenner were doing their research, the link with tainted water supplies had not yet been established.

Such was the state of London in the 1850s that diseases of filth were everyone's problem, not just the poor. In 1858, the city suffered the Great Stink, in which – because of low rainfall and hot weather – the Thames became a vast open cesspool. As the physician William Budd remarked, 'the sewage of nearly three millions of people had been brought to seethe and ferment under a burning sun, in one vast open cloaca lying in their midst.'[307]Another commented a 'stench so foul, we may well believe, had never before ascended to pollute this lower air. Never before at least, had a stink risen to the height of an historic event.'[308] People wrote to the *Times* complaining about the stench, and subscribers to the miasma theory of disease were convinced the smell would produce a terrible epidemic. The House of Commons, enjoying a commanding view of the Thames, was brought to a standstill. Curtains soaked in chloride of lime were hung in the windows, but it did little to reduce the overpowering fumes; 'politicians choked and retched'[309] and threatened to leave London. As the Great Stink didn't create the feared pandemic, anti-miasmatists like Budd felt vindicated. But momentum to tackle London's dirt was gathering pace. One of the most notable achievements in this respect was the design by Sir Joseph Bazalgette (1819–1891) of a sewerage system for London, which prevented further 'great stinks' by diverting waste out of the city. This also represented a huge step forward in the city's fight against typhoid and cholera (see below).

Royalty was also regularly inconvenienced by the Thames. Whenever the river rose, the royal cesspits at Windsor Castle disgorged their contents into the castle grounds. Each time this happened, the groundsmen raked the ordure back into the river. By the summer of 1859 Prince Albert was showing signs of illness, suffering from stomach cramps. The prince was plagued by the symptoms over the next two years. He was gravely ill in December 1861, and Royal Physician William Jenner diagnosed typhoid. Albert died on 14 December.

Cholera

At around the time doctors began to talk of 'tuberculosis' and 'typhoid', a new pandemic came out of Asia. Out of all the filth diseases of the nineteenth century, cholera was one of the deadliest and most feared, and also arguably the disease that most threw into relief the problems of the industrialised, urbanised world. Initially dubbed 'Asiatic' cholera, news of its relentless spread westwards in the late 1820s struck terror into European imaginations, a fear that 'probably exceeded that of any epidemic since the fourteenth-century plague'.[310]

Cholera reached England in late October 1831, when shipping from Hamburg brought it to Sunderland.[311] As with ships bringing yellow fever to the US, attempts were made to quarantine incoming vessels. Business owners panicked, fearing that quarantine would lead to a loss of trade, and a complete collapse of the status quo (shipping was the largest employer in Sunderland – almost everyone had a connection with the docks). As Norman Longmate remarked in his history of the epidemic, those with vested interests put their interests first, and denied that anything untoward was going on in Sunderland at all: 'Not for the last time in British history a lead in greed and stupidity was given by a member of the House of Lords. The Marquis of Londonderry, who had a financial interest in the coal trade from the port [Sunderland], wrote to the London *Standard* that the alarm was false.'[312] The Marquis's supporters enlisted 'the support of what were later described as "some insignificant medical practitioners" who were persuaded to announce that the disease they had seen was only an acute form of the familiar bilious disorder called "English cholera". A group of anti-quarantine business men then succeeded in gaining control of the Sunderland Board of Health.'[313] At a public meeting on 12 November, nearly all the doctors in Sunderland rose one after another to deny that there was any cholera in the town. Their efforts, alas, were in vain. News about the denial spread as fast as news about the impending epidemic, 'and made Sunderland a target for laughter or abuse throughout the medical profession.'[314]

There was little laughter when it became clear that cholera had undeniably reached British shores, producing a reaction that was more redolent of the Middle Ages: 'On 6 February 1832 it was announced that Wednesday the 21st March in England, Wales and Ireland and Thursday the 22nd in Scotland was to be a day of fasting and humiliation, when the nation would acknowledge its sins and plead with God to remove the affliction of the pestilence.'[315] The fasting did no good, and within days people were dying. Cholera claimed around 6,000 lives in London over the coming months, and 55,000 in Britain as a whole. The pandemic reached North America in the summer of 1832, arriving with Irish and German immigrants, and also struck Indonesia, the Middle East, the Caribbean and Latin America.

Cholera is an ancient disease, probably originating in the Ganges-Brahmaputra delta in India, where it had been endemic for centuries. Its earliest recorded appearances are in the first millennium BC, when mention is made of the disease in ancient Sanskrit, Chinese and Greek texts. Caused by the free-swimming bacterium *Vibrio cholerae*, its symptoms include painful convulsions, violent vomiting and uncontrollable 'rice water' diarrhoea. (Perhaps unsurprisingly, the name cholera derives from the Greek *khol*, meaning 'bile', and *rhein* meaning 'to flow'.) Like typhoid, it is transmitted by the faecal-oral route, either through contaminated drinking water, or food. It can kill within hours and, in severe outbreaks, the death rate can be around 50 per cent.

The first cholera pandemic originated in Jessore, Bengal (now in Bangladesh) in 1817. Usually, the disease would affect the likes of pilgrims bathing in the Ganges, but in this year a combination of circumstances spread the disease from its usual stamping grounds across Asia as far as southern Russia, the Middle East and around the Horn of Africa. The circumstances in this instance were floods, crop failures and the movements of the British army.

The spread of the British Empire had been afflicted with disease ever since the first colonists established Jamestown in Virginia. Like the Spanish before them, the British found themselves often paying for their imperial ambitions with the lives of their troops, usually losing far more to disease than enemy action. As Britain's ambitions in India grew, so did the number of her troops on the ground, and an increase in traffic between the two countries. But trade routes and armies, as we've seen with the Black Death and the Antonine Plague, also function as arteries for disease. Factor in improved methods of travel, in the shape of steam ships and trains, as happened in the nineteenth century, and for the first time, worldwide pandemics became a reality. This was the world cholera became exposed to in 1817, and it didn't miss the opportunity to move around the Ganges delta with British troops, before hitching a ride out of the Bay of Bengal to the wide world beyond.

From the outset, cholera was linked to imperialism. Hindus thought it was linked to colonial rule, while in Manila people rioted in 1820, 'convinced that cholera came as a result of a plot to poison the city's water' by 'foreign physicians'.[316] In one of their more ironic interventions, the British army helped spread cholera to Oman, but they had gone there with the best of intentions: to abolish slavery.

Tens of thousands died in the first pandemic, but the figures are almost mediaeval in their unreliability. 30,000 deaths were claimed for Bangkok in 1820 alone, while in the Javanese city of Semarang, 1,225 people were said to have died in just one eleven day period in April 1821.[317] The pandemic seems to have petered out in the Russian city of Astrakhan, possibly stopped by the severe winter of 1823–4.

By the time the second pandemic reached Europe, therefore, there was a great deal of concern that cholera, having been a 'storm over Asia', would be equally calamitous in Europe. Carried by traders, soldiers, sailors, pilgrims, refugees and migrants, cholera first struck Moscow, then moved southwest into Bulgaria, and west into Poland courtesy of the Russian army (Poland then being under Russian control). The Baltic ports were affected, followed by Hamburg, Paris, and London. In Paris, cordons were set up around the city as a preventative measure, and troops were ordered to shoot cordon crossers on sight. Despite these and other precautions, the disease still ran rampant in the city. Parisians rioted. Similar measures in Russia – cordons, quarantine, and restrictions on movement – also caused riots.

In Britain, people rioted too, but more out of fear (or outrage) that doctors were killing people with cholera in order to dissect their bodies in the name of medical research. (This was only a few years after the notorious Burke and Hare had been arrested for murdering people and then selling their bodies on for medical dissection in Edinburgh.) There was also the feeling among disenfranchised rioters across Europe that the disease was a government plot to get rid of troublemakers.[318]

In America, the pandemic was immortalised by Edgar Allan Poe, who witnessed cholera doing its work in Baltimore in 1832. His story 'The Masque of the Red Death' tells of a stranger who appears in the midst of revellers at a masqued ball, whose own mask is that of a corpse, bearing the signs of the 'red death'. In Paris, polite society remained defiant by holding balls of its own, where the poet Heinrich Heine recorded events that could have come straight from Poe's story. He records that on 29 March 1832, during the traditional mid-Lent carnival, one of the costumed revellers was suddenly taken ill:

> ... all at once the merriest of the harlequins felt that his legs were becoming much too cold, and took off his mask, when, to the amazement of all, a violent-blue face became visible.
>
> It was at once seen that there was no jest in this; the laughter died away, and at once several carriages conveyed men and women from the ball to the Hôtel-Dieu, the Central Hospital, where they, still arrayed in mask attire, soon died. As in the first shock of terror people believed the cholera was contagious, and as those who were already patients in the hospital raised cruel screams of fear, it is said that these dead were buried so promptly that even their fantastic fools' garments were left on them, so that as they lived they now lie merrily in the grave.[319]

The deployment of armed guards in Paris – who were ordered to shoot cordon-crossers on sight – reflects both the fear of cholera, and also the political uncertainties in the wake of the recent (1830) revolution. The powers that be were taking no chances, especially as the Paris mob was also on the prowl, fearing the epidemic was being spread by undesirables. Heine's descriptions are reminiscent of Boccaccio witnessing the plague:

> It seemed as if the end of the world had come. The crowds assembled chiefly at the corners of the streets, where the red-painted wine-shops are situated, and it was generally there that men who seemed suspicious were searched, and woe to them when any doubtful objects were found on them. The mob threw themselves like wild beasts or lunatics on their victims. Many saved themselves by their presence of mind, others were rescued by the firmness of the Municipal Guard, who in those days patrolled everywhere; some received wounds or were maimed, while six men were unmercifully murdered outright. Nothing is so horrible as the anger of a mob when it rages for blood and strangles its defenceless prey. Then there rolled through the streets a dark flood of human beings, in which, here and there, workmen in their shirt-sleeves seemed like the white caps of a raging sea, and all were howling and roaring – all merciless, heathenish, devilish. I heard in the rue Saint-Denis the well-known old cry, '*À la lanterne!*'[320] and from voices trembling with rage I learned that they were hanging a poisoner. Some said that he was a Carlist,[321] and that a *brevet du lis* had been found in his pocket; others declared he was a priest, and others that he was capable of anything. In the Rue Vaugirard, where two men were killed because certain white powders were found on them, I saw one of the wretches, while he was still in the death-rattle, and at the time old women plucked the wooden shoes from their feet and beat him on the head till he was dead. He was naked and beaten and bruised, so that his blood flowed; they tore from him not only his clothes, but also his hair, and cut off his lips and nose; and one blackguard tied a rope to the feet of the corpse and dragged it through the streets, crying out, '*Voilà le cholera-morbus!*'
>
> ... It appeared the next day by the newspapers that the wretched

> men who had been so cruelly murdered were all quite innocent, that the suspicious powders found on them consisted of camphor or chlorine, or some other kind of remedy against the cholera, and that those who were said to have been poisoned had died naturally of the prevailing epidemic.[322]

Heine was also in no doubt as to what caused the cholera to spread. It was not suspicious-looking people in the street. Rather, it was the

> vast misery prevailing here... the incredible filth, which is by no means limited to the lower classes, to the excitability of the people and their unrestrained frivolity, and to utter want of all preparation and precaution whatsoever, the cholera laid hold here more rapidly and terribly than elsewhere.[323]

Europe's politicians and religious leaders responded in like manner. There was a sense of clamping down, of getting ready for a siege. Whether the pandemic was the work of God or not, it couldn't be allowed to stoke simmering political tensions. An 'us and them' mentality prevailed: the pandemic was interpreted as a menace from Asia, a pestilence that Asians were most susceptible to. That Europeans died of it too was merely an inconvenience that could be overcome through carefully co-ordinated responses from government, and putting a brave face on things. Some commentators came out with semi-Malthusian arguments, pointing out that the cholera was only affecting members of the lowest social classes in Bengal, and 'was particularly prevalent among the abandoned class of women.'[324]

In Britain, the prospect of an impending pandemic not only inspired days of national prayer and penitence, but also political action. The Central Board of Health was established in June 1831 in anticipation of the pandemic reaching Britain. Fear that densely populated slum areas might spread disease led to the formation of a Royal Commission to investigate the need to reform Britain's Poor Laws which, it was hoped, might then lead to the cleaning up of 'fever districts', the lessening of infection, and any possible unrest. The last thing the government wanted were revolting peasants who also had cholera.

In the shape of Edwin Chadwick (1800–90), appointed to assist the Royal Commission, the government got more than it bargained for. Chadwick and his team meticulously studied urban living conditions, and incidence of infectious diseases. (In addition to cholera, there was also a typhus epidemic in London in 1838, while Chadwick was at work.) The result was a document that would have repercussions far outside the sphere of British public health and Poor Law reform. *The Report on the Sanitary Condition of the Labouring Population of Great Britain* (1842) unambiguously demonstrated the link between overcrowding, filth, pollution, lack of adequate sanitation and infectious disease and low life expectancy. The report also pointed out how the loss of the family breadwinner could lead to crime, prostitution and the poor being led astray by 'anarchist fallacies'. Although Chadwick ascribed the spread of disease to miasmas – he believed that 'all smell is disease' – it was perhaps the threat of 'anarchist fallacies' and other unthinkable horrors that galvanised the British government into action. His biographer was to comment that Chadwick 'drew his respectable hearers to the edge of the pit and bade them observe the monsters they were breeding beneath their feet.'[325]

The Public Health Act of 1848 was one of the report's first major achievements. With another cholera epidemic looming, and fear of political unrest increasing – it was the year of revolutions in Europe – the British government passed a piece of legislation that not only began the long, slow process of cleaning up Britain's cities and towns, but would also inspire action abroad. Chadwick's 'disciples' included the Bostonian Lemuel Shattuck (1793–1859), whose *Report on the Sanitary Condition of Massachusetts* (1850) paved the way for American public health (and Shattuck himself was to inspire the later work of John Shaw Billings in the US). In Germany, the Bavarian chemist Max Pettenkofer designed a new sewerage system for Munich.

Ironically, 'Mr Chadwick's Report', as it was known, also had a direct influence on the kind of political agitators that the British establishment feared – the propagators of 'anarchist fallacies'. *The Condition of the Working Classes in England* (1845) by the German political theorist and philosopher Friedrich Engels (1820–95) was based on research Engels conducted in Manchester in 1842. The book described the overcrowded, dirty and squalid conditions of working people, whose houses were mere 'kennels to sleep and die in.' Piles of offal and refuse clogged the streets; ordure oozed from outside privies.

That Engels had been in Manchester at all was itself an irony. His father, an industrialist, had sent him to work in a mill owned by the family firm in the hope that hard graft would cure the young Friedrich of his 'anarchist fallacies'. Unfortunately for Herr Engels, and conservatives everywhere, it had the opposite effect. Three years later, Engels junior co-authored *The Communist Manifesto* with his friend Karl Marx. 1848 was a year of revolutions across Europe: governments tottered and fell, people flocked to the barricades, and streets echoed with the spirit of '*À la lanterne!*' The same year, Rudolf Virchow managed to light the fuse of another, perhaps more significant revolution: the publication of his *Report on the Typhus Epidemics of Upper Silesia* helped lay the foundations of public health in Germany.

It was among the lower classes of Britain that progress was made against cholera. A young Yorkshire doctor, John Snow (1813–58), treated patients during the 1831–2 outbreak, and came to believe that a miasma could not be the cause of the pandemic. He published his theories in 1849 in a pamphlet entitled *On the Mode of Communication of Cholera*, by which time the third, and probably worst, cholera pandemic, had reached Britain.[326] Snow's ideas fell on deaf ears. Around 14,000 people died from cholera in London alone, twice as many as in the 1832 epidemic. After that, cholera mortality decreased, but did not disappear. Then, in 1854, the pandemic renewed its intensity, becoming 'one of the worst cholera years on record'.[327] It was also the year that Snow made his breakthrough.

Snow had been in London since 1836, working for the Westminster Hospital, where he was able to study the incidence of cholera in Soho. The central London district suffered from the usual litany of urban collapse and decay, when, in August 1854, people began dying from cholera in alarming numbers. The families most affected were drawing their water from the pump in Broad Street; those drawing their water elsewhere suffered fewer cases. In the case of monks from the nearby abbey, there were no casualties at all: the monks only drank small beer they brewed themselves. Snow concluded that cholera must be a water-borne disease, and got the authorities to remove the handle of the Broad Street pump. The death rate dropped significantly. The pump was found to have been built just three feet from a cess pit. Further research found that other affected areas were served by the Southwark and Vauxhall Waterworks Company, a utility company that drew water from polluted downriver sections of the Thames. However, cholera cases were far fewer in neighbourhoods served by the Lambeth Water Company, who drew their water upriver at Thames Ditton, which was uncontaminated by London's sewage.[328]

Snow published his findings the following year in a revised version of *On the Mode of Communication of Cholera*. Medical – and political – opinion remained sceptical, and the handle on the Broad Street pump was put back. By then, the third pandemic had largely run its course, and the government no doubt heaved a sigh of relief that it didn't have to offend public sensibilities by explaining faecal-oral transmission. But cholera remained a problem for politicians as much as the residents of Broad Street: by the time Snow presented his findings to the Houses of Parliament in 1855, Britain was in the process of losing nearly 18,000 troops in the Crimean War (1853–6), almost all to cholera. By contrast, only 2,700 were killed in action, with another 1,800 dying of wounds.[329] (All the belligerents in the war were to suffer heavy losses to cholera and other diseases such as dysentery; disease casualties far outnumbered deaths in action.)

Despite the reluctance of politicians in Britain and elsewhere to accept Snow's findings, Snow was not working on cholera alone. 1849 also saw the publication of Thomas Shapter's study of the 1832 outbreak in Exeter, a pioneering piece of work that inspired Snow during the 1854 epidemic. William Budd and others published their findings on microscopic bodies in cholera excreta, contributing to the emerging discipline of microbial etiology. In 1851–2, the First International Sanitary Conference took place in Paris, which focussed on cholera. More conferences were to follow, and international cooperation in the field of public health began in fits and starts (wars and diplomatic spats permitting). In 1854, the cholera bacillus was first observed by the Italian scientist Filippo Pacini (1812–83) although, like Snow, Pacini was faced with peers who believed in the miasma theory of disease, and his work did not achieve recognition straight away.

Meanwhile, cholera was not idle. Two further pandemics followed. The fourth (*c.*1863–79) was the most widespread yet, reaching Europe, Africa and the Americas. It was particularly bad in the Near East, where 30,000 pilgrims died from cholera in Mecca. 90,000 died in Russia.[330] But the pandemic marked another turning point in the battle against the disease: New York City authorities acted on John Snow's findings and supplied clean drinking water and mounted a disinfecting campaign; the result was a significant drop in cholera deaths. The fifth pandemic (1881–96), however, saw major breakthroughs that would change humanity's relationship to cholera forever.

Receiving news that pilgrims returning from Mecca had introduced cholera into Alexandria in 1883 – 5,000 were dying each week – the powers that be in Europe feared another epidemic reaching them. Britain, France and Germany dispatched teams in a competitive attempt to try and find the cause, and cure, of cholera, before it was too late.

However, the British had a vested interest in keeping the Suez Canal open. By 1880, four-fifths of the tonnage passing through the Suez Canal was British. Journey time to India was halved. While this brought economic advantages, it also meant that diseases could travel to Europe in half the time. The British decided to deny cholera was an infectious disease – i.e. deny germ theory – and instead espouse miasma and tainted soil theory. This would protect British financial interests, and also India. And so the British team comprised men who would find evidence in favour of the miasma and tainted soil theory. As medical historian John Waller noted, 'the government panel that appointed the British medical team was careful to avoid including anyone already sympathetic to the germ theory of cholera. The team selected also lacked experts in microscopy, so that in Egypt it carried out totally inadequate microscopical studies of water supplies and made no attempt to isolate specific microbes.' The British team decided that cholera was due to unusual weather patterns reactivating cholera poisons that were dormant in the soil of Egypt. Therefore, it did not come from India, was not a microbial disease and Britain had every right to continue trading with India (or exploiting it, depending on your point of view). The head of the British team, Dr Guyer Hunter, was honoured with a KCMG. It was, as Waller notes, 'a travesty of investigative science'.[331]

The French behaved more honourably. Louis Pasteur helped organise the expedition, although he remained behind in Paris and did not participate in field work. The team was led by key Pasteur collaborator Émile Roux (1853–1933). The French team struggled to find bodies fit to dissect, as the epidemic was on the wane by the time they arrived in Egypt. Things went from bad to worse when one of the team, Louis Thuillier (who also worked on anthrax vaccines), contracted cholera and died. The French went home. The German team, led by the epidemiologist Robert Koch (1843–1910), had the good grace to attend Thuillier's funeral.

The Germans then got on with the business of performing autopsies on the bodies of some of the pilgrims. Koch was convinced germs, not miasmas or tainted soil, caused cholera, and his team's results were encouraging: in the intestines of the victims they found a bacillus, the comma-shaped *Vibrio cholerae*. But Koch didn't have enough evidence to suggest that *V. cholerae* was the cause of cholera. The following year, Koch and his team were in Calcutta when cholera flared up there, and they found the bacillus again, this time in tanks drinking water was drawn from, and also in victim's stools. The discovery of *V. cholerae* seemed to support John Snow's theory that cholera was a water-borne disease. It was also a major advance for germ theory, as the bacillus now appeared to be present wherever there was an outbreak of cholera. The eminent

British medical journal, *The Lancet*, fumed that 'It seems probable that the discovery of the true nature of the virus of cholera will be effected in England's greatest dependency, but not by an Englishman.'[332]

The Lancet's indignation was slightly premature, as Koch's discoveries were still not conclusive proof, but nonetheless, it was a major blow, not only to British pride but also to miasma theory which, even at this late stage, still had adherents. Perhaps the most colourful of them was the Bavarian chemist Max von Pettenkofer (1818–1901), who also believed that contaminated soil played a key role in the spread of cholera. He clashed frequently with Koch over the latter's new-fangled germ theory. Despite this, Pettenkofer felt that contaminated water probably *was* involved in the spread of cholera, and campaigned for clean water supplies. One of his great achievements in this area was building a modern sewerage system for Munich, the state capital of Bavaria. At the height of his dispute with Koch over the cause of cholera, Pettenkofer went to almost lunatic extremes to prove that germs did not cause cholera: he drank a glass of water containing the cholera bacillus. Remarkably, he survived. This is thought to have been because *V. cholerae* can be killed by stomach acids before it gets a chance to take root in the wall of the gut. Pettenkofer must have been extremely acidic.

While such theatrics were going on, a Spanish doctor called Jaime Ferrán (1851–1929) produced a cholera vaccine. He tested it on himself before inoculating 30,000 people. Independently of Ferrán, Russian scientist (and would-be revolutionary) Waldemar Haffkine (1860–1930) developed a vaccine in Paris while working under Pasteur's assistant Émile Roux. In an echo of Pettenkofer publicly drinking cholera laced water, Haffkine got Roux to inject him with cholera to prove that the experimental vaccine worked. This was nothing if not an age of heroic derring-do in medicine. Haffkine survived after a spell of what John Waller described as 'only moderate discomfort.'[333] When an epidemic of cholera broke out in India in 1894, Haffkine knew this was an ideal opportunity to test his vaccine. Lord Dufferin, the former Viceroy of India, enabled Haffkine to begin vaccinating, perhaps hoping to save some British embarrassment after *The Lancet*'s fear that the cure for cholera would be found, but not by an Englishman. Perhaps Dufferin was hoping that, if Haffkine succeeded, a certain amount of face could be saved. As it turned out, Dufferin's hunch was right. Haffkine worked in a suburb of Calcutta, vaccinating 116 out of 200 residents. All of them survived. He then moved on to work in Assam, where 20,000 people were vaccinated. Of those Haffkine had treated, the death rate fell to only two per cent, compared with 22 to 45 per cent for the unvaccinated.

When Robert Koch heard about this, he said 'the demonstration is complete'.[334] The cure for cholera had been found, proving right Koch's 1883 discovery that the comma-shaped bacillus, *Vibrio cholerae*, was indeed the causative agent of cholera.

The Age of Breakthroughs

The last major European outbreak of cholera occurred in Hamburg in 1892, a city whose port had played a prominent role in spreading the disease during the second pandemic. But the sixty years between the two outbreaks had seen a paradigm shift of almost unimaginable proportions when it came to the understanding – and treatment – of disease. What had started with virtually mediaeval responses – the day of penance in Britain and Ireland, the Paris mob lynching anyone thought to be spreading cholera through 'powders' – had ended with modern: the disease had been shown to be caused by the bacillus *V. cholerae,* spread by water.

The medical, political and social effects of cholera were immense. The likes of Chadwick, Shattuck and Virchow had made an indelible mark on public health, whose development would contribute to a significant drop in disease in the developed world as the nineteenth century turned into the twentieth. In identifying the bacillus, the new sciences of epidemiology and bacteriology had played decisive roles, aided by developments in laboratory technology such as better microscopes, the introduction of solid substances in culture media and the use of industrial dyes to better identify microbes.

Robert Koch also played a pivotal role in science's thinking about disease. Convinced that diseases were caused by germs, he formulated a set of rules that became known as Koch's Postulates:

1. The bacterium must be present in every case of the disease.
2. The bacterium must be capable of being isolated and grown in pure culture.
3. The specific disease must occur when the culture-grown bacillus is injected or inoculated into a host.
4. The bacterium must then be recoverable from the experimentally infected hosts.

These strictures, as John Waller noted, 'soon acquired an authority on a par with the rules Moses brought down from Mount Sinai'.[335] The increased rigour demanded by Koch's postulates meant that, while it might take time for the causative agent of a disease to become proven, such as in the case of cholera, when that agent was found, it was definitive; there could be no going back to miasmas and tainted soil. Humoural theory had at last been laid to rest. It had had a good run, dominating medical thinking since Galen's time. What replaced it was germ theory.

In addition to Koch, the other great name of the period was the Frenchman Louis Pasteur (1822–95). The two men could be regarded as among the principal architects of germ theory, although they did not invent it. As early as the sixteenth century, Girolamo Fracastoro had proposed that diseases were caused by 'seeds', and the invention of the microscope in the following century suggested that the great Italian doctor was correct. Englishman Robert Hooke (1635–1703) and Dutchman Antonie van Leeuwenhoek (1632–1723) reported seeing microbes beneath their instruments, and thus virtually invented the science of microbiology. Nicolas Andry (1658–1742) and Richard Bradley (1688–1732) both believed that the small organisms seen under Hooke's and Leeuwenhoek's microscopes caused disease, although they had no way of proving it.

Silkworms, dead bodies, childbirth and a cattle disease all played an unlikely role in the development of germ theory in the following century. The Italian entomologist Agostino Bassi (1773–1856) discovered that muscardine, a disease that affects silkworms, was caused by a fungus (eventually dubbed *Beauveria bassiana* in Bassi's honour). This was the first time a microbial organism had been shown to cause a disease. And if silkworms could be so affected, Bassi reasoned, why not humans?

In 1843, the American physician and author Oliver Wendell Holmes (1809–94) wrote an article important in the history of germ theory, in which he noted the case of a physician who had examined the body of a man who had died of gangrene of the leg, and then attended a woman giving birth. She, and six other women he had treated, all developed puerperal fever. Also known as childbed fever, it had been known to Hippocrates, and by the early nineteenth century was a frequent cause of mothers dying in childbirth, claiming 5 to 20 per cent of maternity fatalities. In some small hospitals, it was not unknown for epidemics of puerperal fever to break out, killing between 70 to 100 per cent of expectant mothers.[336] Holmes believed that puerperal fever was contagious, and in the case he'd studied, it had somehow been transmitted from the dead man to the mother. Holmes argued that the chance of a woman contracting puerperal fever could be greatly reduced if doctors washed their hands thoroughly before conducting an examination. This simple solution was greeted with outrage in some quarters: Charles Meigs, an obstetrician practising in Philadelphia, countered with a typical response, exclaiming that 'Doctors are gentlemen, and gentlemen's hands are clean!'[337]

Similarly outraged gentlemen greeted the work of the Hungarian Ignaz Semmelweis (1818–65), a doctor at the Vienna maternity clinic. Puzzled by the ten per cent death rate from puerperal fever in the student wards, compared to three and a half per cent in the midwives' ward, Semmelweis was convinced that the disease was transmitted by staff who had carried out autopsies and dissections just prior to working on the maternity wards. He advised hand-washing in a chlorine solution to sterilise the hands, whereupon the death rate fell to less than two per cent in his ward. His colleagues were outraged that Semmelweis was implying their professional practices were below par, and the ensuing row caused Semmelweis to resign and move to a hospital in Budapest. There, he wrote a book in 1861 that linked childbed fever with the autopsy room, and argued that midwives who had not worked in autopsy or dissection rooms had a much lower incidence of puerperal fever and deaths than those who had. Another furore ensued, and this time Semmelweis had a breakdown, being admitted to a mental hospital in 1865 where he contracted the skin disease erysipelas – ironically an infection caused by the same pathogens as puerperal fever – and died.[338] However, Semmelweis was vindicated in 1879 by Pasteur, who, while researching sepsis in surgery (among other things), identified the bacteria (streptococci) responsible for puerperal fever, erysipelas and scarlet fever. During the 1880s and 90s, English surgeon Joseph Lister (1827–1912) would do much to improve surgical safety by sterilising equipment before use.

Around this time, anthrax entered the story of germ theory. Anthrax has a long history. It has been speculated that the fifth and sixth Plagues of Egypt in the Book of Exodus could have been anthrax (see Chapter 2), while Virgil graphically records a virulent animal plague in *The Georgics* (III) that humans were also susceptible to. Anthrax is a disease that affects primarily cattle, sheep and goats. Humans can become infected through contact with animals or animal products, although they can't spread it from one person to another. There are three forms of human anthrax, and they are all at the ghastly end of the scale. The gastrointestinal form is caused by eating contaminated meat, when it attacks the intestines, causing severe diarrhoea and vomiting; the cutaneous form is contracted through cuts or lesions in the skin, and can cause malignant pustules and vivid rashes; or the disease can take hold via the airways, when it settles in the lungs, and causes pneumonia-like symptoms and collapse of the lungs. This pulmonary form is the most lethal, with mortality rates around 80 per cent. Even the mildest form of anthrax, the cutaneous, claims around 20 per cent of those infected. The gastrointestinal form is somewhere between the two. Its effects on animal victims are equally severe.

The causative agent, *Bacillus anthracis*, was discovered by the French physician Casimir-Joseph Davaine in 1863, although Davaine could not prove at the time that the rod-shaped bacillus was definitely the cause of the disease. Davaine also couldn't provide a solution for one of the key mysteries of anthrax – the puzzle of how a herd of cattle or flock of sheep could be healthy one day, but dead the next. Robert Koch agreed with Davaine that the rod-shaped bacillus was the cause of anthrax, and set about proving it.

In the early 1870s, Koch was living in the small Polish town of Wolsztyn (then part of Germany), which was at the time plagued with anthrax. Koch decided that if the elongated corpuscles Davaine had seen were indeed the cause of anthrax, then they must be able to survive outside of an animal's body for long periods of time. Experimenting by injecting infected blood into ox eyes, Koch surmised that the spores produced by the bacillus lie in grass and soil until ingested by an animal. Once in the animal's system, the bacillus is able to feed, grow and replicate itself, killing the animal in the process. Koch injected some of the spores into mice, which quickly developed anthrax and died. He then injected other mice with a different spore-producing microbe, and the second batch of mice remained healthy. Koch was convinced that the elongated bacillus caused anthrax. Now he had to prove germ theory to everyone else.

Koch demonstrated his findings to leading bacteriologist Ferdinand Cohn at the University of Breslau. Cohn was convinced, and word soon spread. Koch published his findings, but still had critics, who pointed out that he had not been able to isolate the anthrax bacillus from the blood. A chance, however slender, remained that the disease was caused by a mysterious *something else* in the blood. In 1876, Louis Pasteur managed to grow *Bacillus anthracis* in a culture of urine, which was then injected into guinea pigs. No blood was used in this experiment; the animals developed anthrax and died. (The use of guinea pigs in these and other pioneering experiments is the origin of the term 'guinea pig' to mean any experimental subject.)

Now all that was needed to prove that a germ caused anthrax was a vaccine, and that is what Pasteur was able to demonstrate in 1881. In May, 25 sheep were given two shots of Pasteur's vaccine, 25 were not. On 31 May, all 50 animals in the experiment were injected with a virulent strain of anthrax. On 2 June, it was found that all 25 of the control group were dead or dying, while all but one of the vaccinated group were healthy. (The vaccine used on the day had been developed by one of Pasteur's team, Charles Chamberland. Pasteur took all the glory, and made further refinements to his colleague's vaccine. The vaccine had really been a team effort, but Pasteur, ever the showman, is the one who is remembered.) As Bassi had wondered about infection, so too did Pasteur (who kept a portrait of the Italian in his office). If germs caused anthrax, then surely the same must hold true for other diseases? Perhaps all?

Less than a year later, on 24 March 1882 in Berlin, Koch delivered his paper 'On the Aetiology of Tuberculosis', in which he demonstrated that he had isolated the tuberculosis bacillus. Koch's audience were stunned. The immunologist Paul Ehrlich recorded that 'All those present were deeply moved and that evening has remained my greatest experience in science.'[339] Koch explained how he had followed the lead of the French doctor Jean-Antoine Villemin who, in 1865, had been almost alone in claiming that tuberculosis was contagious, capable of being passed from humans to rabbits. Probably due to the fact that TB is only mildly contagious, many scientists were unable to replicate Villemin's results. Worse, there was no sign of the TB germ.

As John Waller notes, one of the problems in proving that a microbe was the cause of tuberculosis was that it was very difficult to make the TB bacillus stand out in a culture. Koch began using industrial dyes, first methyline blue and then 'washing' it with another dye called vesuvin, which isolated the 'elongated, wiry but incredibly small germ' that 'seemed to be present in all cases of TB'.[340] Another problem had been the slow rate at which the TB bacteria replicate themselves. Although most bacteria can replicate within 24 hours, thus providing the scientist with a 'healthy' culture overnight, Koch had to wait two weeks for the TB bacillus to produce a colony. (The disease can also have a very long incubation period, making it impossible to tell when a person will actually start to become sick.) Once he had his colony, Koch injected the bacillus into healthy guinea pigs, which developed tuberculosis.

Koch's discovery was a major step forward for advocates of germ theory, and the new discipline of bacteriology. As John Waller notes, 'Everywhere, from the hospital ward to the parlour room and the public house, the danger of the invisible germ began to capture the public's attention.'[341] Germs quickly became the nineteenth century equivalent of mediaeval demons, who were thought to lurk everywhere. But unlike demons, germs could be seen under the microscope.

Pasteur, Koch and their respective teams, together with other scientists around the world, spent the last two decades of the nineteenth century on a crusade. Both men set up research facilities that continue to exist today, the Pasteur Institute in Paris and the Robert Koch Institute in Berlin. Germs were conclusively proven to be the cause of disease in case after case: in addition to cholera and tuberculosis, rabies, puerperal fever, undulant fever, diphtheria, leprosy and tetanus – among others – were shown to be caused by microbes. Vaccines were developed for many. Epilepsy was revealed to be a neurological disease, even if its mysteries still went unfathomed. The historian and explorer William Winwood Reade rhapsodised that 'Disease will be extirpated; the causes of decay will be removed; immortality will be invented.'[342] Although such hubris now seems woefully premature, we can't hold Reade's optimism against him. This was, after all, an age giddy with invention; Victorians and Edwardians thought that they would invent everything, cure everything, conquer all.

The Third Plague Pandemic

Both Koch and Pasteur can claim indirect credit for the victory over one of the most feared diseases in history – plague. The Third Pandemic of plague began in the Yunnan province of China in 1855 and would have probably remained contained there were it not for a rebellion by the Hui

– indigenous Chinese who practised Islam – and other Muslim ethnic groups. This uprising, known as the Dungan Revolt, began in 1862 and lasted for fifteen years. The waves of refugees that the conflict generated took the plague with them, often heading towards more densely populated regions of China and resulting in the pandemic reaching ports such as Shanghai and Canton, where there was a catastrophic outbreak in 1894, which killed 60,000 people in a matter of weeks.

It was while the plague was raging in Hong Kong in the summer of 1894, killing an estimated 100,000 people – 75 per cent of the population – in just two months, that a young Franco-Swiss bacteriologist named Alexandre Yersin (1863–1943), who had studied under Pasteur in Paris, began to examine plague victims in search of the cause of the disease. He had little money or equipment, and worked in a hut he built himself in the grounds of the city's Alice Memorial Hospital. Made to feel unwelcome by the British head of the hospital, Yersin was virtually *persona non grata* and had to acquire cadavers through bribery.

In contrast, a Japanese team that arrived days before Yersin had been extended every courtesy, being given a room in the hospital in which to work, and all the equipment they needed. The Japanese effort was led by Aoyama Tanemichi (1859–1917) and Shibasaburo Kitasato (1853–1931), a former student of Koch's in Berlin, who had also worked on antitoxins for tetanus, diphtheria and anthrax. Within a fortnight of arrival, Tanemichi and two other members of the team had contracted plague (one fatally). Undeterred by the loss of half his team to the disease they were studying, Kitasato continued working, and on 14 June, he announced that he had found the bacillus that caused plague. Within days, Yersin emerged from his hut to announce the same news. It was yet another controversy. Kitasato had made the discovery first, but Yersin's was the better science. The plague bacillus, *Pasteurella pestis*, was eventually renamed *Yersinia pestis* in his honour. Yersin noted that Hong Kong seemed to have more than its fair share of dead rats, and four years later the French bacteriologist Paul-Louis Simond (1858–1947), another Pasteur Institute alumnus, discovered that plague was a rodent disease, and that their fleas, *X. cheopis*, were the main plague vector.

The next major triumph over plague took place in Bombay, where the pandemic claimed 19,000 lives in the space of the six months from August 1896 to February 1897. In the midst of this runaway death toll, Waldemar Haffkine – like Yersin and Simond, a student of Pasteur – was called in to offer what assistance he could in containing the disease. Working in the unlikely setting of a makeshift laboratory set up in a corridor in the city's Grant Medical College, Haffkine spent three months of round-the-clock work trying to find a vaccine against plague. It was a strenuous and difficult task; two of his assistants walked out on him, while a third had a nervous breakdown. On 10 January 1897, Haffkine felt that the vaccine was ready and tested it on himself. He then asked for volunteers from a local jail: all those who had been inoculated survived, while the control group, who had not had the vaccine, lost seven members to the plague.

Despite these scientific breakthroughs, the Third Pandemic proved impossible to stop. As with the Black Death, the disease spread along trade routes. International shipping unwittingly helped to spread the disease more rapidly around the globe, and it struck with particular virulence in India, Australasia, North Africa, South Africa and South America. Hawaii suffered a severe outbreak in late 1899, and the Board of Health decided on the drastic action of burning down Honolulu's Chinatown in a last-ditch effort to stop the disease spreading further. San Francisco was affected in 1900–1904, and again in 1907–1909, the second outbreak being exacerbated by insanitary conditions following the earthquake of 1906. Probably travelling over land, the pandemic also reached Russia, which experienced the last major European outbreak of plague during the last two decades of the nineteenth century. It continued to add to the sufferings of the Russian people, however, well into the 1920s, by which time the country had experienced revolution and was wracked by civil war.

Western Europe looked on aghast as the pandemic seemed to get ever nearer, and medical authorities met in Vienna in 1897 to draw up contingency plans in case the disease travelled any further west. It did, coming in with the ships, but remained contained in ports such as Glasgow, Liverpool, Cardiff and Hamburg where there were only a handful of deaths, mainly among port workers. Sporadic outbreaks continued worldwide for years. The last significant outbreak occurred in Peru and Argentina in 1945. The World Health Organization did not declare the Third Pandemic officially over until 1959, although some researchers believe it has yet to run its course completely.

The White Man's Burden

Disease could still surprise. In January 1875, the Fiji islands were subjected to an epidemic of measles. In Europe, this was a usually harmless childhood disease. But in six months in the Fiji islands, around one quarter of the islands' population of 135,000 died. The same disaster had happened in Hawaii in 1853, just as the Maori in New Zealand were succumbing to measles, smallpox, whooping cough and flu. Between 1840 and 1860, Maori numbers fell from over 100,000 to 40,000.'[343] The Australian Aborigines likewise fell victim to smallpox, cholera, typhus and flu, followed by tuberculosis and leprosy, ending their forty thousand year isolation from the world's diseases.

As Europe's imperial ambitions and desire to trade spread, so did Europe's diseases. Medical historian Mark Harrison has argued persuasively that commerce has played a greater role than war in spreading disease, drawing especial attention to 'The nineteenth century [which] was a period of rapid change and saw an unprecedented redistribution of infections.'[344]

Despite the advances in public health in the 'civilised' world, it was capitalism and imperialism that kept Reade's disease-free utopia strictly in the realm of wishful thinking. As soon as a public health act was passed at home, a new disease would appear from abroad, brought back by troops or trade. A constant flow of pathogens from the tropics was one of the prices European powers paid for dominating other countries. Disease was an unavoidable part of the 'White Man's Burden'.

Indeed, Kipling's 1899 poem from which the phrase is taken saw part of the 'burden' of colonialism being the White Man's duty to bring civilisation to the whole world, which would necessitate 'Fill[ing] full the mouth of Famine/And bid[ding] the sickness cease.' But if so, Kipling's poem was both misguided and ironic. European intervention, far from filling famine's mouth, frequently created or exploited it, and far from 'bidding the sickness cease', all too often caused more. 'The ecological transformation [wrought by imperialism] triggered massive epidemics, in particular sleeping sickness, while the planting of coffee, cocoa, rubber and other cash-crop monocultures led to decline in the nutritional status and general well-being of natives in Africa, Asia, America and the Pacific.'[345]

The colonial powers were well aware of the role disease played in their empire-building. While it claimed the lives of the colonised, it also claimed colonisers (to a lesser extent), and the conquering of disease became another part of the White Man's Burden, inseparable from the stockpiling of European coffers at the expense of the peoples they were colonising. The White Man's Grave was the obverse side of the Burden, a nickname for tropical areas like West Africa where Europeans fell in their droves to disease. As the old slavers' proverb had it:

> Beware and take care
> of the Bight of Benin.
> Of the one that comes out
> there are forty go in.

As Roy Porter notes, 'For Cecil Rhodes, empire meant civilization, and tropical medicine was high among its crowning glories. Joseph Chamberlain (1836–1914), who became Britain's colonial secretary in 1895, viewed disease control as integral to imperialism. Hubert Lyautey (1854–1934), one of the architects of the French colonial medical service, declared "La seule excuse de la colonisation, c'est la medicine".'[346]

*

Despite the embarrassment felt by *The Lancet* that the cause of cholera had not been discovered by an Englishman, the story of British India does include at least one medical triumph. The Scottish doctor Patrick Manson (1844–1922), the so-called 'father of tropical medicine', had a theory that malaria was transmitted by mosquitoes. The theory seems to have been related to Manson's discovery that filariasis (which can produce the unsightly swellings of elephantiasis) was also transmitted by mosquitoes. It was an idea that had further support from the French surgeon Alphonse Laveran (1845–1922), who had discovered the *plasmodium* parasite in human blood in 1880. Laveran believed *plasmodium* causes malaria, and that it was also transmitted by mosquitoes, but almost no one (including the great Robert Koch) believed him.

Manson needed someone to go to India and cut up mosquitoes on his behalf; he couldn't go himself because he suffered from gout. When he read a paper by the British army medic Ronald Ross (1857–1932), who was already in India, Manson knew he had found the right man for the job.

Ross had gone to India in 1895. He wasn't particularly interested in science, malaria or even India, but went to please his father, and to use his copious spare time to write. Ross had already published a novel (in 1889), and wanted to further his literary ambitions. He therefore 'spent his days in pleasant distraction, playing sports and writing poetry, while all the bloody revolts and epidemics of the Raj swirled around him.'[347] But then he became interested in microscopy, becoming something of an enthusiastic amateur. As malaria historian Sonia Shah notes, 'he didn't know half of what he was looking at.'[348] But he had a very keen eye for detail, and that is what Manson needed if he was to prove his theory.

Manson and Ross did not have the support of the British government, despite appealing that someone from 'continental nations, whose stake in tropical countries is infinitely smaller than ours'[349] might make the discovery before them. An Italian team led by the pathologist Amico Bignami was certainly close to pipping Manson and Ross at the post. Although malaria still flared up in Britain occasionally – the last case occurring in the Romney marshes in 1911[350] – Manson was correct in stating that the main problem the disease posed to Britain was in her territories abroad. Unlike the British, Italy's main problem with malaria was at home.

The Pontine Marshes outside Rome had been a malarial black spot since time immemorial, and the disease was still claiming victims all over the country, including high profile figures such as Anita Garibaldi, the wife of the great Italian patriot, and Cavour, the first prime minister of the united kingdom of Italy. The country was losing vast amounts of money due to malarial sickness in both her workforce and army. Something had to be done to ensure the Risorgimento didn't end in the whimper of the sick ward.

Bignami and his team noted that the Indians did not go out at night, and slept under mosquito nets. Convinced the locals knew more about malaria than they did, Bignami questioned them, asked them to participate in experiments, and generally treated them with a certain degree of respect. In contrast, Ross was the typical white man with a burden, treating Indians as might be expected. A number of them ran away after Ross had paid them to be experimental subjects, causing the poet and would-be scientist's progress to slow to a near halt.

It was therefore something of an accident when, in July 1897, Ross discovered the cause of malaria. On a field trip near the town of Ooty, he found some *anopheles* mosquitoes in a forest. Trapping them, he dissected them and found the *P. falciparum* parasite in their guts. In 1898, while researching avian malaria, Ross discovered the parasite in the saliva glands of the mosquito, and he conjectured – rightly – that the act of biting conveyed the disease into the victim.

Bignami and his colleague, Giovanni Battista Grassi, had already arrived at this conclusion. Indeed, Grassi had formulated a simple equation that became known as Grassi's Law: man + *anopheles* mosquito = malaria. But it was Ross who was awarded the 1902 Nobel Prize for medicine for his efforts. Some feel it should have been shared with the Italians. But given the rivalries that dominated the period, such disputes were not uncommon.

The story of British India and malaria didn't end with Ross's

Nobel Prize. As Sonia Shah notes, 'in British-ruled India, the British knowingly worsened malaria' by building dams, 'creating thousands of miles of irrigation canals. The irrigated farmlands were better for wheat, sugarcane, cotton, indigo, and opium – export crops the British authorities could tax – than for the locals' traditional sustenance crops.'[351] Worse, the canals disrupted natural drainage, creating conditions ripe for the *anopheles* mosquitoes to breed. British authorities refused to do anything about the numbers of Indians dying of malaria, even when surveys had highlighted the danger posed to locals by British irrigation. During the last decades of the nineteenth century, hundreds of thousands of Indians died as a result.[352]

Colonial powers sometimes did manage to have a more forward-thinking approach to malaria. When the French began building the Panama Canal in 1881, they were hoping to repeat the success they had enjoyed with the Suez Canal, which had opened in 1869. Both vast projects were seen as aiding international trade, rather than conquest. (Although the two are bedfellows: apparently the first person to suggest connecting the two oceans by means of a 'strait' was a Castilian engineer in the party of the Spanish conquistador Vasco Núñez de Balboa, in 1513.[353]) But the Panama project was beset by malaria almost from the start. With the addition of engineering problems, planning mistakes and bad weather, the company behind the canal went bankrupt in 1889. By that time, some 22,000 workmen had died of disease, principally malaria and yellow fever. Eventually, the United States took over the project in 1904, and President Theodore Roosevelt made certain the US would not repeat the mistakes of the French planners, including not racking up the same huge numbers of disease fatalities.

Colonel William Gorgas, who had pioneered anti-yellow fever efforts in Havana, was appointed chief sanitation officer. He set about implementing similar measures on the canal: anti-mosquito fumigation, draining and filling in stagnant water, swamps and wetlands, and establishing quarantine areas. The anti-malarial drug quinine was also given to workers. Derived from the bark of cinchona trees, quinine was given to Jesuit missionaries in Peru in the seventeenth century by the indigenous Quechua people. It was first used in Europe to treat malaria in 1631. Gorgas's work in Panama enabled the Americans to complete the canal in a decade. By the time it opened in 1914, Yellow Fever in the canal zone was extinct, and malaria under control. The number of the workforce suffering from the disease fell from 82 per cent in 1906 to just eight per cent in 1913,[354] while the death rate dropped from 11.59 per 1,000 in 1906 to 1.23 per 1,000 in 1909.[355] Although workers had died of disease during the US-led part of the project, the death rate had only been a fraction of what the French had experienced in the 1880s. It is thought that Gorgas's campaign saved somewhere in the region of 14,000 lives.[356]

*

If tropical disease didn't directly affect colonial powers, it could still wreak appalling havoc indirectly. As Mike Davis notes, 'Few regions have ever endured such a literally biblical declension of disaster – still known as the *Yakefu Qan* or "Cruel Days" – as did the Horn of Africa beginning in 1888.'[357] A four-year drought began in Ethiopia, accompanied by an epidemic of rinderpest. Rinderpest, unlike anthrax, isn't zoonotic, so humans were not directly affected. But 90 per cent of the cattle died. As wealth was based on head of cattle, with most of that source now dead, the tribal system was greatly weakened and began to disintegrate. The emperor, Menelik II, was said to have lost a quarter of a million head. Social and political structures at a local level were ruined.

With no cattle to trade with, people weren't able to eat. Attempts to import food failed, largely because the country was ravaged by civil wars, and a war with Italy was looming. Prices increased a hundredfold. Villages were abandoned, families torn apart or lost to migration. And with no cattle or oxen, the bush went ungrazed, the fields unploughed. Locusts, caterpillars and rats overran the once verdant fields, aiding the drought in turning them into wastelands. People were left to scavenge, or turned to cannibalism, when they weren't themselves under attack from starving wild animals.

Menelik ordered his people to pray. 'When the animal epidemic was starting, I made a proclamation, saying "Pray to God." The animals are ... all dead ... all this has happened because we have not prayed enough. Now the epidemic is turning to people and has begun to destroy them.'[358] The epidemic and famine permanently altered Ethiopia's tribal power system. Menelik's biographer, Harold Marcus, wrote that 'millions of people died'.[359]

The origins of the rinderpest epidemic were traced to infected cattle imported from India, the beasts being used to provision an Italian army that invaded neighbouring Eritrea in 1889. '"Many Ethiopians," writes Richard Pankhurst, who interviewed survivors of this period in the 1960s, "knowing of Italian ambitions in the country, believed that the disease had in fact been spread deliberately."'[360]

With the country reduced to the condition of a cemetery (as one contemporary account put it), the Italians used the famine as a pretext to invade the country. This suited the British, who reasoned that a strengthened Italian presence in East Africa would keep the French at bay. Menelik protested that Ethiopia needed no one's help except God's. The emperor had few soldiers, and no food to provision them with. But he did have arms supplied by the French. At Adwa on 1 March 1896, Ethiopian forces managed to annihilate the Italians. But it was a temporary lull. The Italians invaded again in 1935, defeating Emperor Haile Selassie's forces. A victorious Mussolini declared that Adwa had been avenged.

*

The high-water mark of European imperialism, the so-called Scramble for Africa, which began in the 1870s, had a lasting effect on the continent. The use of drugs like quinine, Roy Porter points out, was to colonials' advantage. The drug 'gave colonists fresh opportunities to swarm into the Gold Coast, Nigeria and other parts of West Africa and seize fertile agricultural lands, introduce new livestock and crops, build roads and railways, drive natives into mines, and introduce all the disruptions to traditional lifestyles that cash economies brought.'[361] As Mike Davis notes,

> 'Indeed, the century's end became a radical point of division in the experience of humanity. For Europeans and their North American cousins, as David Landes has written, "the wheel turned" in 1896 and the depression that had started with the Panic of 1893 was replaced by a new boom. "As business improved, confidence returned – not the spotty, evanescent confidence of the brief booms that had punctuated the gloom of the preceding decades, but a general euphoria such as had not prevailed since … the early 1870s. Everything seemed right again – in spite of rattlings of arms and monitory Marxist references to the 'last stage' of capitalism. In all of western Europe, these years [1896–1914] live on in memory as the good old days – the Edwardian era, *la belle epoque*."'[362]

Davis argues that such economic exploitation by the European imperial powers, combined with natural disasters like famine and the diseases that followed in their wake, and combined with the diseases created by western interference in local ecospheres (such as the link between British irrigation that exacerbated malaria in India) created what became known as the Third World. 'If Kipling's verse exalted colonizing optimism and scientific racism,' Davis suggests, 'Conrad's troubling stories warned that Europe itself was being barbarized by its complicity in secret tropical holocausts. *La belle epoque*, in his view, was dangerously downriver of the Apocalypse.'[363]

6

The Twentieth Century

In September 1914, with the First World War barely six weeks old, Lord Kitchener announced that no man joining the British army could fight at the front unless he had been vaccinated against typhoid. Although the vaccine had been discovered in 1896 by the British immunologist Almroth Wright (1861–1947), it was still a controversial practice, far from universal. But such was the enthusiasm for war that most new recruits willingly received the jab, and by 1916, almost all British forces were vaccinated. It was one of the most successful, if unlikely, vaccination campaigns in history. But Kitchener had seen what typhoid could do to an army, and wasn't taking chances. For the first time in a conflict, an army lost more men to enemy action than disease. There were only 7,000 cases of typhoid among British troops, compared with 125,000 among the French and 112,400 among the Germans. Given the scale of troop mortality in the Great War, such figures might represent small consolation, but as John Waller notes, 'in a war of attrition, in which marginal advantage was everything, Wright's vaccine might well have been the difference between victory and defeat.'[364]

Almroth Wright was something of a celebrity by 1914, and had been immortalised as Sir Colenso Ridgeon in Bernard Shaw's play *The Doctor's Dilemma*. Wright was an admirer of Waldemar Haffkine's work, although the two men probably couldn't have been further apart politically: Wright was also a vehement anti-Suffragette. The first test of Wright's vaccine had been in Maidstone in the autumn of 1897, when a contaminated water supply led to the largest ever typhoid outbreak in the UK, with 1,847 people becoming infected, 132 of whom died. (As a precaution, the water supply was also sterilised with chloride of lime, a first for British public health.) When an appeal was launched to help 'stricken Maidstone', even Queen Victoria sent funds to help.[365] Among the nurses sent to Maidstone to help with the epidemic was Edith Cavell, later to become a national hero in the Great War. The disease then broke out at nearby Barming Heath mental asylum. 84 of the 200 staff asked for the vaccination. All of them survived. Four of their unvaccinated colleagues didn't. Wright then went to India in 1898 as a member of the India Plague Commission to further test the vaccine, vaccinating any member of the British army who was willing to receive it. Many army doctors were convinced that the vaccine was effective.

Wright's vaccine had its first major test during the Boer War (1899–1902). At the Siege of Ladysmith (November 1899–February 1900), around 17 per cent of British troops had been vaccinated. Out of this number, the mortality rate was 1: 213, whereas in the other soldiers, it was 1: 32. 22,000 British soldiers died in the Boer war – 65 per cent of them died from disease. Even if the Boer War had damaged Britain's reputation – among other things, the war was notable for the widespread use of concentration camps by the British – most doctors were now convinced of the germ theory of typhoid, and of the need for vaccination.

Long before hostilities on the Western Front and the Cape, armies had frequently been victims of disease as much as enemy action, from the Achaean army in *The Iliad*, afflicted with plagues by the god Apollo, to the Roman army that brought the Antonine Plague back with them from Persia in 165 AD. 'Camp fever' became the nickname for any troop-related sickness. Typhus, transmitted by the human body louse, accompanied armies as faithfully as whores in the camp. When the Spanish besieged Granada in 1489 – one of the earliest known typhus epidemics – the Spanish lost 3,000 men to enemy action, but 17,000 to typhus. During the English Civil War (1642–51) and the Thirty Years War (1618–48), typhus was rampant, and Napoleon's 1812 march on

Moscow had been defeated by the disease. Typhoid had afflicted both sides in the American Civil War, with tens of thousands of fatalities. In the first Sino-Japanese War (1894–5), nearly 12,000 Japanese troops died of typhoid, while in the Spanish-American War of 1898, more American troops died of typhoid than enemy action; vaccination became compulsory in 1911. During the Great War, typhus rampaged along the Eastern Front, being especially busy in Serbia, where it claimed 150,000 lives, including 30,000 Austrian prisoners of war and just over a quarter of the country's doctors.[366]

But typhoid was not just afflicting military personnel by the time the British army sent thousands of vaccinated men to the front in 1914. One of the most celebrated cases was that of the Irish cook, Mary Mallon, better known as Typhoid Mary. Mallon (1869–1938) was arrested in 1907 on suspicion of causing a number of typhoid outbreaks in the families she had worked for as a cook in and around New York City. These had resulted in several deaths. After examination, it was found that Mallon's gallbladder was riddled with typhoid bacteria, although Mallon herself was in perfect health; due to some quirk of her immune system, the microbes did not affect her. She was kept in quarantine in Riverside Hospital on North Brother Island in the East River, before being released in 1910 on the condition that she gave up being a cook.

Despite her ordeal, Mallon believed that she didn't have anything wrong with her, and went back to her former profession. History repeated itself. More outbreaks followed, but each time the authorities tried to track Mallon down, she had left her employers (who were often in hospital by that stage) and had gone to ground, only to reappear working under false names elsewhere. She was eventually re-arrested in 1915 and sent back to Riverside Hospital, where she spent the last 33 years of her life in quarantine. Given the number of aliases she had used, the precise number of Mallon's victims remains unknown, but she could have been responsible for up to fifty deaths. Mallon was what is known as an asymptomatic carrier, the first known to medical science. The precise nature of her immunity is still being researched.

The Spanish Lady

Ironically, quarantine could have saved Mary Mallon's life. On 11 August 1918, a Norwegian ship, the *Bergensfjord,* entered New York City's harbour. Eleven of her crew and ten passengers were sick with a new, and very deadly, form of influenza.[367] Other ships followed in the coming weeks, bringing what became known as the Spanish Flu with them. As the First World War entered its final, bloody months, soldiers and civilians alike were struck down in the deadliest pandemic the world has ever seen. Up to fifty million people died, more than had perished in the Great War. Perhaps due to war fatigue, perhaps due to shock, people stoically accepted the devastating losses and, by the end of 1919, it was all over. There were no memorials, no eulogies, no parades of remembrance.[368] It has become 'a global calamity the world forgot'.[369] As Mark Honigsbaum notes, 'Why this should be so puzzled commentators at the time and has continued to puzzle historians ever since. "Never since the Black Death has such a plague swept over the face of the world," commented *The Times* in December 1918 "[and] never, perhaps, has a plague been more stoically accepted"'.[370]

No one knows exactly where the pandemic began. It could well have had several points of origin. Spain was the first country to report outbreaks, in May 1918. As she was a neutral country, her news was not censored, and so the epidemic became known as the Spanish Flu, or the 'Spanish Lady'. Some think it might have begun on the Western Front, where it was known as 'Flanders grippe' among the British; the Germans dubbed it *Blitzkatarrh.* China or Hong Kong have also been proposed as points of origin. Other theories hold that it began in American army camps in the midwest in the spring of 1918, when America was preparing to send troops to Europe.

The earliest report seems to have come from Camp Funston, a newly built training facility in the grounds of Fort Riley, in central Kansas. On 4 March, Camp Funston's cook, Albert Gitchell, reported sick. 'Today many scientists believe that Gitchell was the Great Flu's patient zero.'[371] If so, Gitchell didn't have to wait long for others to join him in the sick ward. By noon the same day, 107 men had fallen ill. Within weeks, it had spread to other American camps, and when American Expeditionary Force troops landed in France in April and May 1918, they brought the flu with them. There were initial outbreaks in Brest, Marne and Vosges.

Places like the huge British army field hospital at Étaples demonstrated how closely troops and microbes mingled on a continual basis, and could well have played a part in spreading the flu. Despite ostensibly being a hospital, Étaples was rife with tetanus, dysentery and typhoid, as well as conditions particular to the Western Front, such as trench foot and trench fever. Trench foot was the result of prolonged exposure to cold mud, and causes the toes to become gangrenous until they rot and fall off. Trench fever was a form of relapsing fever transmitted by a louse, *Pediculus humanus*, that was endemic to the trenches. Other soldiers were suffering the effects of mustard gas attacks. Add to this panoply of infections the sheer number of men in the camp – more than a million soldiers passed through Étaples between June 1915 and September 1917 – and the presence of horses, chickens and pigs, and you have 'the perfect conditions for the emergence of pandemic influenza.'[372]

There were three waves of flu. The first occurred in the spring and early summer of 1918, being active in Europe by April, but also appearing in China the same month. In Spain, the first country able to report on the epidemic, up to one third of the population was affected (about eight million people). People taken ill included the King, the Prime Minister and the Minister of Finance. *The Times* reported that 700 people had died in Madrid in May and that the disease had 'passed the joking stage'.[373] In May, influenza appeared in India, although there is almost no way it could have reached there from Europe in so short a time. Over the course of the summer it reached Australia, Southeast Asia and South America.

Its initial effects seemed to have been military. The pandemic quite possibly crippled the major German spring offensive, which ground to a halt just 40 miles from Paris before the numbers of soldiers falling sick forced them to turn back. The Allied Powers were not in much of a position to exploit the German weakness: by June, the American Expeditionary Force was experiencing 'phenomenally high' rates of illness. It was not unknown for battalions to have 80 to 90 per cent of their fighting men incapacitated by the flu, while 5,500 British troops died in the pandemic's first wave, and a further 226,000 were taken ill.[374] In addition, around ten per cent of the British navy was sick. Many of those returning home to recuperate spread the disease on the home front.

Attacks could be very sudden. Initial cold-like symptoms could suddenly deteriorate into full-blown pneumonia. People died quickly, often within 48 hours, drowning in their own phlegm. Doctors performing autopsies on dead servicemen noted that the victims' lungs were like 'red currant jelly' they were so destroyed by the virus. Victims could also bleed from the nose, ears and lungs. Some literally dropped dead in the street without warning. It was not unknown for people to go out wearing tags that bore their names and addresses and those of their next of kin, in case they never returned home.

In many cities in Britain, America, and elsewhere, public gatherings were temporarily banned, and the wearing of white cotton face masks advised. (Although they weren't terribly effective against flu germs, it was better to be seen doing something rather than nothing.) Spitting was banned in New York City; while in Prescott, Arizona, even shaking hands became a criminal offence. In Britain, soldiers sent home to convalesce were banned from public places such as cinemas and concert halls. Similar troop bans and quarantines were enforced in other countries, too. Industry suffered. *The Times* reported that a textile house in Lancashire, employing 400, had 100 off sick. One third of Wigan mine workers fell ill, and in Newcastle collieries, the absentee rate was 70 per cent.[375] It's possible that these rates were so high because people in these areas were already suffering from ill health caused by the effects of industry. In the US, industrial cities such as Pittsburgh suffered similarly high rates of illness.

The second wave of the pandemic struck in the autumn of 1918. Normally a typical winter wave of flu will hit the old and children hardest, but the Spanish Lady's second visit was unusual in that young adults between the ages of 20 and 40 also proved highly susceptible. The flu was also no respecter of social class or position: British Prime Minister Lloyd George was bedridden in September, and 'he was ill to such an extent that his valet, Newnham, considered it "touch and go" as to whether he would survive.'[376] The Prime Minister's illness was kept out of the papers in the name of the war effort.

Schools and factories were closed. Public services were affected: in Philadelphia, the telephones were knocked out because most of the operators had contracted the flu. There were too few police to patrol the streets in some cities, and streets became choked with uncollected refuse. Letters went undelivered. Temporary hospitals were set up in schools, town halls and other municipal buildings; doctors and nurses were in constant demand. In India, 'rivers became clogged with corpses'[377] because there was so little firewood left available for funeral pyres. In Enfield, one funeral director had to turn work away, due to having 97 funerals to conduct in one week.[378] In Sheffield, people lay dead at home for up to 10 days sometimes, due to the lack of hearses. In Philadelphia, the dead were collected in taxis.[379] In Central Africa, villages of 300–400 families were 'completely wiped out, the housing having fallen in on the unburied dead.'[380]

Despite the rising death toll in the autumn of 1918, people tried to carry on regardless. Schoolchildren made light of the calamity with a playground rhyme:

I had a little bird
Its name was Enza
I opened the window
and in-flu-Enza.

Even when the war ended in November – itself an event possibly hastened by the pandemic – people still celebrated by throwing parties and attending dances, despite the fact that these celebrations continued to spread the virus. 1918 was the first year on record in which the death rate in Britain exceeded the birth rate.

Numerous folk remedies were tried against the flu. Potatoes and cucumbers were thought to possess medicinal properties. Other folk remedies included garlic, sulphur, Lifebuoy soap, Oxo stock cubes, incandescent gas burners, aspirin, quinine, opium, ammonia, camphor, eucalyptus, iodine, creosote, turpentine, snuff, cinnamon, salt water, tobacco, beef tea, cocoa, disinfectant and alcohol. (Champagne was very popular in France in this respect.) Among the most bizarre was bathing in cat's urine.

Such folk beliefs are part of an age-old tradition of quack medicines whose ancestors may have made an appearance every time influenza did. The disease itself is certainly age-old, although there seem to be no definite identifications prior to the sixteenth century. What is known for certain is that influenza is an ancient zoonotic virus: Dorothy Crawford notes that flu has been with us 'ever since the Chinese domesticated water fowl and pigs some 9,500 years ago.'[381] It was unknown to Hippocrates. Mary Dobson suggests the first European epidemic occurred in 1173, and that Columbus and his men might have caused an epidemic on Hispaniola in 1493, a form of swine flu which the natives are thought to have caught from the ships' pigs.[382]

Flu produces several pandemics every century, and the 1510 European outbreak is the most reliable early date we have for its appearance. Due to its apparent ability to appear everywhere, it was thought to be caused by malign astrological influences, hence the name *influenza*, from the Italian. The English physician Thomas Willis (1621–75), whom we met thrashing patients in Bedlam in Chapter 5, remarked of the 1658 epidemic that it was 'sent by some blast of the stars'.[383] Another epidemic began in 1557, when it was referred to in Edinburgh as 'the newe acqayntance' that had affected Mary Queen of Scots, and which

> passed also throughe her whole courte, neither sparinge lordes, ladies nor damoysells, not so much as ether Frenche or English. It ys a plague in their heades that have yt, and a sorenes in their stomackes, with a great coughe, that remayneth with some longer, with others

> shorter tyme, as yt findeth apte bodies for the nature of the disease. The queen kept her bed six days. There was no appearance of danger, nor manie that die of the disease, excepte some olde folkes.[384]

The next epidemic, in 1580, spread from the Mediterranean to the Baltic and 'deserves the title of pandemic'.[385]

The 1781–82 epidemic, known as 'la Russe' due to its supposed origins in Eastern Europe, even reached the Americas. That influenza could produce high fatality rates among Native Americans, as it did during the seventeenth and eighteenth centuries, is a strong indicator that the virus originated in the Old World. Lower mortality in Europe, Africa and Asia suggests the populations of those continents had developed some degree of immunity due to repeated exposure to the virus over many centuries. These were also the parts of the world where the domestication of animals was practised longest, another significant factor when the virus in question is a zoonosis. By the time la Russe struck, it also had the industrial revolution to help it on its way. As Alfred Crosby remarks, 'It was the most impressive of the early examples of what population growth and improving transportation systems could do in extending the reach of influenza.'[386]

'Russian' flu returned again in 1889–90. Originating in Bokhara in Tsarist-controlled Uzbekistan, it spread westwards via railways and commercial and diplomatic travellers. It killed an estimated quarter of a million people in Europe, and probably several times that in total. 27,000 people died in Britain, which did force the authorities to regard it as something more than a nuisance. But, as FB Smith notes in regard to this epidemic, '[British] government action was precluded by the uncertainties in early diagnosis and the cost and resistance to official meddling with everyday business to contain what the public regarded as a minor illness.'[387] Being such a 'minor illness' – it was an annual visitor each winter – meant that the Russian flu didn't elicit the same kind of panic in Britain that the 1831 approach of cholera had done. Familiarity had clearly bred contempt. Also, such had been the success of medical science that, 'By the 1890s many Britons had lulled themselves into thinking that the wonders of medical science could vanquish any foe, no matter how microscopic. In Germany Robert Koch had isolated the bacilli of tuberculosis and cholera while in Paris Louis Pasteur had developed vaccines against anthrax and rabies and discovered the process of pasteurisation. But, for all their achievements, neither had the least notion of what a virus was.'[388]

Notions about what a virus was had not progressed when the Spanish Flu appeared in 1918. A third and final wave swept the world in the spring of 1919, but by May, it had run its course. A study conducted in 1927 thought the pandemic had killed 20 million people, more than had died in the Great War, which 'only' claimed 15 million lives. But the figure for the Spanish Flu is now thought to be around 50 million, making it the deadliest pandemic in history. Some experts even think that figure is far too low, and that the true death toll may be around 100 million.[389] Around 675,000 Americans died; in the UK, the death toll was 228,000. In India, 12 million died – around ten per cent of the population.

What caused the Spanish Flu to be so virulent is still a matter for research. One of the reasons for influenza's success as a disease is that it mutates after every pandemic. So far, the 1918 strain, a variant of the H1N1 flu virus, has not reappeared, despite great efforts to find it. Bodies of victims who died on Spitsbergen and in Alaska in 1918–19 have been exhumed from the permafrost of their Arctic graves in the hope that their bodies may still contain the virus that killed them. So far results have not been conclusive. Other theories posit a link between the Russian and Spanish Flus. Could survivors of the former have been immune to the latter? Again, without evidence in the form of preserved tissue samples, the theory remains unproven. Or was the Spanish Flu a form of swine flu? Before the outbreak at Camp Funston in Kansas, local farms had experienced an outbreak of swine flu which disappeared in mid-March, around the time the first human cases were reported. Or had the Spanish Flu virus in fact been around for a number of years before 1918, with the pandemic being triggered by an unfortunate combination of events?[390] (Army doctors at the British field hospital at Étaples, for instance, thought they had seen similar flu-like symptoms in 1916.[391]) Latest research suggests it was a form of bird flu that by-passed pigs and other susceptible hosts entirely, going straight into humans. Scientists fear that the Spanish Flu – or a variation of it – will return (see avian flu and SARS, below).

Perhaps the suddenness of the pandemic, and people's seeming acceptance of it, makes it unique. As Andrew Nikiforuk notes, 'The flu's impeccably modern persona (brief, global and anonymous) made it a simple event to accept. A quick and easy death is a twentieth century ideal and the flu, so familiar and so fast, performed to expectation.'[392] But its reputation as a catastrophe the war-weary world wanted to forget continues. When Mark Honigsbaum was researching his book on the pandemic in 2005, he found one of the few remaining British survivors, 93–year-old Ada Darwin. 'Tragically, both Darwin's baby brother and both parents died in the pandemic but nearly 90 years on she still had perfect recall, telling me she could "see" the triple funeral cortege passing by a street near her school "like a film" in her head.'[393] Ada Darwin's memories sound for all the world like a piece of forgotten newsreel that no one has seen in a very long time.

Medical Advances

Newsreels of a very different sort were seen by cinema audiences at the end of the Second World War in Europe. On 12 April 1945, before British forces liberated the Nazi concentration camp at Bergen-Belsen, they were met by a German officer, who warned them of conditions inside. A typhus epidemic had been raging in the camp since February, and thousands of inmates had died. A quarantine zone around the camp was established, with white flags and signs reading *Danger – Typhus*. The Germans surrendered, and the British entered the camp. When BBC journalist Richard Dimbleby sent his report back to London, his superiors at Broadcasting House didn't believe him. They were sure conditions at Belsen couldn't possibly be as bad as he had claimed. As one eyewitness wrote of the liberation, 'Even the most hardened warriors were crying, vomiting and cursing at this never-imagined depth of human depravity.'[394]

Belsen, initially a POW camp, had been designed to hold around 10,000 inmates. In 1943, its status had been changed to that of a concentration camp. Ironically, conditions were quite good by concentration camp standards to start with: there were no gas chambers, no forced labour. People got regular meals. Then, as Germany began to lose the war, the situation began to unravel. Belsen was designated an *Erholungslager* [Recovery Camp], where prisoners from other camps too sick to work were brought, although none received medical treatment. Over the course of 1944, more and more people were evacuated to Bergen-Belsen. Conditions, already bad, became even worse. Supplies of food and clean water ran low, and sanitation broke down. Although new arrivals were disinfected, in February 1945, the disinfecting process was abandoned, probably for want of supplies. Typhus quickly tore through the camp which, by then, held around 60,000 people. Among its victims was Anne Frank.

As bulldozers dug mass graves in the main camp, a field hospital was set up at Belsen's satellite camp a mile away. Typhus was the main problem, although tuberculosis, gangrene and various skin diseases also had to be treated. All the patients were severely malnourished, being little more than skin and bones. There was even evidence that some had resorted to cannibalism prior to the liberation. A shortage of equipment in the hospital caused constant problems with hygiene. Instruments could not be properly sterilised. 80 per cent of the patients had diarrhoea, and would attempt to get up in the middle of the night to relieve themselves. They would often be found dead in their own filth the next morning, 'in all kinds of grotesque positions [that] reminded one nurse of the terrible stories told to her of the Black Death in the Middle Ages and the cries of "Bring out your dead!"'[395] As nurses worked in conditions they had never imagined encountering, the last hut at Belsen's main camp was burned to the ground on 21 May 1945 to stop the spread of disease.

*

By the time images of Bergen-Belsen were appearing in newspapers and on cinema screens, a vaccine for typhus had been in existence for several years. The story of its development was inextricably bound up with the Second World War.

In 1928, French bacteriologist Charles Nicolle (1866–1936) was awarded the Nobel Prize for his discovery that the human body louse was the vector for typhus. Nicolle had made the discovery nearly twenty years earlier, when he had been the director of the Institut Pasteur in Tunis, noting that patients who were stripped, shaved and washed before entering the hospital didn't go on to infect others. Although the louse is the vector, the disease is caused by the bacterium *Rickettsia prowazekii,* discovered in 1916 by the Brazilian Henrique da Rocha Lima (1879–1956), who named it after his colleague Stanislaus Josef Mathias von Prowazek (1875–1915), and the American Howard Taylor Ricketts (1871–1910), both of whom died of typhus while trying to find the cause of the disease. Rickettsia are microorganisms midway between bacteria and viruses. (Despite the similar names, rickettsia do not cause rickets, which is caused by vitamin D deficiency.)

Typhus had been almost endemic on the Eastern Front during the First World War, as we've noted, but it was in Russia that the disease found its most fertile feeding grounds. As Arthur Allen remarks, 'Typhus epidemics occur when a population is at the end of its tether. Starvation, cold, fear, and exhaustion are the normal prerequisites. Typhus corresponds with social collapse.'[396] All of these elements were doing their work in Russia in the late nineteenth century, where typhus found an amenable home. The disease reached catastrophic proportions during the Revolution of 1917 and the subsequent civil war between reds and whites. Some twenty-five million Russians contracted typhus, and about three million died, possibly more.[397] It was the worst outbreak of typhus in history. And then, with the disaster scarcely over, in the early 1930s typhus came back, 'undoubtedly associated with the dislocations caused by Stalin's industrialization and collectivization drives, and the ensuing famines.'[398] Both under the tsars and the Bolsheviks, history had shown that typhus will rage 'whenever human stupidity and brutality give it a chance.'[399]

Charles Nicolle was unable to produce a vaccine, although it was not for want of trying. Polish bacteriologist Rudolf Weigl (1883–1957) continued the work at his laboratory in Lviv, Ukraine. Weigl managed to develop an effective vaccine by growing lice, injecting them with typhus and then grinding their guts into a paste. When the Nazis occupied the city, they forced Weigl to increase production of the vaccine for Wehrmacht troops, typhus still being a major problem on all sides in the conflict. Weigl told the Nazis he needed more human guinea pigs for his trials, and was able to save thousands of intellectuals and resistance fighters from deportation to the camps by getting them to take part in laboratory tests. Each person was required to become a human breeding ground for lice, which meant allowing hundreds of lice to crawl all over their legs and feed. (The lice were in cages attached to the legs, thus preventing them from venturing further afield.) Weigl then gave the Nazis a watered-down version of the vaccine which was not very effective, while sending the full-strength version to Jewish ghettos in Poland. Weigl's former assistant Ludwik Fleck (1896–1961) did the same, although in far more precarious circumstances. A Jew, he was arrested and deported first to Lviv's ghetto, and then to Auschwitz and finally Buchenwald. Far too valuable to be exterminated, Fleck was forced to work in the laboratories of both camps on typhus. The vaccine he produced pleased the Nazis, although it saved no lives. The vaccine Fleck had given them was a placebo.

Meanwhile, in the USA, bacteriologist Herald R Cox had found a way to cultivate *rickettsiae,* a discovery that led to the manufacturing of a vaccine that was given to Allied troops when war broke out in 1939. Nobody wanted a repeat of what happened on the Eastern Front and in Russia. Dusting the body with the insecticide DDT (dichlorodiphenyltrichloroethane) also proved an efficient anti-typhoid measure. This was especially good news when it became clear that Cox's vaccine wasn't as good as initially thought: it didn't completely prevent the disease, but merely ensured that the vaccinated person only got a milder form of typhus. The combination of the two procedures worked: among American troops, there were only 104 cases of typhus in the whole war, and no deaths.[400] DDT also saw frontline action, being used to stop a typhus epidemic in Naples in the winter of 1943–4.

Typhus is now treated with antibiotics, whose discovery and manufacture is perhaps the main stride forward against disease that occurred during World War II. It began with a story everyone heard at school: how Alexander Fleming came back to his laboratory after a summer holiday to find mould growing in one of his culture dishes. The mould had the ability to kill a number of pathogenic bacteria, and Fleming christened it *penicillin*, from its genus *penicillium*. Fleming published his findings in the *British Journal of Experimental Pathology* in 1929, but no one paid much attention to the would-be miracle drug. Unsure of how effective penicillin might be, and also of the practicalities of its manufacture, Fleming's interest waned. The baton was then taken up by two scientists at the Radcliffe Infirmary in Oxford, Howard Florey and Ernst Chain. Together with Edward Abraham, Norman Heatley and others, they managed to isolate and concentrate penicillin. Owing to the privations of wartime, conditions in the lab were makeshift: cultures of penicillin had to be grown in bathtubs, buckets, milk churns, food tins and bed pans. With funding from the American and British governments, who were clearly aware of its use in wartime, the Oxford team were able to get penicillin mass-produced by early 1942. With various pharmaceutical companies now involved, mass-production was ramped up in early 1944 in time for the Normandy Landings on 6 June, where antibiotics played a major role in saving the lives of Allied troops at an absolutely crucial moment in the war.

*

The discovery and development of antibiotics – of which penicillin was the first and most well-known – marked a turning point in humanity's struggle with disease. The years immediately following the end of the Second World War were loud with pronouncements that echoed the Victorians in their optimism. US Secretary of State George C Marshall declared in 1948, at the Fourth International Congress on Tropical Medicine and Malaria in Washington DC, 'that the conquest of all infectious diseases was imminent.'[401] The same year, the World Health Organization was founded to promote health and medical research around the globe. The concept of international cooperation to combat disease had taken its first hesitant step at the 1851 sanitation conference in Paris, when cholera was on the agenda. Now, with Marshall's ambitious objectives on the table, international cooperation would be vital if some of them were to be achieved.

(It's no coincidence that George C Marshall also put his name to the Marshall Plan, another child of 1948, which was intended to spread American culture, values and industry across the world in the name of de-Nazification and post-war reconstruction. Its real aim, however, was not to make the world safe, but to make the world safe for America. As with Victorian campaigns against disease, which were inextricably bound up with imperialism and capitalism, so too was the post-war drive to eradicate disease. However, it wasn't just the West that was optimistic in the battle against disease: the Chinese communist party 'waged a peasant-based war on infectious diseases' during the 1950s and 1960s.[402])

'For Western physicians, the 1950s and 1960s were a time of tremendous optimism', Laurie Garrett notes. 'Nearly every week the medical establishment declared another "miracle breakthrough" in humanity's war with infectious disease.'[403] It was the era in which 'the end of' a particular disease would be regularly trumpeted. Many of these breakthroughs were in the fields of vaccines and other treatments, making good on the discoveries of Fleming and the Oxford team. By 1965, more than 25,000 antibiotic drugs had been developed. 'The term "miracle drug" entered the common vernacular.'[404]

Among the triumphs was the development of a vaccine for polio. A disease whose provenance stretches at least as far back as ancient Egypt, when it appears to have been depicted on funerary stelae (see Chapter 2), polio became a major problem in the early twentieth century. The reasons for its sudden appearance as an epidemic, rather than endemic, disease are unknown.

Poliomyelitis is a virus that, although asymptomatic in 90 to 95 per cent of cases, can cause paralysis, paresis and even death if the respiratory system is attacked. Quite why the disease progresses to these more serious stages in such a small percentage of cases still remains a matter for research. Polio derives its name from the Greek for 'grey matter' – a reference to the spinal cord, which can be seriously affected by the disease. It was first recognised as a 'debility of the lower extremities' by the British physician-apothecary Michael Underwood (1736–1820), followed by the German doctor Jacob von Heine (1800–79), who dubbed it 'infantile spinal paralysis'; in 1908, the Austrian biologist Karl Landsteiner (1868–1943) discovered polio to be contagious. Following a few sporadic nineteenth century outbreaks (England, the USA and, of all places, St Helena, were affected in the 1830s), the worst epidemic occurred along the Eastern Seaboard of the USA in the summer of 1916. 9,000 cases were reported in New York City alone, almost all of which were children under five years of age. In the sort of mass panic we might more readily associate with Orson Welles's later *War of the Worlds* radio broadcast, 50,000 children from New York and New Jersey were evacuated to the countryside in an attempt to stop the disease spreading further. Rumours spread that the disease had been started by Italian immigrants, causing riots. The rich fled to their summer homes, and schools were closed. Infected families were quarantined in their own homes, and in Hoboken, New Jersey, police rounded up stray children at train, subway and ferry stations. In all, the epidemic claimed around 6,000 lives across the country.

As with cholera and typhoid, polio is a disease that flourishes in poverty-stricken urban neighbourhoods, being transmitted by unwashed hands or faecal contamination of drinking water (the faecal-oral route). However, it was also able to strike the rich and well-to-do: the most famous victim from Ivy League circles was future US president Franklin Delano Roosevelt, who contracted polio in 1921 at the age of 39. Again, no one is quite sure why this should be so, as FDR was clearly not living in a dirty tenement in Hell's Kitchen when he was taken ill.

One theory regarding polio's ability to cross social boundaries was that, prior to the great late nineteenth and early twentieth century improvements in public health and hygiene, children had more or less become immune to polio, due to constant exposure to the virus over the course of centuries. And then, ironically, the great drive to improve public health and hygiene left children vulnerable to the virus once more.

Various treatments were devised over the succeeding decades. These included hydrotherapy (favoured by FDR); the use of leg braces, which became closely associated with the disease; the Kenny regimen (a course of physical therapy devised by Australian nurse Elizabeth Kenny); and the development of the iron lung, first used to treat polio patients in 1928. These machines, although expensive to build and as cumbersome as a First World War tank, saved thousands of lives by enabling collapsed or otherwise disabled lungs to breathe using the process of negative pressure ventilation. The patient would be put into the iron lung flat on their back, leaving just the head visible. The British writer JG Farrell (1935–1979), himself an adult victim of polio, described the experience of being inserted into one of the machines in his novel *The Lung* (1965):

> Feeling as horizontal and as petrified as a stone crusader, Sands discovered with dismay that the fountain of joy spurting up in him so suddenly at those first, deep lungfuls of air had now subsided to virtually nothing. How much longer was he likely to be in the bloody thing? This was something about which he had not the faintest idea. Was one in an iron lung for a matter of days, or weeks, or years? He felt that he had already been in the lung for far too long... a matter of three minutes or so. And what if...? But he knew that he must abandon the future and remain always in the present, wobbling

dangerously, as if it were a difficult and dangerous bicycle from which he was unable to dismount without the risk of total calamity.[405]

The calamity Farrell feared began to be a thing of the past with the development of effective vaccines against polio in the 1950s and 60s, the first by American doctor Jonas Salk, and then a second by his rival, Albert Sabin, which could be administered orally. Salk was hailed a national hero in the USA at the unveiling of his vaccine on 12 April 1955. As BBC broadcaster Alastair Cooke reported at the time, 'Nothing short of the overthrow of the Communist regime in the Soviet Union could bring such rejoicing to the hearts and homes in America as the historic announcement last Tuesday that the 166-year war against polio is almost certainly at an end.'[406] Although the battle against polio did not end in 1955, the vaccination campaigns were extremely successful, a model of post-war public health policy in action: cases in North America and Western Europe dropped from 76,000 in 1955 to under 1,000 in 1967.[407]

Two other campaigns were even more ambitious than the one to eradicate polio: the attempts to rid the world of malaria and smallpox. A campaign of pesticides and drugs was waged against malaria from 1955 onwards, and by 1970 the disease had at least been eradicated from most of Europe, North America, much of the Middle East and the coastal regions of the Mediterranean. But it proved ultimately impossible to rid the world of the disease: there were simply too many mosquitoes.

The campaign against smallpox began at the request of the Soviet Union in 1958. The disease was endemic in many of the Soviet Asian republics and was killing around two million people across the world each year. The issue was discussed at the WHO, and received almost unanimous support. They had a head start, as there had been a vaccine since 1796 thanks to Edward Jenner, and the disease was also easy to diagnose. The fact that only humans are susceptible was a further factor that helped the projected eradication programme: there was no vector such as the ubiquitous mosquito to deal with. The campaign finally began under the auspices of the American doctor Donald Henderson in 1967, who headed the WHO's Smallpox Eradication Unit. The various teams under Henderson's supervision were to administer millions of vaccinations over the next decade. They also set up a system for containing the disease. If an outbreak occurred, quarantine measures would be put in place to ring-fence the disease and thereby break the chain of infection. This was easier said than done, as it transpired that 95 per cent of cases of smallpox worldwide didn't come to the attention of health authorities in the country affected, or to the WHO. This resulted in the occasional use of force to vaccinate people, with Henderson's units operating more like special forces teams, breaking into people's homes with the local police in order to make sure people were treated. In another instance, a WHO team had to forcibly vaccinate armed robbers in Bangladesh, who were spreading the disease in the course of their activities. Gunshots were exchanged before shots of vaccine. But the robbers surrendered.

Such tactics were deemed necessary in what seemed to be an impossible task. War and religion frequently provided additional obstacles. Either teams could not get vaccines to war-torn areas, or religious observances prohibited treatment. Sometimes, as had happened with cholera, religious pilgrims spread the disease unwittingly. This was how Europe experienced its last outbreak of smallpox in 1972, when a pilgrim returning from Mecca brought it back to Yugoslavia. The last case reported anywhere occurred in Somalia in October 1977. Then, in December 1979, the WHO felt cautiously confident in believing that its work on smallpox was done.

HIV/AIDS

On 8 May 1980 the World Health Organization made a momentous announcement: they 'Declare[d] solemnly that the world and its peoples have won freedom from smallpox'.[408] For the first time, one of the major diseases in history had been consigned to laboratory vaults and would no longer be claiming lives. No one involved in the smallpox campaign could have suspected that a new pandemic was already upon the world.

Later that year, a 30-year-old man went to see Dr Joel Weisman, a Los Angeles doctor who specialised in gay men's health. Weisman noted his patient 'had painful eczema, persistent diarrhea, and endless fevers.'[409] The man was clearly very unwell, but the symptoms puzzled Weisman. A colleague had reported a similar case just a month or two before, of another young gay man, who had a 'strikingly similar disarray in his immune system.'[410] The man was suffering from a 'constellation of diseases [that] was startling. White fungi grew around the man's fingernails, fluffy candidiasis was sprouting all over his palate, and he too was suffering from rashes, prolonged fevers, swollen lymph glands, and low white blood counts.'[411] By December, Weisman's colleague had also diagnosed immune deficiency.

By the end of 1980, there would be 55 reported cases in the USA, four of them fatal. The one thing that linked them was the fact that all the men were gay. Doctors such as Weisman and his colleague, the Centers for Disease Control and Prevention in Atlanta (the CDC), the National Cancer Institute in Maryland, and elsewhere began to fear that something was going on. 'If something new gets loose here,' commented the San Francisco Department of Public Health's Dr Selma Dritz – a specialist in gay health and STDs – 'we're going to have hell to pay.'[412]

Something indeed was getting loose. On 5 June 1981, the CDC's *Morbidity and Mortality Weekly Report* – a journal sent to hospitals, public health institutions, doctors and anyone working with infectious diseases – ran a report on five young male patients with an unusual immune deficiency, who were all suffering from a rare form of pneumonia called *Pneumocystis carinii pneumonia* (PCP). All were gay. The author of the paper, Dr Michael Gottlieb, commented, 'The fact that these patients were all homosexual suggests an association between some aspect of homosexual lifestyle or disease acquired through sexual contact and *Pneumocystis* pneumonia in this population.' The *San Francisco Chronicle* ran a story on the report, 'A Pneumonia That Strikes Gay Males', the following day. It was the only mainstream newspaper to carry the story.

PCP wasn't the only thing afflicting the men with the mystery illness. Many of them were also suffering from a rare form of skin cancer called Kaposi's Sarcoma, more commonly seen in old Mediterranean men. One of the first cases had been reported to the CDC on 24 April. Ken Horne, a young San Franciscan former ballet dancer, was suffering from Kaposi's Sarcoma, and also cryptococcus, a fungal yeast infection. The *New York Times* ran an article on the Kaposi's Sarcoma cases on 3 July, 'Rare Cancer Seen in 41 Homosexuals'. The following day's issue of the *MMWR* also reported on the prevalence of Kaposi's Sarcoma among gay men. Many of them were also suffering from PCP.

News of the 'gay plague' spread fast. As with leprosy, the Black Death and cholera, some commentators were quick to ascribe moral blame for the new mystery illness, dubbed GRID – gay related immune deficiency. Just as lepers had been blamed in the Middle Ages for their condition, on the grounds that it was the result of sin, sexual sin in particular, just as the Black Death was the result of everyone's sins, and cholera afflicted the poor because they were morally weak and had committed the sin of being poor, so GRID was seen by some rabid conservatives as the fruits of the 'sin' of homosexuality. The religious right foamed at the mouth. Newspapers ran headlines such as 'Exterminate gays' and called for victims to be placed in quarantine.[413]

Doctors such as Joel Weisman and Selma Dritz knew full well that gay men were certainly on the front line of health issues in places like San Francisco in the 1970s. Gay liberation meant sex, lots of it, in bathhouses, private cinemas, the back rooms of bars, men's rooms, alleyways, etc. Such liberal sexual practices – central to gay identity at the time – had led to gay men suffering from abnormally high cases of hepatitis B, as well as amebiasis – a deadly parasitic disease that causes dysentery and diarrhoea and is often transmitted by faecal-oral route or, as was common in gay bathhouse culture, the anal-oral route (rimming, in other words) – shigellosis, a bacterial disease that causes diarrhoea, cramps, fever and vomiting, and a condition known as 'gay bowel syndrome'.

The more the new illness was studied, however, it became clear that there were other susceptible groups. Along with homosexuals, haemophiliacs, heroin addicts and Haitians were suffering. They were dubbed the '4 H Club'. It was clear that, whatever the disease was, it was not just affecting gays, and GRID became AIDS – acquired immune deficiency syndrome. To the chagrin of the anti-gay fearmongers, a fifth 'H' group was identified in a 1984 article in *The Lancet*: heterosexuals.

Peter Piot, one of the authors of the piece in *The Lancet*, was a Belgian clinical microbiologist who worked at Antwerp's Institute of Tropical Medicine, 'the go-to doctor for people arriving from Africa with embarrassing tropical infections.'[414] But the patients were increasingly suffering from diseases that were strange rather than embarrassing. One case, from 1979, stuck in Piot's mind. A Greek fisherman, who had lived and worked on the shores of Lake Tanganyika in eastern Zaire, was suffering from a number of severe infections that eventually killed him. But the autopsy results proved startling to Piot: the man's internal organs had virtually been destroyed by an unusual mycobacterial infection. Like American patients suffering from Kaposi's Sarcoma and PCP, the Greek had had a condition that under normal conditions should not prove fatal, but, in his case, it had.[415]

Hearing about the 'gay plague' in America, Piot wondered whether this might be the same illness that his African patients were suffering from. Colleagues in Brussels had reported numerous similar cases. If there were 100 sick Africans who could afford to be treated in Belgium, what might the number be back home? Piot and his team began taking blood samples in gay bars and clubs, noting higher incidences of syphilis and hepatitis B than would normally be found.[416] In 1983, Piot and a team of European and US doctors visited Zaire. They encountered conditions in Kinshasa's Mama Yemo Hospital that would not have looked out of place in one of Goya's paintings of a madhouse: some parts of the building had collapsed, there were piles of rubbish rotting in the courtyard, and the wards were full to overflowing. The sick were two to a bed, with more ailing on soiled mattresses on every available bit of floor space.

Piot recalled his first impression of the wards in Mama Yemo:

'They were mostly twenty-five- to thirty-five-year-olds, with enormous weight loss, intractable diarrhea, and that ghastly, glassy-eyed look. Many of them had dramatic itching, with skin symptoms that had not been described in the literature. They had a lot of sores in their mouths – yeast infections and very ugly herpes sores – and eye infections. A few had Kaposi's Sarcoma markings, especially on their legs, and many were breathing very superficially; perhaps the respiratory distress stemmed from tuberculosis. There was also quite a bit of cryptococcal meningitis, which we knew was a marker of AIDS... their symptoms were remarkably aggressive: they progressed with startling speed and seemed not to respond to treatment.

'We were all silent and staring at each other... When we got out of there, I took a deep breath, as I was nearly breathless. I remember it well – a physical sensation that was so strong, I wrote it down. It wasn't the happy tingling energy of scientific discovery... [but] the overwhelming feeling that we were facing a truly momentous catastrophe.'[417]

When published in *The Lancet* the following year,[418] Piot et al's findings from Kinshasa 'clearly demonstrated that HIV [see below] was well established in central Africa where it affected both men and women and was spread by heterosexual contact.'[419] Alarmingly, the prevalence of AIDS was higher in Kinshasa and Rwanda's capital, Kigali 'than in San Francisco or New York,' clearly 'dispelling any lingering notions that AIDS was a disease restricted to ethnic or sexual minority groups.'[420]

While Piot was at work in Africa, an American team of researchers led by Robert Gallo at the National Cancer Institute, and a French team led by Luc Montagnier at the Pasteur Institute in Paris, both announced that they had discovered the cause of AIDS. The human immunodeficiency virus, or HIV, is a retrovirus that attacks the immune system, making normally routine diseases suddenly fatal. There are two main types, HIV-1 and HIV-2. HIV-1 is the more deadly, and is now thought to derive from SIV – simian immunodeficiency virus – which affects chimpanzees. HIV-2 is related to a virus of the sooty mangabey, a monkey found in West Africa. Within HIV-1, there are various subtypes, and it is only HIV-1 group M that causes the pandemic. The incubation period can be anything up to ten years, but when it develops into AIDS, it is fatal. Drugs were powerless to stop it. HIV is transmitted through sexual intercourse, contaminated needles, infected blood or from mother to baby in the womb. Three of the '4 Hs' were covered – but what about the fourth, Haitians? Why had the virus seemingly attacked Haitians, out of all the ethnicities in the USA?

In trying to answer that, doctors inevitably faced the challenge of trying to discover where HIV/AIDS had originally come from. Given that the incubation period can be anything up to ten years, what were then thought to be the first victims – 1975–78 in Kinshasa, 1978–80 in Europe, 1979/80 in the US – could have picked up the virus at any time from the late 1960s onwards. A report published in July 1982 suggested Haiti as the possible source of the epidemic. Between 1980 and 1982, 20 Haitians had been admitted to hospital in Miami, suffering from AIDS. It transpired that all of them had been working in West and Central Africa before being taken sick, and it was towards Africa that scientists began to look for the origins of HIV.

Mystifyingly, scientists began to uncover cases even earlier than the ones already noted. The earliest they found both came from the Democratic Republic of Congo. A man had died of HIV in 1959, and a woman the following year. In 1987, tissue samples were tested of a young African American from St Louis, Robert Rayford, who had died from a mystery illness in 1969. Rayford had been suffering from immune system collapse, and had also developed Kaposi's Sarcoma. The 1987 tests showed he had died from AIDS. It is thought he might have worked as a rent boy, been sexually abused, or both. Given that Rayford had been ill since late 1966, it seems HIV may have first entered the USA around that time, but didn't start to become epidemic until the late 1970s, possibly due to a reintroduction of the virus into the country.

Then there was the case of the 'Norwegian Sailor', whose identity was initially hidden to protect his family. He was eventually named as Arvid Noe.[421] When samples of his blood and tissue were tested in 1988, it was found he had died of AIDS in 1976. As a sailor in the Norwegian merchant navy, it was thought Noe had been infected by a prostitute in Cameroon at some point between 1961 and 1965. He returned home in 1966, and found work as a truck driver. It was around this time that Arvid Noe began to fall ill. Doctors didn't know what was wrong with him. Noe's wife also began to suffer from the same cluster of illnesses; she died in December 1976, eight months after he did. Tragically, it was their 8-year-old daughter who died first, in January 1976. She was the first European to die of AIDS, and the first known case of mother-baby infection.

While these early cases were coming to light, the number of cases in the USA continued to rise, going from 55 in 1980 to 7699 in 1984, of which 3665 had died. In the UK, 108 cases had been reported, resulting in 46 deaths.[422] The World Health Organization launched its Global Programme on AIDS in 1987, and public health campaigns to stop the disease were launched in Europe and the USA. The first International AIDS conference was held in Atlanta, Georgia (home of the Centers for Disease Prevention and Control), and the first antiretroviral drug for HIV/AIDS, AZT (azidothymidine), was approved by the American FDA. AZT was then rolled out for use in Europe. In the UK, a needle exchange programme was started, and safe sex messages appeared across the media. Organisations such as the Terrence Higgins Trust in the UK and the San Francisco AIDS Foundation became well-known for their work in fundraising, providing palliative care and raising awareness. These were all timely measures: by 1987, there had been 40,051 AIDS cases in the USA, with 23,165 deaths,[423] and in 1988, it was announced that AIDS cases worldwide had jumped by 56 per cent.[424] The possibility that AIDS could become the worst pandemic ever known was being mooted.

Film icon Rock Hudson was the first major celebrity to announce that he was suffering from HIV, in July 1985; he died from AIDS that October. His death helped boost funding for AIDS research, as Hudson was seen as a 'respectable' actor (his homosexuality was not widely known), and if someone respectable could get AIDS, it was clearly a disease that could affect everyone, and not just minorities (Haitians, haemophiliacs) or 'deviants' (gays, intravenous drug users). The same issues resurfaced when tennis champion Arthur Ashe (1943–1993) announced he had HIV in 1992. Ashe was among the first high profile non-gay victims of the disease, who is thought to have contracted HIV as the result of a blood transfusion. Ashe's admission that he had contracted HIV in hospital became a high-profile case, and Ashe, who was also a vigorous activist, used the glare of publicity to ask the UN for more funding into AIDS research.

But in the early 90s, HIV/AIDS was still seen mainly as a disease affecting gay men; the escalating numbers of heterosexual casualties in Africa made the news less often. As with the Spanish Flu, it was a classic case of third world (i.e. black) lives mattering less to first world media corporations. (Asked if getting AIDS was the hardest thing he had ever had to face, Arthur Ashe replied, 'No, the hardest thing I've ever had to deal with is being a black man in this society'.[425]) When British writer and journalist Ed Hooper visited East Africa to research the effect of AIDS, he was met with some frightening facts. The disease was known as 'Slim' because of the weight loss and wasting it caused. No one knew exactly what caused it, or where it had come from. Its prevalence among the general population in Uganda was alarming. One doctor remarked that there were no high-risk groups for the disease except 'being Ugandan'.[426] Hysterical patients received minimal treatment in overcrowded hospital wards, where the nurses were too terrified to touch the patients (the conditions Peter Piot and his team encountered at Mama Yemo Hospital in Kinshasa in 1983 were clearly not unique). People resorted to witchcraft remedies, such as eating dog's liver soup, in an attempt to get well. Others killed themselves. Whole villages lay abandoned. The situation that confronted Hooper was 'one of very high levels of infection, increasing numbers of people with full-blown AIDS, and of a quite inadequate government response.'[427]

> Heading back to Kampala, we picked up a hitch-hiker who was eager to talk about the epidemic. He himself knew of two cases of Slim, one a woman who now had skin 'like a frog's'. He told us that Slim was not caused by 'free sex', but by sharing needles for injections, or the straws that were commonly used for drinking *malwa*, the local beer. The prostitutes in Kyotera, he added, were telling people that Slim disease was not AIDS, but a special type of poisoning caused by certain Tanzanian tribes who were expert in witchcraft. When we questioned him further, he told us that a local priest had said at the funeral of a 'Slim victim' that the disease was like one of the plagues of Egypt, striking down the immoral.[428]

Drugs were initially too expensive to be widely distributed in the West, let alone Africa. HAART (Highly Active Antiretroviral Therapy) was developed in the mid-1990s, and proved effective in subduing the effects of the disease. Over the next decade, the cost of these drugs came down and did eventually reach Africa. The problem with developing vaccines has been that HIV doesn't behave like any other known infection: it mutates rapidly, resulting in a genetically diverse group of subtypes and forms. If a drug works for HIV-1, for instance, it may do nothing for HIV-2, and within those two strains, there are the M, N, O and P groups, and further distinctions within some of those (such as HIV-1 group M subtype C), and so on.[429]

Vaccines have also played an intermittent role in the search for the origins of HIV. One theory proposed that HIV had been accidentally created by scientists when they were developing anti-polio treatments for the developing world in the 1950s. These early vaccines had used monkey kidney cells which, when administered in the Congo in the late 50s and early 60s, had accidentally kick-started the AIDS pandemic. This theory, known as the Oral Polio Vaccine theory, has been largely discredited, although the earliest known cases of HIV do seem to have come from the Democratic Republic of Congo, as we've seen.[430] What remains a possibility is that the re-use of hypodermic needles in the campaigns against polio and smallpox helped spread HIV, but this remains conjectural. If true, it would be one of the more horrible ironies in the story of humanity's battle with pandemics.

Current medical thinking on the origins of HIV suggests that it first appeared in southeast Cameroon at some point between 1884 and 1924.[431] Both main types of HIV are now known to be related to Simian Immunodeficiency Virus (SIV), which affects chimpanzees and sooty mangabeys respectively. At some point, the virus made the species jump between monkeys and humans, possibly when hunters became infected from either eating bushmeat, or from cuts sustained while butchering the meat.

The date of 1884 is significant because that was the year in which the Germans took over Cameroon and began developing the country's infrastructure, building road and rail networks, 'with a view to exploiting the country's potential wealth – ivory, rubber, timber, coffee and cocoa – to the full.'[432] The result of this was twofold: new roads and railways disrupted traditional Bantu hunting grounds, and cities began developing. The crucial species jump may therefore have happened when the Bantu were seeking new areas in which to hunt, territories not being disrupted by German expansion; or conversely, it could have been the monkeys who were displaced. Either scenario is conjecture, and we must also remember that the species jump could have happened on more than one occasion before the virus was established as a human disease. But this is where the railways, roads and expanding cities came in: as a way for the new disease to travel and multiply.

HIV seems to have been active in Kinshasa in the 1920s, when the country was under the control of the Belgians. A combination of a large population, a million migrant workers passing through each year, a thriving sex trade and good transport connections meant that Kinshasa became a disease factory.[433] Then, around 1960, additional expansion of the railways spread HIV even further afield. And this was around the time when Arvid Noe was known to have visited Africa; a few years later, Robert Rayford was thought to have become infected, by person or persons unknown who had (presumably) recently been in central Africa. Both men seem to have been early victims of what would become the AIDS pandemic, as the disease slowly made its way out of Africa.

In its first quarter century, AIDS has infected around 65 million people, with around 25 million dead. The disease's devastating effects make for grim reading. Nearly 40 million people are living with the disease, half of them women. Young people under the age of 25 account for half of all new infections worldwide. The majority of people living with HIV today are in sub-Saharan Africa. The disease still kills around 3 million people a year, half of them children. Around 6,000 people become infected every day. Africa has 12 million AIDS orphans. In North America, 1.4 million people are living with AIDS. HIV also has links to tuberculosis: people are more likely to get TB if they already have HIV. Between 1986 and 2006, there was a five-to-ten fold increase in TB cases worldwide.[434] Just over half of all AIDS deaths have been in Africa.[435]

As the chief epidemiologist at Kampala's Mulago Hospital said, 'It all started with a rumour. Then we found we were dealing with a disease. Then we realized it was an epidemic. And, now, we have accepted it as a tragedy.'[436]

Lifestyle Diseases

In 1967, the US Surgeon General William H Stewart 'would be so utterly convinced of imminent success [in public health campaigns against disease] he would tell a White House gathering of state and territorial health officers that it was time to close the book on infectious diseases and shift all national attention (and dollars) to what he termed "the New Dimensions" of health: chronic diseases.'[437] If AIDS could initially have been seen as a gay lifestyle disease, then many of the chronic diseases Stewart wanted to see action on in 1967 could also be seen as lifestyle diseases. The latter half of the twentieth century saw a huge rise in the incidence of cancer, heart disease, diabetes, obesity and a cornucopia of allergies, all linked to the sedentary consumer culture of the developed world. Our comforts are killing us.

The prominent Canadian physician William Osler, whom we met in Chapter 5, noted in 1892 that coronary heart disease was 'relatively rare'.[438] The concept of a heart attack was unknown, the phrase first being used in the early twentieth century. By the 1940s, a study conducted in Framingham, Massachusetts, found that heart disease was linked to smoking, lack of exercise, diets rich in saturated fats and or salt, heavy alcohol consumption, stress, obesity, type 2 diabetes, high blood pressure and high cholesterol levels.[439] By the end of the century, cardiovascular disease (heart disease accompanied by a stroke) was the leading cause of death worldwide.[440]

Many of these problems had, of course, been known in earlier times. The effects of obesity and heavy drinking were certainly known in eighteenth century Britain, as was the danger of stress: After performing an autopsy on a person who had died in a fit of anger, Scottish surgeon John Hunter (1728–93), who knew Edward Jenner, commented, 'My life is in the hands of any rascal who chooses to annoy me.' Hunter's words proved prophetic: he died of a probable ruptured aortic aneurysm after having an explosive argument with a colleague at St George's Hospital, London.[441] Obesity was clearly a problem, too, as Mary Dobson notes: 'It was frequently noted that "gross" individuals of "corpulent living, ruddy complexion, hard drinking and overindulgence" ran a high risk of disease and death, as did those who had "a want of fresh fruit and greens and the disadvantages of a low diet".[442]

Doctors themselves could be just as guilty of these errant lifestyles as their patients. George Cheyne (1671–1743), spent so much time eating and drinking with his patients – who included the writers John Gay, Alexander Pope and Samuel Richardson – that, at one time, he weighed 32 stone. Cheyne's servant walked behind him with a stool so that he could rest frequently, as he was 'excessively fat, short-breath'd, lethargic and listless'.[443] Cheyne eventually converted to vegetarianism, took exercise and fresh air, and cut down on visits to the tavern. His weight went down, and his health improved dramatically. Health advice manuals in the eighteenth and nineteenth centuries followed Cheyne's example in recommending a good diet, lots of exercise, moderate alcohol consumption, and a balanced diet.

As Mary Dobson notes, 'there were few specific recognizable clinical descriptions of heart disease prior to the twentieth century'.[444] Diagnoses that are possibly heart-related can be gleaned from journals, mortality records, doctors' case notes, diaries, letters and newspapers. *The Gentleman's Magazine* ran a story in 1796 about a servant girl who had dropped dead while reading a letter from her beau, a fellow servant. It transpired he had run off and married someone else; the girl was said to have died of a 'broken heart'. Other possible heart-related demises were said to be from the deceased being 'sad', 'weak', 'infirm', or suffering from an 'oppression of the spirits', a 'pining sickness' or an 'iliac passion'. Some died 'suddenly' or 'untimely', while others were 'planet-struck', inflicted by the 'visitation of God', or 'the work of the Devil'. Some died because they were 'worn out', 'frenzied', 'distracted' and 'short of breath' or declined through 'exhaustion', 'grief' or 'old age'. 'Decay' or being 'bedridden' were often cited as causes of death in the elderly. As Mary Dobson remarks, 'How many such sudden or slow deaths were related to heart disease is impossible to tell.'[445]

One of the first descriptions of what we can now say was heart disease came from English physician William Heberden (1710–1801). In 1768, he coined the term 'angina pectoris' – a term related to chest pains, 'a most disagreeable sensation in the breast, which seems as if it would extinguish life, if it were to increase or continue'.[446] What constituted heart disease continued to be refined by nineteenth-century authorities like August Hirsch, who saw heart problems as mainly causing diseases in other parts of the body. By the early twentieth century, actual irregularities, such as a heart murmur, were automatically seen as evidence of heart disease. During the First World War, a condition known as 'Soldier's Heart' was common.

Its symptoms of 'breathlessness, fatigue, and a feeling of impending doom'[447] were treated with extended stays in hospital, until the ailment became one of the most common causes of military discharge. After the authorities realised that keeping so many soldiers in hospital because of suspected heart conditions was costing Britain a huge amount of money, as well as weakening her militarily and putting a huge strain on hospitals, 'Soldier's Heart' was re-diagnosed as 'Effort Syndrome'. This new, less serious condition, was to be treated with a regimen of exercise, freeing up much-needed hospital beds and saving the British war chest considerable amounts of money. 'All of this demonstrates that some notions about what constitutes heart disease are informed by social needs.'[448]

Even if some instances of heart disease could be thus reassigned to lesser categories, technological developments in the early part of the twentieth century certainly aided the detection of genuine heart problems. The invention of the polygraph and the electrocardiograph before the First World War helped doctors monitor heart disturbances and the pulse with better clarity than the stethoscope. By the time of the Framingham study in 1948, therefore, doctors had a pretty good idea of what heart disease was, and what was likely to be causing it.

Likewise, type 1 diabetes was rare until the second half of the twentieth century. Type 2 diabetes has become 'predominantly a disease of older and fatter people and has become increasingly common as a result of increased life expectancy, urbanization, lifestyle changes, and population growth.'[449] As Robert Tattersall notes, 'An observer in 1900 would have been amazed by the magnitude of these figures [that, in the year 2000, an estimated 171 million people worldwide suffer from diabetes] but not by the concept that diabetes was a product of wealth, dietary change, and urbanisation. A Victorian physician had even described diabetes as 'one of the penalties of advanced civilization.'[450]

Diabetes was probably known to the ancients, who recorded a disease that produced large amounts of 'honey-tasting' urine. Diagnosed by drinking the said honey-tasting beverage, it was treated with dietary and lifestyle changes, such as an increase in physical exercise and vegetables.

Many writers noted the sweet taste of the patient's urine, although Paracelsus, never one to mince words, ridiculed 'pisse prophets' who claimed they could explain disease solely through studying urine, and suggested that chemical analysis should be employed if the cause of diabetes was to be found.[451] Paracelsus recognised that diabetes could be a serious disease. Thomas Willis (1621–75) wrote in *Diabetes or the Pissing Evil* that the disease was rare among the ancients, and that the urine was 'exceedingly sweet' or 'wonderfully sweet like sugar or honey' but did not consider this to be because there was sugar in it.[452] Matthew Dobson (1735–84) disagreed with Willis, believing that the sweetness came from sugar. In 1772 he evaporated two quarts of urine from a patient who was passing 28 pints (15 litres) of urine a day. The white residue that was left could not 'by the taste be distinguished from sugar'.[453]

Progress was made by William Cullen (1710–90), who identified two kinds of the disease: *diabetes mellitus* and *diabetes insipidus*. Army physician John Rollo (d.1809), who studied under Cullen, tried to eliminate the production of sugar. He thought it was formed in the stomach from vegetables, and treated patients with a meat diet. Although he was wrong, as Tattersall notes, it was at least 'an attempt to treat diabetes rationally by preventing the formation of sugar.'[454] In 1815, the sugar was identified as glucose.

John Camplin, a doctor, wrote what is possibly the only autobiographical account of suffering from the disease in 1858. He noted the first symptoms in 1844, when colleagues predicted that treatment would be 'smoothing my path to the grave'. Camplin was initially advised to eat fat meat and eggs, but this produced 'great biliary derangement'. He was later advised to add fish to his diet, and also took to eating bran cakes 'by no means a pleasant composition but one which acted powerfully on the bowels.' Camplin survived his ordeal with diabetes and his doctor's prescriptions; indeed, his book is entitled *On Diabetes and its Successful Treatment*.[455]

Dobson and Cullen had both believed that glucose was formed in the stomach. Josef von Mering (1849–1908) and Oskar Minkowski (1858–

1931) discovered that it was in fact the pancreas that played the crucial role. In experiments in 1889, they removed dogs' pancreases and found that the animals developed all the signs of diabetes; the animals answered calls of nature on the laboratory floor. In 1910, the English physiologist Sir Edward Albert Sharpey-Schafer (1850–1935) proposed the lack of a single chemical normally produced by the pancreas as the cause of diabetes. He dubbed it *insulin*, after the Latin word for island, a reference to the insulin-producing regions of the pancreas, the islets of Langerhans. It wasn't until 1921 that an effective treatment for diabetes was developed by Frederick Banting and Charles Best at the University of Toronto, who discovered a method for extracting insulin from the islets of Langerhans. The discovery led to a Nobel for Banting but, in another controversy, not for Best. (Banting did at least share his prize money with him.) Shortly afterwards, the Canadian pharmaceutical firm Eli Lilly began to produce insulin for general practice.

It was a well-timed discovery, as what was probably the first reference to an epidemic of diabetes came in 1921 from American doctor Elliott Joslin (1869–1962), who became one of the first modern authorities on diabetes. He noted that six of out seven people in adjoining houses to his own in his hometown of Oxford, Massachusetts, had died of diabetes. 'He pointed out that, had they died of cholera, the public health authorities would be round like a shot. As it was diabetes, nobody was particularly bothered.'[456] Joslin established that the main risk factor in developing diabetes was being overweight, and the principal reason for an increasingly heavy population was that it was doing less manual work. Mechanisation, wrote Joslin, 'has made industrial workers mere tenders of machines, has lightened the burden of farm workers, transferred large numbers into clerical and sales jobs, reduced hours of labour. The amount of energy expended in work, therefore, has been drastically cut down for the majority of the working population.'[457] The problem with weight was backed up by a contributor to the *British Medical Journal* in 1932 who wrote: 'should the national overweight continue to grow unchecked, the mortality from the degenerative non-bacterial diseases will diminish the average expectation of life.'[458]

Such sedentary habits were not solely confined to factory workers who were being replaced by machines. The English physician Robert Saundby noted in 1897 that 'diabetes is undoubtedly rare among people who lead a laborious [manual labour] life in the open air, while it prevails chiefly with those who spend most of their time in sedentary indoor occupations… there is no doubt that diabetes must be regarded as one of the penalties of advanced civilisation.'[459] As Robert Tattersall points out, diabetes was proving to be a dashed nuisance to members of the English aristocracy in India. 'Much of the evidence that diabetes was a disease of the rich came from India. At a meeting on tropical diabetes in 1907, it was said that "what gout is to the nobility of England, diabetes is to the aristocracy of India" and "exercise, as a rule, is disliked by the gentleman class of Bengal after a certain age."'[460] It seems parts of the Raj were being run by men who were increasingly rotund due to a diet rich in starches and sugars, topped off by a complete lack of unbecoming exercise. Gentlemen's subalterns could also fall victim to diabetes, such as one 'Bengali babu' (a clerk who could read and write English), 'whose girth had a great tendency to increase in direct proportion to any increment in his pay.'[461] In contrast, Hindu widows, who lived ascetic lives in comparison to their white 'superiors', were never known to get diabetes.

Bound up with both heart disease and diabetes is the phenomenon of an increasingly heavy population. 'Obesity is not itself a disease,' Sander L Gilman notes, 'but rather a phenomenological category that reflects the visible manifestation of body size, which potentially can have multiple… causes.'[462] Being overweight has long been synonymous with ill health, although the boundaries between the two constantly shift. Obesity doesn't meet Koch's postulates, as Gilman comments. 'No one dies from obesity. One dies from the pathologies that may result from extreme overweight. It may lead to diabetes, which may lead to vascular disease.'[463]

Body weight (and shape and size) were important to the ancients, and 'control of the body and its weight was an intrinsic part of religious belief. The ancient Greeks saw food as part of a complex web that connected human beings and the gods through the humours.' Hippocrates and Galen discussed obesity, seeing it, unsurprisingly, as an imbalance of the humours. Of course, seeing the body in an ideal state, with perfect health, was more Platonic form than reality. Despite being overweight himself, the philosopher Thomas Aquinas (1225–1274) eloquently railed against overindulgence, proclaiming, 'Let us not give our minds to delights, but to what is the end of delights. Here on earth it is excrement and obesity, hereafter it is fire and the worm.' But when he entered the hereafter suddenly at the age of 49, his weight was such that, 'fat as he was, the monks were unable to carry his body down the stairs.'[464]

Obesity has now become such a problem that the World Health Organization coined the word 'globesity' in 2001 to reflect what is now an international problem. As with the Victorian idea that diabetes is one of the 'penalties of advanced civilisation', so with obesity; but the civilisation is decidedly of the corporate-consumer-fast-food-instant-gratification kind. As Gilman comments, 'Obesity is dangerous to society as well as to the individual because it is now globalized: in complex ways obesity is now (as smoking was) a sign of the deleterious effect of the modern (read: the American) influence on the body.'[465]

As civilisation advanced through a combination of mechanisation, overindulgence and sloth, cancer likewise saw an upsurge in the twentieth century. Although 'canker' had been in the English language since probably the fourteenth century,[466] early cases are mainly identifiable through the mention of 'cankers' or tumours. One early example is the story told about Raymond Lully (1232–1315), the Majorcan scholar, alchemist and crusade apologist. He had fallen in love with a beautiful young woman by the name of Ambrosia de Castello, but she continually refused his advances. Exasperated by Lully's persistence, she revealed the reason that she could not return his love: she bared her breast, and Lully could see that it was eaten away by a tumour. (As to what happened next, accounts differ: in one version, Lully realised the folly of carnal desire and pledged to devote his life to serving Christ; in other accounts, Lully gallantly travelled to Mauritania to seek out the alchemist Geber, who was said to possess a cure for cancer.)[467]

Advances in microscopy in the nineteenth century meant that doctors could see evidence of cancer, other than tumours visible to the naked eye. Starting in the late 1820s, the microscope enthusiast Joseph Lister (1786–1869, father of the Lister of antiseptic surgery fame) made improvements to the instrument, principally by having better lenses ground that reduced the amount of optical aberration. With better optics, it became possible to detect the abnormal cells that are cancer's hallmark. Within a few years of Lister's improvements, Thomas Hodgkin (1798–1866) described cancer of the lymph nodes (Hodgkin's lymphoma), using one of Lister's new microscopes. Lister got himself elected to the Royal Society for his work, and histology took a huge step forward. Just as the discovery of the lymphatic system in the seventeenth century had helped end the humoural theory, so now the new work being done on lymphs helped pave the way for cell theory, which revolutionised our understanding not only of cancer, but also of life itself.

German physician Johannes Peter Müller (1801–1858) built on Hodgkin's work, theorising that cancer develops when new cells form, while Theodor Schwann (1810–82) and Matthias Jakob Schleiden (1804–81) suggested that cells are fundamental to all life. Schwann and Schleiden's new cell theory proposed that all living organisms are composed of one or more cells, and that the cell is the most basic unit of life. In 1855, Rudolf Virchow added a third tenet to the theory, that all cells arise only from pre-existing cells (the Latin form, *Omnis cellula e cellula*, became something of a cell-theoretician's motto). Virchow suggested that cancer sprang from abnormal cellular changes, having noticed that leukaemia was indicated by the proliferation of white blood cells. No one took Virchow's theory seriously at the time, but he has since proved to be in essence correct. As we now know, abnormal cell division is the common feature to all forms of cancer.

Research into cancer continued, aided by further advances in technology, such as the discovery of X-rays by Wilhelm Röntgen in 1895, which could detect deeper tumours; of radium by Marie and Pierre Curie in 1898, which could be used in treatment; and the development of another treatment, chemotherapy, by Paul Ehrlich in the first decade of the twentieth century (whose laboratory also developed salvarsan, the first effective modern treatment for syphilis). Some discoveries were accidental. It was found that soldiers who had been the victims of mustard gas attacks in the First World War had significantly lower white blood counts than those who had not, the so-called Krumbhaar effect. Research was conducted at Yale University in the 1940s into nitrogen mustard (the active ingredient of the gas) as a possible cancer treatment. Although it wasn't used as a prescription treatment, it did assist in the development of new forms of chemotherapy.[468] Cancer, of course, was one of the diseases included in the post-war public health drive, and thousands of potential drugs were tested in the 1950s and 60s for potential anti-cancer properties use.

(While no miracle drug for cancer was found, such campaigns can sometimes lead to useful pharmaceutical discoveries, when a drug developed for disease A actually turns out to be effective against disease B. Its subsequent use against disease B is known as repurposing. One such discovery was that thalidomide, while notoriously causing birth defects in babies in the 1960s, has properties that have been successfully used in treatment for leprosy. It is also effective against certain aspects of HIV infection.[469])

Scientists are still trying to work out why cancer occurs in the first place. Galen thought people developed the disease due to a melancholy humour, an excess of black bile. Victorian doctors viewed the wearing of corsets with suspicion.[470] Later thinkers believed it to be contagious; others, that too much excitement or insufficient exercise was to blame. More recent research suggests that poor diet – especially the diabetes-friendly western kinds – is now thought to account for around one third of all cancers. Processed food, a lack of fruit and vegetables, too much salt and alcohol, are all viewed with the same suspicion that corsets were once subjected to, but with stronger scientific data to back up their possible links to cancer.

Although the list of modern carcinogens is long – more extensive even than anything the Victorians could have thought up – one thing in particular has long been linked to cancer. A paper published as long ago as 1923 highlighted the dangers of smoking, and research conducted in the 1940s found that deaths from lung cancer had gone up exponentially since 1900. Further studies appeared in the 1950s, the era of mass public health initiatives, linking smoking not only to lung cancer, but also to other types of cancer, such as throat, mouth and stomach cancer, and also leukaemia and heart disease.

While doctors were increasingly vocal in their condemnation of smoking, cigarettes were advertised as being good for you, complete with medical endorsement. 'More doctors smoke Camels than any other cigarette!' the ads proclaimed. Lucky Strike were advertised as being effective against throat irritation and coughs, and also apparently had weight loss potential ('To keep a slender figure'); Philip Morris cigarettes were 'born gentle', depicting a mother coddling her newborn baby; L&M filters were 'just what the doctor ordered'. Other brands linked smoking to manliness. Marlboro, after ditching the newborn baby campaign, switched to the rugged Marlboro Man, which became arguably the most iconic of all cigarette campaigns, while Tipalets promised to boost a man's powers of seduction to almost mesmeric levels: 'Blow in her face and she'll follow you anywhere.'

The Marlboro Man was leading a fulfilling life ranching in Idaho, the tobacco companies wanted people to believe. (Perhaps the less said about Tipalets Man, the better.) But from the 1950s tobacco manufacturers knew that cigarettes are addictive and cause cancer, yet spent millions on denial, hiring PR firms, passing the buck and even lying under oath when the matter came up in front of the US Supreme Court. But the truth emerged. As Clive Bates and Andy Rowell note, 'Thousands of internal tobacco industry documents released through litigation and whistleblowers reveal[ed] the most astonishing systematic corporate deceit of all time.'[471] One has to wonder, if corporations can lie for so long about tobacco, what else might they be lying about? But hey, why tell the truth and protect the public's health, when there's a lot of money to be made? It's one of the penalties of an advanced civilisation, after all.

7

New Diseases

Marburg virus

In August 1967, three employees working on vaccines for the pharmaceutical giant Hoechst AG in Marburg, Germany, were taken sick with flu-like symptoms, and were taken to the University Hospital. By the following day, they had enlarged spleens, bloodshot eyes, skin tender to the touch, and 'sullen, slightly aggressive… behaviour'.[472] Other workers from the pharmaceutical plant began to fall ill and, like the original three patients, they had been working on monkey kidney cells. By September, 23 people were very ill, with six more ill in Frankfurt; a third outbreak of the mystery illness occurred in Belgrade. Whatever it was, it was clearly not flu.

Described as agonising, the symptoms of the strange disease progressed from the initial flu-like stage to acute viremia (a physical response to the flood of newly made viruses in the bloodstream): large tender lymph nodes, inflamed spleens, a drop in the number of disease-fighting white blood cells, and a sudden shortage of blood platelets and other factors that are required to stop bleeding. By the sixth day the patients were covered in red rashes, and their skin was too sensitive to be touched. They had raw throats and couldn't eat, requiring them to be hooked up to intravenous drips. Acute diarrhoea set in by the end of the first week. By the eighth day, microscopic blockages had developed under the skin, giving the patient the appearance of a crimson glow. Red blood cells were immobilised, oxygen not getting through, causing intense pain. By day ten they were vomiting blood. After three weeks of this, the patients' skins began peeling off as oxygen- and nutrient-starved cells died by the millions. The most intense pain was around the genitals. The disease appeared to be skinning the patients alive at the same time as bleeding them to death. It appeared to have similarities to acute haemophilia, in that the patients' blood wasn't coagulating properly. As one of the Frankfurt doctors noted, 'Blood is pouring from all apertures'.[473]

By December 1967, six of the patients were dead. Some had become demented and had fallen into comas from which they never emerged. Two of the patients died of massive heart attacks. Several had permanent liver damage, leaving them with chronic lifelong hepatitis. One became psychotic. Several men became impotent.

The new disease was christened Marburg virus, and was classified as an acute viral haemorrhagic fever. The World Health Organization gave Marburg its highest rating in its risk group categorisation of disease, group 4, which means a disease is highly contagious, and requires the full protective suit to be handled safely. There are no known cures. In other words, Marburg is just about as dangerous as a disease can get; plague is only group 3.

The common factor between the Marburg, Frankfurt and Belgrade outbreaks was that all the victims had been working with monkeys from Uganda, a species of vervet monkey called *Cercopithecus aethiops.* The animals had been shipped first to Belgrade, and then on to Germany. When the monkeys arrived in Belgrade, 49 of the shipment of 99 were dead. All had died of massive haemorrhages. A week later, the vet who examined them also contracted Marburg. Then his wife, who had looked after him, also fell sick.

With a clear major medical emergency on their hands, a WHO team flew to Uganda to find the source of the monkey virus. Although they found more infected animals, the WHO team could not find where the virus came from. The mystery of Marburg intensified in 1975, when two Australian backpackers contracted the disease in Rhodesia (modern Zimbabwe). The woman survived, but her boyfriend died. No one knew how the man could have contracted it: he initially thought he'd been bitten on the leg by something. He'd slept outdoors in Rhodesia on zebra-grazing land, handled raw meat in Bulawayo, touched monkeys near the Great Zimbabwe ruins, and hand-fed monkeys caged in the lobby of his hotel in Natal. But scientists couldn't answer the question: how had the man contracted Marburg. And how had it moved from Uganda in 1967 to Rhodesia in 1975?

Lassa fever

In between the two Ugandan and Rhodesian outbreaks of Marburg, another new disease appeared. On 12 January 1969, Laura Wine, a 69-year-old nurse at the Church of the Brethren Mission Hospital in Lassa in eastern Nigeria noticed that she had a bad back. A week later, she also had a sore throat. Penicillin didn't help. Then she became feverish and severely dehydrated. Her heartbeats became irregular, and she began to suffer from unusual blood-clotting; there was a complete lack of proteins in her urine. On 25 January Wine was flown to a bigger hospital, in the town of Jos. But after a day of convulsions, she died. Then Charlotte Shaw, a nurse who had tended Wine in Lassa, became ill. She also died.

When Wine's body was autopsied, the doctors 'gasp[ed] when they saw the devastation; every organ of Shaw's body was seriously damaged. The heart was stopped up, with loads of blood cells and platelets clogging up the arteries and veins. Fluids and blood filled the lungs. Dead cells and fat droplets clogged the liver and spleen. The kidneys were so congested with dead cells and protein that they had failed to function.'[474] There were also no white blood cells in her lymph nodes.

A week later, Lily Pinneo, the assistant at the autopsy, also fell ill. She was transferred first to Lagos, and then to New York City, where she was placed in isolation. Staff in the hospital were afraid of whatever it was Pinneo had; some were 'highly agitated, some clearly fearful'.[475]Her temperature went up to 107° F, her throat filled with lymphatic fluid, and her lungs and chest also filled with fluid. Then

Pinneo developed malaria, followed by spasms and convulsions. The disease began attacking her central nervous system. Doctors thought that she had contracted Marburg, but tests proved negative. Then Jordi Casals, the scientist at Yale who was studying the Lassa microbes, also became ill. He had no idea how he had become infected, having followed every safety precaution in the book. Remarkably, the disease seemed to burn itself out in Pinneo, and by May she had recovered. Casals received plasma from Pinneo, and he too recovered.

Jordi Casals continued to research Lassa, although he was now under threat of being closed down. Although his work was potentially lifesaving, the university felt extremely uneasy at the thought of a lethal disease of unknown provenance getting loose in downtown New Haven. As Laurie Garrett notes, Casals was used to these kinds of problems facing the researcher: 'Ever since he and Karl Johnson had travelled all over the Soviet Union investigating strange haemorrhagic diseases [in the spring of 1965], the pair had discovered that the real danger was not the viruses, but politics.'[476] They had been researching Omsk haemorrhagic fever, Crimean-type fever and Central Asian haemorrhagic fever, and the trip proved very useful for all the scientists. But every time Casals and Johnson returned to the US, they were hounded by the CIA, who clearly had an eye on the biological warfare potential of these new diseases.[477]

With the added pressure of closure and the interest of the CIA, Casals was able to make progress on Lassa. He found that the virus could be spread four ways: by inhaling viral particles, by contact with contaminated urine, through blood to blood contact, 'or by some less clear method involving laboratory mice.'[478] This led Casals to think that the reservoir could be rodents, but he had no proof. And then, somehow, a lab technician, who had not been working with Casals, died of Lassa. It was the excuse the university needed to shut Casals down, and research switched to Level 4 labs at CDC in Atlanta.

The hunt for Lassa's reservoir continued. There was a serious outbreak in Nigeria in January 1970, when 28 people contracted the disease. Blood serum from Lily Pinneo, which had saved the life of Jordi

Casals, was sent but did not get through due to the Biafran war, which was still ongoing at the time. Thirteen died. Scientists managed to get to Sierra Leone in September 1972 when Lassa broke out there. While serum was administered to patients, a large trapping operation was mounted. It was thought that the Lassa reservoir was a common African animal, and so the team set about collecting more than 640 animals, including mice, bats, rats and shrews. One type of common African rat, *Mastomys natalensis*, tested positive for Lassa. Further analysis revealed that Lassa was spread to humans through its droppings. As the rat was a common visitor to people's homes, seeking warmth or food, Lassa could potentially be spread easily. And the disease could already be well established. Scientists didn't know, and waited for the next outbreak.

Ebola

The next major outbreak in Africa was not of Lassa, but of yet another deadly and previously unknown disease, one that would eclipse its two elder siblings. On 28 August 1976, at the Catholic Mission Hospital in Yambuku in northern Zaire (now the Democratic Republic of Congo), a man was admitted, suffering from severe diarrhoea and a nosebleed. The Sisters had no idea who he was, or where he had come from, and were puzzled by his symptoms. After two days, the man discharged himself, and they never saw him again. Another of their patients was a 16-year-old girl, Yombe Ngongo, who was receiving treatment for what appeared to be severe anaemia. Naturally, the nuns didn't link the girl with the man from the bush. Their health problems seemed entirely different.

And then on 1 September, Mabalo Lokela, the headmaster of the local school, appeared, suffering from what was thought to be malaria. He was given shots of quinine, the antimalarial drug, and went home. Four days later, he was back. This time, he was vomiting and had acute diarrhoea, had pains in his chest, his skin was tight and dry, his eyes sunken by serious dehydration. He was also bleeding from the gums, his nose, and there was blood in his diarrhoea and vomit. The Sisters injected him with further shots, but his condition worsened. They gave him aspirin, nivaquine, blood coagulants, calcium, cardiac stimulants, caffeine, camphor and antibiotics. Nothing worked. Mabalo Lokela died on 8 September. A day earlier, Yombe Ngongo had died in her home village.

And then things began to escalate at the Mission Hospital. Over the next two weeks, 21 people died, all showing similar symptoms to Mabalo's. They were suffering from pains in the abdomen and chest; were feverish; had headaches and sore throats; were nauseous and vomited – some were vomiting blood; had diarrhoea but also the inability to pass urine (anuria); joint and muscle pain; general weakness and loss of appetite; had sore, red eyes and suffered from rapid breath. Some developed rashes and suffered from hiccups and experienced a constant ringing in the ears. In addition to the vomiting of blood, some experienced bleeding from the gums and anus. It was not uncommon for patients to go into shock. As Laurie Garrett notes,

> The horror was magnified by the behavior of the many patients whose minds seemed to snap. Some tore off their clothing and ran out of the hospital, screaming incoherently. Others cried out to unseen visitors, or stared out of ghost eyes without recognizing wives, husbands, or children at their sides.[479]

The disease began to spread to the neighbouring villages as terrified patients fled the hospital, taking the disease with them. Huts belonging to dead villagers were burned to the ground in a frantic attempt to stop the disease spreading.

Blood samples were sent to various labs. The one that arrived at the Institute for Tropical Medicine in Antwerp came in a thermos flask. When it was opened, Peter Piot – who was to witness early AIDS cases – recalled, one of the test tubes inside had cracked in transit. Blood was swishing around freely. Piot and his colleagues had no real idea at the time just how much danger they were in. 'Indeed, the Belgians laboured under conditions no more sophisticated or secure than might be found in a typical high school biology lab... all concerned would later express astonishment that they suffered no ill consequences from such frivolous disregard of the potential hazards of the microbes.'[480] Initially suspecting the Yambuku disease to be yellow fever, they performed the necessary tests, but they turned up negative. There was also the possibility that Yambuku was experiencing an outbreak of Marburg, as the symptoms were similar. But when Piot examined blood taken from one of the Sisters, he found something no one had seen before – strange viruses shaped like question marks.

By the time an international team, comprised of people from the CDC, the WHO and a team of Belgians, including Piot, arrived in October, they found that the Yambuku Mission Hospital had closed, as most of the staff had either died from the disease, or were sick. The case fatality rate was 88 per cent, making it one of the most lethal diseases ever known. One of the team admitted that he was 'no Marlboro Man' and was 'scared shitless... I'm really frightened. As, I think, we all should be.'[481] They would not only have to make a thorough inspection of the mission hospital, but also visit every village that had been infected, all of which were now under quarantine. They put on their protective suits and began work.

Blood and tissue samples were sent to Europe and the US for analysis, where the new disease was found to be a virus, somewhat similar to Marburg. In the quest to find the virus's reservoir, hundreds of animals were tested to see if they were the reservoir: 818 types of bug went under the microscope, as did mosquitoes, ten pigs, one cow, six monkeys, two duikers, seven bats, 123 rodents, including 69 mice, 30 rats, and eight squirrels. None of them carried any signs of the disease.[482] The lab work was also not without its risks: just as Jordi Casals had fallen victim to Lassa while studying it at Yale, so one scientist at Porton Down in the UK became ill while examining samples from Zaire. The team of experts warned 'No more dramatic or potentially explosive epidemic of a new acute viral disease has occurred in the world in the past 30 years.'[483]

Peter Piot decided the new disease should not be named Yambuku, to spare the village the stigma of being associated with the horrific outbreak, and so it was named Ebola, after the river some sixty miles from the Yambuku Mission Hospital where Mabalo Lokela had been immediately prior to becoming ill, and possibly where he had also contracted the disease.

After further outbreaks in Zaire and Sudan, Ebola had effectively disappeared by 1979. Its next reported case occurred in very different circumstances. In 1989, in echoes of the 1967 Marburg outbreak in Belgrade, a shipment of lab monkeys from Luzon in the Philippines died of Ebola in a quarantine facility in Reston, Virginia, in the Washington DC metro area. The animals appeared to have died of an airborne variant of the disease, and panic ensued. The building was locked down and sterilised by the US Army Medical Research Institute of Infectious Diseases (USAMRIID). Luckily, none of the staff in Reston developed Ebola. Further research into the virus determined it was a different strain to the one that had proved so fatal in Yambuku, and was christened Reston virus. Despite fieldwork in the Philippines and Indonesia, the source of the outbreak was never found, and no one knows how the virus got to the Philippines in the first place. Alternatively, the virus could have been endemic, but only broken cover when the monkeys were caught and sent to the labs for research. Reston remains one of Ebola's puzzles. As David Quammen noted, 'the good news about Reston virus, derived both from the 1989 US scare and from retrospective research on Luzon, is that it doesn't seem to cause illness in humans, only in monkeys. The bad news is that no one understands why.'[484]

Scientists have, however, been able to piece together how Ebola gets transmitted to humans. As with the animal to human jump that HIV made, Ebola is passed to humans by close contact with infected animals. This usually means animal blood or other secretions entering the human body, or the eating of meat from an infected animal. Chimpanzees, gorillas, fruit bats, monkeys, forest antelope and porcupines are all susceptible to Ebola. (Some scientific studies have focussed on die-offs in these animal populations, in an attempt to predict Ebola's movements and incidence.[485]) The disease is spread between people through direct contact with bodily fluids, or clothes or bedding contaminated with them. Anyone coming into contact with an infected person, such as a nurse or person preparing a body for burial, is at extreme risk. But even shaking someone's hand might pass on the disease. People remain infectious for as long as the virus remains in their blood and bodily fluids, although men who have recovered can still transmit Ebola in their semen for up to seven weeks after recovery.

Further strains of Ebola have been found. In 1994, Taï Forest ebolavirus affected a Swiss scientist in Côte d'Ivoire (she survived); and in 2007 the Bundibugyo ebolavirus emerged in Uganda. The two original strains of the disease have remained active, the Yambuku strain (also known as Zaire ebolavirus), which has remained the most widespread and lethal, and the Sudan strain (Sudan ebolavirus). The Sudan variant is actually the 'original' form of Ebola, breaking out in a cotton factory in Nzara, in what is now South Sudan, and then affecting neighbouring areas between June and November 1976. This outbreak wasn't quite as bad as Yambuku, with a mortality rate of 'only' 53 per cent.[486]

One of the major problems scientists have had in finding Ebola's reservoir is that outbreaks were sporadic until the mid-1990s, when they began to increase in frequency. Indeed, apart from the 1989 outbreak of Reston virus, there was a 15-year silence (1979–1994) from the Zaire strain. A major outbreak in Kikwit in the Democratic Republic of Congo in 1995 became an immediate emergency: Kikwit is a city with a population of over 300,000, the first time Ebola had struck an African city. It was the worst since Yambuku, with 254 deaths – a case fatality rate of 81 per cent. There was a massive trapping operation to find the reservoir: thousands of small mammals, birds, reptiles and amphibians were caught, killed and sampled. Blood was also taken from dogs, cows and pet monkeys. In total, 3,066 samples were sent to the CDC for analysis.[487] The Ebola virus wasn't found in any of them.

Despite this result, the team at CDC were able to make some assumptions: that the reservoir is a mammal, possibly one with a forest habitat – all Ebola outbreaks in Africa had been in or near forests – and that, due to the sporadic nature of the outbreaks, either the reservoir is a rare animal, or it's one that only rarely makes contact with humans. The importance of reservoirs is that if you know where the reservoir lives, you know where the outbreak is likely to occur. But the more scientists studied Ebola, the more blanks they drew.

Studies of Ebola have not focussed exclusively on the science. The American medical anthropologist Barry Hewlett visited areas affected by the 1994 outbreak in Gabon, and also the 2000 outbreak in Gulu, Uganda. Hewlett learned from the local people in Gabon that they believed Ebola to be *ezanga*, meaning a vampire-like evil spirit. One villager told Hewlett that *ezanga* are '"bad human-like spirits that cause illness in people" as retribution for accumulating material goods and not sharing.'[488] (A possible reference to the fact that one of the epicentres of the 1994 outbreak in Gabon was a gold mine.) For those sufficiently versed in magic, *ezanga* could be summoned and directed at an enemy. The effect of *ezanga* was to eat away a person's insides until they died. In Uganda, the Acholi people told Hewlett they thought Ebola was caused by supernatural agency. They called the spirit *gemo*, and it arrived periodically to cause sickness and death. The *gemo* did not cause just Ebola, but also measles and smallpox, which the Acholi had also suffered. Hewlett learned that the disrespect of nature spirits could awaken the *gemo* and make it decide to pay a visit.

Hewlett discovered that once a *gemo* was known to be present in a community, the sick were quarantined, and could only be nursed by a survivor of the same illness (if there were any); people were not allowed to travel to other villages; had to abstain from sex; could not eat rotten or smoked meat; and ordinary burial practices – which included not only washing the body but voiding the stomach and bowels of the deceased – were proscribed. Dancing was also forbidden. Given that most of these activities can put a person in danger of contracting Ebola – even dancing, given that the disease can be spread by sweat, spittle, and expectoration – David Quammen speculates that these cultural practices may have helped contain the 2000 outbreak in Gulu.[489]

The 2014 outbreak of Ebola was the worst yet recorded, and marked the first time the disease has reached epidemic proportions.

It also marked the first time Ebola cases had been reported in West Africa. The epidemic began in the Guéckédou prefecture of southern Guinea in December 2013, with the death of a two-year-old child and his mother. The virus spread throughout the family, and seems to have been disseminated further at the various funerals, and also by doctors treating the sick, who then themselves died of Ebola. On 10 March 2014, the local health authorities reported the crisis to the Guinean Ministry of Health, at which time the epidemic came to the notice of international health bodies. On 8 August, the World Health Organization declared the epidemic to be a Public Health Emergency of International Concern (PHEIC), the WHO's equivalent of a red alert.

Despite heroic efforts to contain the epidemic, there were serious problems in getting aid to the sick. Much of this had to do with the poor infrastructure in the affected countries. Liberia, Guinea, and Sierra Leone were all countries recovering from decades of civil wars, unrest and instability. As might be expected, levels of public health care were very low, and none had much in the way of immediate resources to throw at the crisis. Unlike the Acholi in Uganda during the 2000 outbreak, people were reluctant to abandon traditional burial practices and stay put. The relative closeness of affected areas to big cities, and their transport networks, meant that the epidemic spread easily. And international aid, when it came, was too late to stop the situation getting out of control.[490] By the start of 2015, the World Health Organization had recorded over 24,000 cases and around 10,000 deaths. The case fatality overall was in the region of 70 per cent.[491]

Studies published during the epidemic noted some important features. A paper published in *The New England Journal of Medicine* found that the virus was not Taï Forest virus, which was the 'local' form of Ebola (Côte d'Ivoire, where Taï Forest virus had broken out in 1994, shares a border with Guinea), but was a variant of the Zaire strain. A second study, published in *Science Express* (a satellite publication of the journal *Science*), noted that the Ebola virus is mutating, and that the 2014 epidemic was probably the result of a single spillover from the animal reservoir to humans. Five of the co-authors of the *Science*

Express paper had died of Ebola before publication, giving it, as David Quammen notes, 'a certain extra gravitas.'[492]

Both papers agreed that Ebola's reservoir could be bats. A large number of diseases are known to come from bats, including Marburg, rabies, SARS (see below), Nipah (see below) and a group of relatively little-known viruses such as Kyasanur Forest virus, Menangle virus, Hendra virus, Tioman virus and Australian bat lyssavirus. Bats make good reservoirs because they have existed in their present form for around fifty million years, meaning that their association with disease is of extremely long standing, more than enough time to develop possible immunity to just about everything, or at least a higher level of resistance. Bats are also very social, and live in close proximity to each other, meaning that any disease one picks up is very easily spread within the community. Bat communities are also sufficiently large for a disease to remain within them, rather than die out. (Known as Critical Community Size: see Chapter 1.) There are also many bats in many species: one in four mammals is a bat. Bats can also cover surprisingly large distances each night on their forages for food.

It seems possible that Ebola has been spreading through the bat colonies of central and west Africa for decades, mutating as it goes. How many bats are infected, no one knows. As to where it will strike next, that too is unknown. And, perhaps most remarkably of all, scientists still don't know exactly *how* Ebola kills people. The most likely route is by causing immune system collapse, and then flooding the body with replicating viruses. As David Quammen notes, 'The current scientific understanding of ebolaviruses constitutes pinpricks of light against a dark background.'[493]

Other New Diseases: The Coming Plagues

Ebola, Lassa and Marburg are – along with HIV/AIDS – perhaps the most well-known of the new diseases that have appeared since the 1960s. But there are many more. Arno Karlen lists another twenty-four that have appeared since 1951, among them: Korean, Dengue, Bolivian, Argentine and Venezuelan haemorrhagic fevers, Kyasanur Forest disease, Chikungunya, Human babesiosis, O'nyong-nyong fever, Oropouche, LaCrosse Encephalitis, intestinal capillariasis, Pontiac fever, human toxoplasmosis, Lyme disease, Rift Valley fever, toxic shock syndrome, Brazilian purpuric fever and human ehrlichiosis. Karlen notes that this list is only a fraction of the new diseases that have appeared.[494]

Not all new diseases have come out of the forests of Africa. Legionnaires' disease first appeared in 1976, striking a convention of the American Legion at a hotel in Philadelphia. Caused by the bacteria of the *Legionella* genus, unknown prior to 1976, the disease can cause fatal pneumonia. Initially thought to be caused by toxic chemicals or even sabotage – American authorities were on high alert at the time due to fears of a possible swine flu epidemic – it transpired that the bacteria had been spread by the hotel's air conditioning.

Intensive factory farming methods are also implicated. Bovine spongiform encephalopathy (BSE, otherwise known as mad cow disease) first appeared in the UK in 1984. BSE is a neurodegenerative condition that is thought to have been caused by feeding cows – normally herbivorous beasts – all manner of refuse from slaughtered animals. Some of this fodder – brains and spinal cords in particular – are thought to have been infected with the sheep disease scrapie, which then made the species jump into cattle. Because of the forced feeding of other animals to cows, BSE has been dubbed 'high-tech cannibalism'.[495] BSE can cause new variant CJD in humans, sometimes called the 'human mad cow disease', through eating the meat of infected animals. It causes the rapid onset of dementia and death, and is incurable.

The study of CJD led to the discovery of a new form of infection – the prion – in 1982, by the American neurologist Stanley Prusiner. An aberrant form of protein, the prion is able to self-replicate and causes a number of diseases in animals aside from BSE. In humans, prions cause the various forms of CJD (including new variant CJD), Kuru, fatal familial insomnia and the extremely rare Gerstmann–Sträussler–

Scheinker syndrome. The discovery of prions won Prusiner a Nobel Prize in 1997.

Factory farming also spread Nipah virus, which first appeared in Indonesia in 1999. As noted above, this disease originally came from bats. Initially causing fever, vomiting and flu-like symptoms, Nipah then attacks the nervous system, and can cause brain damage and hallucinations before death occurs. One pig farmer who survived the 1999 outbreak reported seeing pigs running around his hospital bed.[496] The outbreak caused 257 cases in humans, 100 of them fatal. Over a million pigs were culled to stop Nipah spreading.

Intensive farming is also linked to the first pandemic of the twenty-first century, SARS (Severe Acute Respiratory Syndrome). It began simply enough, with a man visiting the hospital in the Chinese town of Foshan, in Guangdong province, with flu-like symptoms on 16 November 2002. The doctors were puzzled by his condition, but as he didn't die, no one was worried. The man was discharged after treatment, and was never heard from again. But he seems to have inadvertently set up a chain of infection that started working immediately. Then, in January 2003, a seafood merchant in the province's capital, Guangzhou, was taken ill. Retrospectively, the World Health Organization realised he was what's known as a 'super-spreader' – a modern-day equivalent of Typhoid Mary, capable of infecting many more people than would normally be the case. The seafood merchant infected staff in three hospitals, and also infected a professor who was travelling to Hong Kong. The professor then turned the ninth floor of the Hotel Metropole in Hong Kong into a locus of disease, before dying in early March. Other people staying at the Metropole spread the infection across Hong Kong, while others flew abroad, to Vietnam, Canada and Singapore, carrying SARS with them.

The World Health Organization had first been alerted to the new disease in late February by their man in Hanoi, an Italian doctor by the name of Carlo Urbani. He had been rushed off his feet by the new disease, reporting to Geneva that it produces initial flu-like symptoms before developing into pneumonia. Urbani reported that the disease was also affecting hospital staff at an alarming rate. One of his patients had been staying at the Metropole hotel in Hong Kong. By the end of March, both the man from the Metropole and Dr Urbani himself had died from the new disease.

Alarmed at how fast 'atypical pneumonia' was spreading around the world, the WHO issued an emergency travel alert on 15 March 2003. Cases had been reported in Canada, Spain, Germany and the UK, and there were fears it could spread further. Screenings at airports were introduced, some people were placed in quarantine, and the white cotton face mask – so much a feature of the Spanish Flu of 1918 – became a common sight in China.

The WHO believed 'atypical pneumonia' might be an influenza-type disease, as it was marked by similar symptoms – a high temperature, aching muscles, chills and a sore throat. Some even thought it might be pneumonic plague. Tests soon showed that the new, as yet unnamed disease caused severe damage to the lungs, and didn't respond to antibiotics. The WHO coordinated an international team of experts to study the new disease, which was christened SARS. It was found to be a coronavirus, of the same family as the common cold. No one was able to explain why SARS should be so much deadlier, or why it appeared. In June 2003 an international conference on SARS was held in Kuala Lumpur, Malaysia, with 900 participants from 44 countries. By the end of the month, the pandemic was declared officially over.

As with its origins, SARS had an equally sudden and mysterious end. 32 countries had been affected, with 8000 cases and more than 900 deaths.[497] The speed of SARS shows how modern travel has sped up the development of pandemics to 'fast forward'. It took the Black Death over ten years to travel along the Silk Road to the West; now it would arrive in ten hours (or less) on a plane. The pandemic also demonstrates how seriously the WHO and international health authorities took the outbreak, with work starting on analysing the virus immediately. The first paper on SARS – identifying it as a new, deadly coronavirus – was published on 8 April 2003, less than six weeks after Carlo Urbani had first reported the Hanoi outbreak.

Aside from its rapid international spread, SARS became a red alert because scientists have long been expecting another influenza pandemic, and have been expecting that pandemic to possibly start in pigs (as the Spanish Flu might have done in 1918) or birds. SARS is now known to have originated in bats, which then spread to birds and then to humans via intensively-reared poultry sold in Chinese markets. Something similar had happened in China only a few years earlier, in fact. A new strain of flu, H5N1, had appeared in Guangdong province only in 1996, when it affected geese. This avian influenza (bird flu) then spread to Hong Kong, where it made the species jump in the city's poultry markets and killed six people (out of a total of eighteen infected). The authorities reacted quickly and drastically, killing all the city's poultry – over a million and a half birds – and closing the markets down while large-scale disinfecting operations took place.

The appearance of H5N1 in 1996 was only the latest in a line of influenza mutations stretching back to the Spanish Lady herself. That pandemic had been a variant of the H1N1 strain, and scientists have long wanted to find this exact strain in order to try and work out why it was so lethal. Whenever well-preserved tissue from 1918 victims has been found – sometimes in the permafrost of Arctic or Alaskan graves – they have put the samples under the microscope hoping for some clue into why the Spanish Flu was the deadliest pandemic in history, well aware that the influenza virus continually mutates. There have been further flu pandemics: the Asian Flu in 1957, which was the H2N2 strain; the 1968 Hong Kong flu, another new variant, H3N2 (the strain currently circulating in humans); and then in 1977, there was a brief re-emergence of H1N1. (The previous year in the USA, H1N1 had also reappeared in Fort Dix, New Jersey. Although it only killed one soldier, it was similar enough to the 1918 strain to spark a mass immunisation programme; even President Ford got himself vaccinated.)

Part of the problem with the 1996–7 outbreak of H5N1 had been the growth of the Chinese poultry market. Not only were there more birds than ever before, but they had been intensively reared in factory farm conditions, meaning that they had been pumped full of chemicals to make them bigger, and therefore more profitable. In the quest for profit, the birds are kept in tiny spaces, and are injected with cheap vaccines. The result is 'another unadvertised by-product of globalization', as Andrew Nikiforuk has dubbed it.[498] The principal cause of bird flu outbreaks has been

> our gluttonous appetite for cheap, industrially produced meat. Crowded bird factories, rampant bird smuggling, bad vaccines, and duplicitous governments have all played a role in fouling the proverbial nest. Medical professionals may not like to admit it, but avian flu is a fairly predictable man-made plague or what scientists cryptically call a "deliberately emerging microbe". Even the UN Food and Agriculture Organization has repeatedly concluded that avian flu owes its global reach to "the intensification and concentration of livestock production in areas of high density human populations."[499]

Factory farming and globalisation both, it could be argued, fall under William McNeill's definition of macroparasitism.[500] The simplest analogy for this is taxation: governments tax their populations, but leave them just enough money to continue subsisting. (Microbes behave the same way with their hosts: if they are too virulent, they will kill their host and in doing so, probably also themselves.) In globalisation, the desire for profit pushes all else aside, including public health concerns. It happened in Sunderland in 1831, when the Marquis of Londonderry didn't want quarantine restrictions against cholera imposed so that he could continue making money; quarantine opponents in the USA cited the same reasons whenever yellow fever threatened to dent their pocketbooks; it happened in India in 1883, when the British sent a team of 'experts' to tackle cholera, knowing that their results would not hamper trade; the British knew their Indian canals would exacerbate malaria, but that didn't stop their irrigation programme. The list could go on. In sucking up every last cent and penny, capitalism behaves as the most blatant form of macroparasitism. Indeed, if war is a mass psychosis, as Cartwright and Biddiss suggest in their survey of the effect of disease on history, then it is probably not wishful thinking to suggest that capitalism is also a disease that has reached pandemic proportions.

The Return of Pandora's Box

In addition to new diseases, numerous diseases that were once controlled or limited through drugs or containment strategies are now making a comeback. Among them: cholera, diphtheria, genital herpes, giardiasis, viral hepatitis, malaria, measles, pertussis, pneumonic plague, syphilis, tuberculosis and viral encephalitis.[501]

In many cases, these diseases are making a comeback because they have outsmarted the vaccines that were developed to control them. Tuberculosis is a case in point. After effective treatments were developed in the early 1950s, TB had been on the decline. The so-called Edinburgh Method, pioneered by John Crofton and his team, in which the patient was treated with three drugs simultaneously, was seen as one of the great miracle cures in an age of miracle cures. With further developments in treatment over the next few decades, tuberculosis seemed to have been beaten.

But then TB began to fight back. Since the late 1980s, there has been a worldwide increase in the number of new cases. The rise is linked to several factors. After the development of anti-TB drugs, research into the disease became less of a priority in the developed world, as it was thought to have been conquered. But TB was evolving all the time, becoming resistant to the existing treatments. The AIDS epidemic also played a part in TB's renaissance: people with HIV are more susceptible to TB. In Africa, the incidence of TB has tripled or quadrupled since the 80s, while in some countries, as many as 70 to 80 per cent of their TB patients are also HIV positive. In the former Soviet Union, the collapse of communism was accompanied by a rise in TB, as living standards fell and healthcare systems made the faltering transition to western, market-led models. Cases of tuberculosis also rose in affluent countries. In New York City alone, cases of TB almost tripled between 1978 and 1992, particularly among the homeless (who did not have access to free medical care). The worldwide resurgence of the disease led the WHO to declare tuberculosis a global emergency in 1993. The emergency is still ongoing, with around 60 per cent of the cases of multidrug resistant TB occurring in Brazil, China, India, Russian Federation and South Africa.[502]

Microbial evolution has also led to the appearance of the so-called 'superbugs', of which MRSA is perhaps the most widespread and best known. When Alexander Fleming discovered penicillin he had been working on a bacteria called *Staphylococcus aureus*, a common cause of skin complaints, respiratory diseases and food poisoning. It also became resistant to penicillin in the 1950s, forcing the development of a new class of antimicrobial drugs called methicillin, introduced in the 1960s. The bacteria, however, evolved quickly and soon became resistant to methicillin also. The first outbreak of MRSA – methicillin resistant *Staphylococcus aureus* – occurred at Queen Mary's Hospital for Children at Carshalton in Surrey, spreading to eight of the 48 wards, infecting 37 patients and killing one. It quickly went global, favouring hospitals. As Michael Shnayerson and Mark Plotkin put it, MRSA 'was like a feasting hyena that saw no need to range beyond the watering hole where its most vulnerable prey gathered.'[503] It is, in some ways, a twenty first century equivalent of typhus, which preferred jails and the courtrooms of the Black Assizes. There are now at least eleven different strains of MRSA[504], and the disease has now spread to nursing homes, day-care centres, schools, sports centres and fitness clubs, military bases and jails.

MRSA is a bacterium that can live on any surface and 'is almost as hardy as anthrax'.[505] Around 30 per cent of people carry the bacterium in their nostrils (its main home in the human body), or on their skin, in their armpits or perineum. It is thought that about 20 per cent of the population are lifelong carriers of MRSA, with 60 per cent doing so intermittently, and 20 per cent never. MRSA skin infections can cause painful, pus-filled boils and conditions like cellulitis; sometimes a pus-filled lump can form under the skin. If the bacteria get into the bloodstream via a break in the skin – a surgical incision, for instance

– they can cause life-threatening infections such as blood poisoning, heart problems, pneumonia, urinary tract infection, septic arthritis, osteomyelitis and septic bursitis (an inflammation of the bursa, small fluid-filled sacs that lie under the skin and in joints). If it penetrates the bone, MRSA may ultimately require the amputation of the affected limb. MRSA can also cause toxic shock syndrome, itself a relative newcomer to the disease canon (the first case being reported in 1978).

Outbreaks of MRSA in the UK in the 1990s, verging on an epidemic, highlighted the problems faced in combatting the disease. It broke out in three hospitals in Kettering, Northamptonshire, in April 1992, infecting 400 patients and 27 staff. It quickly spread to 15 hospitals and 845 patients in neighbouring counties, and then to London and other parts of the UK. By September 1994 it had infected 21 London hospitals, and four others. MRSA had spread via a combination of patient and staff transfers between hospitals, and by the year 2000, 'was common everywhere in Britain.'[506] Part of the reason hospitals have become MRSA's favoured hunting ground is related to the 'Five Cs', posited by the CDC as greatly increasing the risk of MRSA: crowding, contact, cleanliness, compromised skin and contaminated personal care items. If a hospital is overcrowded or dirty, and also does not have enough to staff to either care for patients or clean the place, then MRSA will thrive. Cuts to the funding of the UK National Health Service by succeeding governments, leading to chronic shortages of beds, nurses, and also contracting cleaning duties out to poorly-regulated private sector companies, have all been manna from heaven as far as MRSA is concerned.

While evolution has played an undoubted part in the resurgence of some diseases, another factor has been the over-prescribing of medication, antibiotics in particular. We are simply popping too many pills. As Sally Davies, the Chief Medical Officer of England, notes, 'We have taken antibacterial and other anti-microbial drugs for granted for too long. We have misused them through overuse and false prescription, and as a result, the bugs are growing in resistance and fighting back.'[507] Repeated use of antimicrobial drugs can reduce the number of good bacteria in the body, weakening the immune system. In taking a pill for everything, we might be keeping the bad bacteria at bay, but we are often killing the good ones off, as well. We are collectively suffering from the proverbial 'too much of a good thing'. The overuse of antibiotics might also be linked to the lifestyle diseases we looked at in the last chapter. Microbiologist Martin J Blaser believes that overuse of antibiotics has also played a part in what he calls our modern plagues: the rise of obesity, asthma, allergies, diabetes, and certain cancers.[508]

It's not just in over-prescription that antibiotics present a danger, but also through their overuse in agriculture and the food industry; they are used, for instance, to fatten animals up, and in pesticides. Macroparasitic capitalism and Big Pharma are not without blame here. Indeed, as James Le Fanu has written that drug companies 'have orchestrated this massive upswing in drug prescribing to their advantage'.[509] The upshot of this limitless greed could have disastrous consequences. Sally Davies warns that:

> if we do not change the course of history, and if we allow resistance to increase, in a few decades we may start dying from the most commonplace of ailments that can today be treated easily. We will regress to the point where, in twenty years' time, when I need a hip replacement, the operation may be deemed too dangerous to even attempt due to the risk of catching an untreatable infection.[510]

Some diseases have been helped through human intervention of a different kind. Fearing that certain vaccines might lead to conditions like autism, many parents have refused to get their children vaccinated, and an anti-vaccination movement has grown up in the United States and elsewhere. While a concern for side-effects and an aversion to corporate big bucks might be understandable (also fuelled by the fear that vaccines cause conditions like autism), it has also contributed to the needless rise of preventable diseases like measles.[511] If we're going to count capitalism as a disease for the sake of argument, then we should probably also label stupidity as one.

Climate change could also bring old diseases back, and introduce new ones. As Jolyon M Medlock and Steve A Leach note in a paper published in *The Lancet* in March 2015, 'the early part of the twenty-first century [has seen] an unprecedented change in the status of vector-borne disease in Europe'.[512] Although malaria has been absent from the UK since 1911, warmer temperatures could tempt the disease-carrying mosquitoes back; the early twenty first century has seen malaria reappear in Greece. West Nile virus, which also has the mosquito as a vector, could also make an appearance. West Nile has already been confirmed in parts of Eastern Europe, and tick-borne diseases such as Lyme Disease continue to increase. As Medlock and Leach point out, 'These changes are in part due to increased globalisation, with intercontinental air travel and global shipping transport creating new opportunities for invasive vectors and pathogens. However, changes in vector distributions are being driven by climatic changes and changes in land use, infrastructure, and the environment.'[513]

*

Speaking of infrastructure and the environment, before we go, biological warfare and bioterrorism deserve a mention. Biological warfare is certainly not new: one theory suggests that the ancient Hittites deliberately set rams infested with tularemia, a devastating bacterial infection that remains deadly even today, on their enemies.[514] If this were true, then it would mark the first time humans had deliberately used disease as a weapon. And when a plague-infested Tatar army attacked the city of Kaffa in the Crimea in 1346, the corpses of the dead soldiers were catapulted over the walls into the city. Plague broke out in Kaffa, and when Genoese merchants in the city decided that the coast was clear, they returned home, and brought the Black Death with them.

In 1942, the small Scottish island of Gruinard was infected with anthrax. It was part of a test to see how well the disease might work as a biological weapon against Nazi Germany. The anthrax proved so virulent – all the sheep on Gruinard were dead within days – it was decided that if it was used against Germany, millions of innocent Germans might die. Furthermore, large swathes of the German countryside might be out of bounds for years. Having such an apocalyptic wasteland in the heart of post-war Europe would, it was felt, hamper reconstruction and de-Nazification efforts, and the plan was scrapped. Pyres were lit on Gruinard for the dead sheep, and the island was left under strict quarantine for forty-five years. It was finally declared safe in 1990. (Although it had become something of a tourist attraction in the meantime, with local boat owners offering tours around – but not landing on – 'anthrax island'.)

In 2001, just after the 9/11 attacks, anthrax spores were sent in the post to several US media companies as well as two Democratic senators. Five people died, and seventeen others were taken ill. A disaffected former government scientist was thought to be behind the attacks, although some doubt has been cast on this.[515] The anthrax attacks highlight the continual security threat posed by deadly diseases stored in research facilities, and the blurred lines between bioweapons and public health. USAMRIID, which cleaned up the Reston incident in 1989, was founded as a bioweapons lab, but was rebranded to fight disease. And when the next pandemic strikes – be it SARS, bird flu, or an act of terrorism – it may well need coordinated might the size of the US military to defeat it.

*

SARS, as Thomas Abraham argues, offered valuable lessons on how to fight the threat of global disease in the twenty first century:

> It demonstrated the importance of early, transparent disease reporting, without which a new disease can spread rapidly across the world. It showed us that global cooperation on many levels is required to control a disease. Scientists and doctors need to share information and collaborate to find the best ways of treating a new

> disease and preventing its spread. Governments have to recognize that a disease in any one part of the world is a threat to every other part of the world, and work together to fight common threats. The test of how well these lessons have been learned will be when the next new disease emerges in the not too distant future.[516]

But, Abraham cautions, politicians need to get their priorities right. 'If SARS has helped to awaken people and governments across the world, particularly in Asia, of the devastation that a new disease can cause, then at least some small good would have come out of the epidemic. But it is not apparent that this has happened.'[517]

Andrew Nikiforuk ends *Pandemonium*, his study of emerging twenty first century diseases, by noting that 'waiting for governments to do the right thing can be a hazardous enterprise and a test of patience.'[518] He suggests that we can do something useful while we wait, by changing how we eat, buy and live. 'If unrestrained global trade in all living things has created unparalleled biological mayhem, then maybe it's time to act and think more locally… to return to personal and local virtues that question bigness and power. Maybe it's time to learn a new canticle for creation that encourages, as Saint Francis did, humility.'[519] Nikiforuk's 'Canticle for Local Living' suggests buying locally grown, organic food, and in doing so, he harks back to the Hippocratic ideal that 'food shall be our medicine'. Both Nikiforuk and Sally Davies remind us that we can all take a stand in the fight against disease, simply by washing our hands regularly and taking fewer antibiotics.[520]

Hippocrates stressed the importance of diet, exercise, and the airs, waters and places in which we live, for maintaining good health. Health was a matter of balance, and disease appeared as a consequence of living out of balance. Hippocrates was revolutionary in his simplicity. He may have been wrong on the four humours, but he was right in broad stroke terms about so much else. Similarly, the cures for some of our modern ailments could lie in other ancient sources. As I was completing this book, a team from the University of Nottingham claimed to have found a cure for MRSA in *Bald's Leechbook*. The recipe, originally for an eye salve, involves onions, garlic, wine and cow's bile that has been 'astonishingly' effective against the superbug in laboratory tests.[521]

Perhaps we will somehow maintain a better balance between health and disease through a combination of Hippocrates' advice, further research into old texts, and a greater emphasis on open source – rather than corporate – research and drug repurposing. (As we've seen from Bald's apparent cure for MRSA, the drugs in question don't have to be modern, expensive or synthesised in a laboratory.)

Meanwhile, in high security vaults, supposedly extinct diseases continue to slumber. One such dweller in the vaults is smallpox. Although officially eradicated in 1980, the disease now spends its leisure hours in Fort Detrick, Maryland, and elsewhere. Pandora's Box has moved underground, and gone high-tech. Let's hope it's never opened again. Once, back in the age of myth, was enough.[522]

Afterword: COVID-19

Scientists had been warning for years that there would be another pandemic. The consensus held that it would likely be a new form of influenza, a Spanish Flu for the twenty-first century. So when the long-feared pandemic turned out to be a virus related to SARS, the world – or at least, the West – was unprepared.

We still do not know precisely how COVID-19 began. What we do know is that on 30 December 2019, Li Wenliang, a doctor at Wuhan Central Hospital, in the Chinese province of Hubei, warned colleagues on WeChat, the Chinese social media platform, about seven cases of what Li initially thought was SARS. All the infected people had had contact with Huanan Seafood Market in Wuhan. He warned his colleagues to get ready to take precautions in case the outbreak spread, and not to circulate the information. But word got out fast: ProMED, a non-profit online bulletin board run by the International Society for Infectious Diseases, reported the new disease as 'undiagnosed pneumonia' on the same day, and requested further information.

Further information was not immediately forthcoming. The Chinese authorities, perhaps fearing a revival of the criticism they faced over their handling of SARS (whose outbreak they had initially denied), were maintaining a strict silence about what was going on in Wuhan. But by 31 December, 27 people were in hospital in Wuhan, all suffering from the new mystery disease, seven of them critical.[523] The health authorities disinfected the seafood market, and told its employees to wear masks. In the early hours of the following day, 1 January 2020, the Huanan Seafood Market was closed down permanently. But had the new virus actually originated there?

The Huanan Seafood Market was close to the Wuhan Centre for Disease Control and Prevention (indeed, one of the CDC's offices was a few minutes' walk away), which had been researching the origin of SARS. Some nine miles away on the other side of the city, across the Yangtze river, is the Wuhan Institute of Virology, also involved in SARS research. SARS is a coronavirus, so-called because the virus is haloed by spikes, giving it the appearance of a crown. Teams from Wuhan had been making regular trips to a copper mine in the Mojiang region of southern China, the source of a mystery pneumonia-like illness that had killed several miners in 2012. The virus that caused this illness was a novel coronavirus, related to SARS, but not identical to it; it was thought to have originated in bats that lived in the mine. The scientists regularly took field samples of bat blood and faeces back to the labs in Wuhan for examination. Could a leak from one of these samples have triggered the new mystery illness that was now filling Wuhan's hospitals to capacity? We will probably never know. The SARS pandemic had been a wake-up call for the Chinese authorities: although there were only some 8,000 infections, it had a mortality rate of 10%, leading to 774 known fatalities across 29 countries, and required an unprecedented level of international co-operation to bring it under control. China's leaders were criticised for the way in which they handled the outbreak, preferring secrecy in an attempt to maintain face. When the new disease appeared in Wuhan in December 2019, the same secrecy prevailed. At least initially.

On 3 January 2020, China formally admitted that a pneumonia-like disease had broken out in Wuhan. What the Chinese didn't say was that – perhaps worried the new disease was a mutation of SARS – they had also forced Li Wenliang to retract his earlier social media warnings, accusing him of scaremongering.

On this day, the BBC ran their first story on the outbreak.

On 4 January, the United Nations incident management system went into stand-by mode, ready to assist in an international response should one be called for. (And it looked increasingly likely that one would.)

On 6 January, the Centre for Disease Control in Beijing announced that there was no evidence for person-to-person transmission.[524] Still trying to control the narrative, officials in Beijing were incensed when a team of researchers, who had been working round the clock, posted some of the new virus's genetic sequence on the online platform GenBank.[525] International concern at the outbreak was growing, and so was a sense of alarm in the international medical community. The Chinese authorities were still keeping largely silent on what exactly was going on in Wuhan.

And what was going on in Wuhan was catastrophe. The city's hospitals were filling fast with people suffering from the new illness. Patients at first suffered a fever and a dry cough, a loss of taste and smell, aches all over the body (including headaches), progressing to difficulty breathing, blood clots, pneumonia, organ failure and death.[526]

On 9 January, the Chinese authorities confirmed that the 'Wuhan pneumonia' was a coronavirus. The first reported death came on 11 January, a 61-year-old man who had visited the Seafood Market. By 12 January, respiratory wards in Wuhan were close to reaching capacity. The following day came the first report of a case outside China, from Thailand, where a 61-year-old woman visiting from Wuhan had fallen sick.

On 11 January, the virus's entire genome sequence was published online. The new virus was initially given the name 2019-nCoV (which simply means novel coronavirus, first reported in 2019).

On 16 January, Japan reported its first case. The following day, Thailand reported a second case.

On 20 January, human-to-human transmission of the virus was confirmed; the United States confirmed its first case.

On 21 January, the World Health Organization (WHO) began issuing daily situation reports, which were to make for increasingly grim reading. It noted that there had been 278 cases, including two in Thailand, one in Japan and one in South Korea.

On 23 January, Wuhan and other cities in Hubei province went into lockdown in an attempt to contain the spread of the virus. Lockdown is a strategy designed to break the chain of transmission. As it was clear that the new disease was contagious, limiting the movement of people and person-to-person contact became a major way to break the chain of transmission, and because the virus had an approximate two-week lifespan, a lockdown of more than two weeks would in theory be enough to stop the spread of the disease. The WHO praised this extraordinarily drastic move, calling it 'unprecedented in public health history'.[527] Sadly, it would be the first of many such precedents.

On 24 January, two papers were published in the medical journal *The Lancet* that detailed the clinical effects of the new virus.[528] It was clear that it was not SARS, but something similar: not only could it spread between humans, but it could do so sometimes asymptomatically. Its reproduction number was later estimated to be between 2 and 3,[529] which means that every infected person could infect up to another three people, meaning the spread of the disease would be exponential: on 2 January, there had been 41 reported cases;[530] by 24 January, this had risen to 835;[531] by 11 February, the tally was up to a staggering 42,708 confirmed cases in China, with more than 1,000 deaths.[532]

On 30 January, the WHO announced a Public Health Emergency of International Concern (PHEIC), stating that:

> all countries should be prepared for containment, including active surveillance, early detection, isolation and case management, contact tracing and prevention of onward spread of 2019-nCoV infection, and to share full data with WHO.[533]

The announcement could not have come a moment too soon. By the end of January, cases of 2019-nCoV had been confirmed in a further 23 countries: the United States, Taiwan, Hong Kong, Macau, Singapore, Vietnam, France, Nepal, Australia, Canada, Malaysia, Cambodia, Germany, Sri Lanka, Finland, the United Arab Emirates, India, Italy, the Philippines, Russia, Spain, Sweden, and the United Kingdom.

On 7 February, Li Wenliang, the Chinese doctor who had first raised the alarm about the new disease, died from it in hospital in Wuhan.

On 11 February, the virus received a new name: SARS-CoV-2, to establish its genealogy with the earlier disease (SARS itself is officially known as SARS-CoV-1). The disease caused by the virus was named COVID-19.

By the end of February, a further 37 countries had reported cases. By the end of March, it was everywhere.

The International Response

Countries around the world followed China into lockdown. The virus had been confirmed in Italy on 31 January, when a Chinese couple from Wuhan were hospitalised in Rome. COVID-19 erupted in Lombardy in February, and then spread to Veneto and Emilia-Romagna. It didn't remain in the north for long, forcing the government's hand. And so, on 9 March 2020, Italy became the first European country to go into lockdown. The same day, the Italian Prime Minister, Giuseppe Conti, declared a state of emergency, and all flights from China to Italy were suspended.

Spain went into lockdown on 14 March, followed by France three days later. Germany took a slightly different approach, phasing in its restrictions from 13 March, when it began closing schools, bars and clubs, and places of worship; university terms were postponed, and visits to nursing homes prohibited. Sweden's government did not impose a lockdown, on the grounds that it would be unconstitutional. The WHO announced that Europe was now the epicentre of the pandemic, a position it would hold until May, when the epicentre shifted to the Americas.

While countries around the world were shutting down, scientists were racing to develop vaccines. The challenge was immense. Vaccines normally take years to develop and receive approval for use; a vaccine against COVID-19 was needed in a matter of months. To make matters worse, there had never been a successful vaccine for human use against a coronavirus (including SARS and MERS). The WHO stated in

February 2020 that it would probably take eighteen months to develop a safe vaccine. Remarkably, the first vaccines to get approval did not take the year and a half the WHO predicted: in June, China approved the use of vaccines that had not, at that point, completed all their clinical trials (a risk deemed worth taking), while in Russia, the Sputnik V vaccine was given approval for limited use in August, followed by a full roll-out in December. On 2 December, the Pfizer-BioNTech vaccine was approved for use in the UK, with the US following suit nine days later. On 30 December, the Oxford AstraZeneca vaccine was approved for use in the UK.

The most widely distributed vaccines were, broadly speaking, of two kinds: messenger RNA vaccines (mRNA), such as Pfizer-BioNTech and Moderna, and adenovirus vector vaccines, such as Oxford-AstraZeneca and Sputnik V. Traditionally, vaccines had used a version of the pathogen against itself, as in the classic case of Edward Jenner's vaccine against smallpox, which worked by essentially giving his patients cowpox. A vaccine instructs the body to produce an immune response, which it remembers and is able to use against further exposure to the disease in question. Vaccines against SARS-CoV-2 needed to do the same thing, but do so using different methods. Messenger RNA vaccines use mRNA to help stimulate the body's immune response, rather than using the pathogen itself. Messenger RNA teaches the body how to make proteins, which then counteract the virus's spike protein (from the spike of the corona). Adenovirus vector vaccines use a modified adenovirus (the group of viruses that cause the common cold) to introduce the vaccine into the body. The modification is the removal of one gene in the adenovirus, which causes it to become what is known as *replication-deficient*: the vaccine makes the virus unable to reproduce itself. Another key modification is the addition of another gene – creating what is known as a *recombinant* virus – that tricks the virus into replicating a protein, rather than itself. This strengthens the replication deficiency, and makes the vaccine more effective. These vaccines were not all invented from scratch in 2020: research into the use of mRNA in vaccines had been ongoing for over a decade before the pandemic struck (indeed, BioNTech was founded in 2008 to develop mRNA research), while work on adenovirus vector vaccines had been in process since 2012 at the Clinical BioManufacturing Facility in Oxford.[534]

Richard Horton, editor of the medical journal *The Lancet*, argues that merely viewing COVID-19 as a disease that needs to be cured through vaccination and cutting lines of viral transmission (lockdowns, social distancing, wearing masks) is too narrow an approach:

> The reality is that two categories of disease are interacting together and within specific populations: infection with a coronavirus is causing particular harm among those who are older and those who are living with chronic diseases, such as obesity, diabetes and hypertension. Worse, these interactions are clustering within particular social groups according to patterns of inequality deeply embedded within our societies. The aggregation of these connecting conditions – viral infection and chronic non-communicable diseases – on backgrounds of social and economic disparity is worsening the adverse effects of each separate illness. COVID-19 is therefore not a pandemic. It is far worse. It is a syndemic – a synthesis of epidemics. The syndemic nature we face from COVID-19 means that a much more nuanced approach is needed if we are to protect the health of our communities.[535]

The term syndemic was coined in the 1990s by American medical anthropologist Merrill Singer, and can be defined as a cluster of pre-existing systemic weaknesses and inequalities – such as poverty, robustness of (or lack of access to) healthcare services, discrimination – that can worsen the effects of a disease. Singer noticed that AIDS impacted African-American communities in the U.S. with especial severity. It often seemed to do its work alongside diseases like tuberculosis and hepatitis, all of which existed in 'precarious social and economic conditions. These diseases and their associated risks did not simply exist side by side. Each made the other worse.'[536]

To the list of systemic problems we must add government: how quickly they acted, and how widely they were trusted by their people, also played a significant role in combatting COVID-19. While scientists around the world developed vaccines, a number of world leaders were dubbed the 'ostrich alliance'[537] for their denial of the pandemic. The Belarusian dictator, Alexander Lukashenko, described the pandemic as a psychosis, and announced that no one in his country would die from it. The best way to remain healthy was to play sports, drive tractors, and drink vodka (although not, presumably, at the same time). Needless to say, Lukashenko did not order a lockdown. In Brazil, far-right president Jair Bolsonaro remarked 'What do you want me to do about it?' when told that a pandemic was sweeping across the world. Another ostrich, Gurbanguly Berdymukhamedov, the president of Turkmenistan, claimed to have found a method of combatting the pandemic that was reminiscent of preventive measures taken against the Black Death in the fourteenth century: burning the herb yuzarlik. Berdymukhamedov ordered government buildings, offices, markets, schools and, bizarrely, cemeteries, to be fumigated with the herb's smoke twice a day to ward off the virus.

There were honorary ostriches. President John Magufuli of Tanzania did not implement lockdowns or mask wearing; instead, he claimed that his country had fought off COVID through prayer. He then disappeared from view, while government ministers denied that anything was wrong. But the reality was that Magufuli had died from the disease he denied.[538] And of course, Donald Trump managed to outdo himself with remarks and actions that varied between colossally stupid and outright criminal. Trump initially described the pandemic as 'the new hoax',[539] asserting a few weeks later that it would 'go away.' When finally forced to admit that the pandemic was indeed real and was indeed happening, Trump blamed China, by calling it 'the Chinese virus',[540] and then blamed the WHO. Trump cut US funding to the WHO in April 2020, an act that has been described as a crime against humanity.[541]

Plague Island

Swift, decisive action was conspicuous by its absence in Britain. Indeed, the UK was singled out as the country that exemplified how *not* to handle the pandemic, earning the nickname 'plague island'[542] in the process, and suffering the highest death toll (and worst recession) in western Europe.

There is not enough space in a short afterword such as this to exhaustively detail the UK government's shambolic, criminally inept response to COVID-19. Despite claiming that the UK had the best disaster response plans in the world, the country was utterly unprepared for the pandemic, exacerbated by having the worst government and worst prime minister in living memory. The reasons for this colossal failure are multifaceted – indeed, very British – but can be sketched out briefly.

The UK *did* have one of the best disaster-response plans in the world, but that was in 2010, not 2020. A decade of austerity policies had greatly weakened the UK's preparedness, as the 2016 pandemic simulation, Operation Cygnus, made clear. The UK 'could not cope' if a new pandemic struck.[543] The government chose to ignore this. To make matters worse, Brexit happened. Touted by politicians and the press as 'the will of the people', this deeply dishonest referendum can now be seen for what it was: a far-right coup led by self-serving politicians who, quite astonishingly, did not have a plan and did not understand the ramifications of what the UK leaving the EU actually entailed (such as how it might damage the economy, or affect peace in Northern Ireland). Instead, they trumpeted meaningless soundbites such as 'Brexit means Brexit' and fixated on 'getting Brexit done' – the slogan that helped Boris Johnson win the 2019 General Election – even though this was an act of calamitous national self-harm. Such trivia was, naturally, brushed under the carpet, as all great national embarrassments are, and the ideology of hard Brexit came to dominate British politics as the 31 January 2020 deadline for leaving the EU loomed.

When news of the outbreak in Wuhan reached London, Johnson and his government did nothing. (In fact, Johnson spent crucial weeks in February 2020 on holiday.) Johnson was obsessed by Brexit to such an extent that he missed the first five COVID-focussed meetings of COBRA, the UK's crisis advisory committee. Such an approach, if it can be called that, speaks volumes about the British ruling elite's inherent exceptionalism and tacit racism: if a nasty disease is happening in China, then it can't possibly affect an English gentleman. Finally forced to announce something, the prime minister said that the country might have to 'take it on the chin'.[544] This reflected the UK government's initial belief that herd immunity would solve the problem. Let the *hoi polloi* become infected, and the disease would burn itself out. As most of the rest of Europe went into lockdown in March 2020, Johnson continued to do nothing. Major sporting events, such as the Cheltenham Gold Cup, still went ahead, presenting opportunities for the virus to spread rapidly through crowds; Johnson, childishly, went out of his way to be photographed shaking hands with people, announcing on 2 March that life should carry on as normal.[545] With the numbers of infections doubling every three to four days, any delay in announcing a lockdown would cost thousands of lives. SAGE, the UK's scientific advisory group for emergencies, urged Johnson to lock down immediately. He ignored them.

But diseases are no respecters of weak leaders, and the spread of COVID in March 2020 was little short of apocalyptic. When Johnson realised he had no choice and had to finally announce a UK lockdown on 23 March, it was already too late. The virus had been reported in the UK on 31 January, and officially claimed its first life the day Johnson announced the country would take it on the chin.[546] By not locking down a week earlier, when government scientific advisors urged, it is estimated that 20,000 Britons lost their lives.[547] From 23 March until the approval of the Pfizer-BioNTech vaccine on 2 December, the actions of Johnson and his government were a litany of lies, failures, U-turns, double standards, and scandals.

There was the Test and Trace scheme, which saw Baroness Dido

Harding – who had previously worked for supermarket chains and mobile phone companies before working for the NHS – waste in the region of £22 billion on a scheme that Boris Johnson announced would be 'world beating'. The scheme, notable for its use of vastly overpaid consultants and a mobile phone app that didn't work, failed to provide any tangible results in bringing down rates of infection.[548]

Then there was the scandal of the shortage of personal protective equipment (PPE). Frontline healthcare workers often did not have any, forcing them to dress in bin liners and plastic bags.[549] Doctors and nurses wrote of failures of leadership and staff shortages. Richard Horton at *The Lancet* received hundreds of despairing, shocked and angry messages from frontline healthcare workers: 'There is a huge mismatch about how the situation is presented publicly and the reality.' 'It's terrifying for the staff [...] Still no access to PPE.' 'There's been no guidelines, it's chaos.' 'We feel completely abandoned.' 'How will we protect patients and staff? I am speechless. It is utterly unconscionable. How can we do this? It is criminal. We feel completely helpless.' Even worse, healthcare workers were not allowed to speak out about the crisis. One message Richard Horton received read, 'Colleagues have to attend disciplinary meetings for speaking out... I never thought I lived in a country where freedom of speech is discouraged.'[550]

By way of tackling the disaster, the government handed an estimated £18 billion[551] of taxpayers' money to friends and donors, many of whom were – just coincidentally, of course – setting up PPE-supplying companies. If there is anything in the British government's response to COVID-19 that screams 'syndemic', it is this.[552] The High Court later ruled this use of the 'fast lane' to award contracts to the government's friends and supporters to be unlawful.[553]

Then there was the care home crisis. Infection ran rampant in Britain's care homes, leading to the deaths of at least 25,000 of the UK's most vulnerable citizens, the elderly and infirm. *Sunday Times* journalists Jonathan Calvert and George Arbuthnott spoke to doctors who believed the government considered care home residents 'dispensable'. One doctor commented that the government's 'lack of empathy and humanity was chilling'.[554] Boris Johnson later blamed care homes and GPs for the huge death toll.

Then government ministers and advisors were spotted not following their own lockdown rules. Most notoriously, Johnson's chief advisor Dominic Cummings flouted the stay-at-home rules by driving from almost one end of England to the other while suffering from symptoms of the infection. It also later transpired that parties had been held at 10 Downing Street regularly throughout the pandemic.[555] The UK government behaved throughout the crisis as if it was above the law. When the government was criticised for not wearing facemasks during debates, the leader of the House of Commons, Jacob Rees-Mogg, explained that Tory MPs didn't need to wear masks because they knew each other. In doing so, Rees-Mogg was exhibiting the same kind of elitist stupidity shown by Charles Meigs in 1855 when he protested that a gentleman's hands were always clean (and therefore doctors, being gentlemen, didn't need to wash their hands before delivering babies). Within days of Rees-Mogg's Meigism, the House of Commons was closed due to an outbreak of COVID-19.

When Johnson announced that England's lockdown would be lifted on 4 July 2020, the tabloid press announced 4 July as 'freedom day'. But infections were still high; it was too soon to lift lockdown. Not only had Johnson's delay in announcing the start of the lockdown in March come too late – costing thousands of lives – he was lifting the lockdown too early. Thousands more would die unnecessarily. One source described the government's policy as 'utterly insane'.[556] As soon as the lockdown was lifted, infection rates began to rise again. A second wave was inevitable. It became clear as the summer wore on that a two-week circuit-breaker lockdown would be necessary. According to Dominic Cummings, the prime minister told him in the summer of 2020 that he didn't believe any of the scientific reasons for lockdown, that it was 'all bullshit'.[557]

But it was clear that delaying a second lockdown would have serious consequences. Johnson and his Chancellor of the Exchequer, Rishi Sunak, seemed more concerned with protecting the economy than with saving lives, and consulted right-wing libertarian 'experts' whose views have widely been condemned, such as the fact that, according to these 'experts', there was no second wave, that herd immunity was a viable strategy, and that Sweden's policy of not locking down had been a success, when in fact it was proving to be a disaster.[558] When it became clear that Johnson was once again dithering, the government's chief scientific advisor, Sir Patrick Vallance, and chief medical officer, Chris Whitty, held their own press conference in an attempt to put pressure on Johnson to announce the circuit-breaker.[559]

Johnson ignored them. Instead of a circuit-breaker, Johnson announced a system of tiered restrictions. Not only was Johnson ignoring scientific advice, he was also going against the findings of the World Bank, which indicated that the best way to protect a country's economy was to lock down early.[560] But the system of tiers was chaotic and ineffective, and cases continued to rise. At another meeting, on 30 October 2020, the subject of lockdowns once more came up. An enraged Johnson was heard to shout, 'No more fucking lockdowns! Let the bodies pile high in their thousands!'[561] But the next day, Johnson was forced into one of many U-turns, by announcing a second lockdown in England that was set to last until 2 December.

Perhaps fearing that his poll ratings might slip, Johnson then looked at ways to ensure that Christmas would not be impacted by health regulations. The fact that a new and deadlier variant of the disease, named Delta, was becoming dominant appeared not to faze Johnson. He had ignored scientific advice throughout the pandemic, so why start now? 'Boris Johnson battles experts to save Christmas' the tabloids announced.[562] Boris's battle to save Christmas resulted in a welter of confused announcements on what could and couldn't be done over the festive period, but the regulations were sufficiently relaxed for January 2021 to see the UK suffer its highest monthly death tolls of the whole pandemic.[563] Not only did Boris's battle to save Christmas cause tens of thousands more unnecessary deaths, a third lockdown in England had to be ordered, beginning on 6 January 2021.

The one glimmer of hope in this ongoing catastrophe was the

authorisation by the UK health regulator of two COVID vaccines, the Pfizer-BioNTech on 2 December, and the Oxford-AstraZeneca on 30 December, making the UK the first country in the world to authorise vaccines for unlimited use. The roll-out began immediately. That they were so successfully administered across the whole of the UK speaks volumes for the efficiency, dedication, and unremitting hard work of the NHS. Naturally, Johnson and his government tried to take the credit.[564]

A report published by the House of Commons in October 2021 declared that the UK government's response to the COVID-19 pandemic had been the worst public health failure ever.[565] Although the report[566] claimed that it did not seek to apportion blame, early drafts were far less critical, seen by some as an attempt to let those most culpable off the hook: Boris Johnson, health secretary Matt Hancock, and his predecessor, Jeremy Hunt.[567] Although Johnson has promised a full public enquiry, it has been delayed, a move described by director of the Wellcome Trust, Sir Jeremy Farrar, as a 'disgrace' motivated by nothing other than 'political manouevring'.[568] Farrar has stated that the decisions made by Johnson and his government in the second half of 2020 were 'unforgivable'.[569]

What Needs to Happen

The novelist and activist Arundhati Roy wrote that 'pandemics have forced humans to break with the past and imagine their world anew. This one is no different. It is a portal, a gateway between one world and the next.'[570] But will it be to a new world, or a world that tries to carry on as it was before 30 December 2019? If the world is to emerge in any way better from the pandemic, urgently needed changes must be fought for; the alternative is what the philosopher Slavoj Žižek calls 'a new barbarism whose first signs are already clearly discernible'.[571]

As I write (January 2022), the pandemic is still far from over. The Omicron variant is dominant, causing a huge surge in infections and hospital admissions worldwide. How things will play out, and how we recover, are very much up in the air.

There is still much we don't know about COVID-19. We don't know why people of some ethnicities appear to be more susceptible to infection than others. We don't know why it mainly affects older people. We don't understand the condition known as long COVID. We don't understand how COVID-19, a respiratory disease, is so effective in affecting other organs of the body. We don't know what effect the pandemic will have on children, whose education has been disrupted. We don't know what the long-term psychological effects of the pandemic will be. In addition to being described as a syndemic, COVID-19 should also be thought of as a collective trauma.

The pandemic has also exposed fault lines in societies around the world, and threatens to create new ones. As Peter Baldwin notes, there has been vigorous debate about how far the state can go in intervening in people's lives,[572] as can be seen in the rift between those who have been vaccinated, and those who, for whatever reason, have not. COVID-19 has been described as a syndemic,[573] as already noted, but the extent to which it is so is debatable: in countries with fewer systemic problems, COVID-19 is perhaps less classifiable as a syndemic.[574] These countries include New Zealand, South Korea, Taiwan, and Singapore, whose governments acted swiftly and decisively against the disease, resulting in far fewer deaths. Conversely, the countries that have suffered the highest death tolls – such as the USA, Brazil, India, and the UK – have also been countries with major systemic problems, where healthcare systems are broken or threatened, where there are divisions along class or race lines, where inequalities of wealth and opportunity perpetuate divided and dysfunctional societies.

When restrictions were lifted prematurely in parts of the US such as Texas and Mississippi, it led to a rise in cases in early 2021.[575] These states were unwittingly repeating history. Lockdowns, social distancing, and wearing masks had all been features of the Spanish Flu in 1918–19. San Francisco lifted its lockdown after only four weeks in the autumn of 1918, resulting in a huge surge of deaths in the early months of 1919, making it one of the worst-hit American cities.[576] Similarly, Philadelphia shut down for 51 days during the same period, resulting in 250 excess deaths per 100,000 of population, while St Louis opted for a hard lockdown, 143 days of closures, resulting in only 30 excess deaths per 100,000.[577] In both pandemics, there was an understandable concern for the economy, but also pressure from those who objected to what they saw as governmental interference in their lives.

Effective response to COVID-19 has been affected by distrust of government, manifesting in the anti-vax movement, opposition to lockdowns, masks, and social distancing; to say nothing of the use of quack cures such as bleach or ivermectin. The fact that people who adopted such positions frequently then died of COVID-19 didn't seem to act as a deterrent to others. This is, sadly, yet another aspect of covid-as-syndemic: when governments repeatedly dithered in their responses to the pandemic, continuing to work in the interests of global capitalism rather than the people who elected them, such distrust and opposition is hardly surprising.

Disinformation has also played a part. Some of this has been deliberate, probably originating from far-right groups, and Russian troll farms. Then there is good old-fashioned lunacy – such as the conspiracy theory that 5G mobile phone masts can somehow spread the disease, or that the pandemic was deliberately engineered by the Chinese government. People who subscribe to these, and other conspiracy beliefs, are unknowingly repeating the folly of mediaeval people who believed the Black Death was spread by Jewish communities, and lepers.

Richard Horton observed that 'Our museums are filled with the relics of ancient peoples who once thought their societies were stable and robust.'[578] COVID-19 has shown us that our societies are just as fragile as any that have come before us. Things must change. What is needed is, as Horton puts it, 'historically unrivalled coordination between nations'.[579] This will not be easy. Even while the pandemic continues to do its work, political tensions worsen in countries like Ukraine and Kazakhstan. Politicians will pay the price for playing their games while people continue to die from COVID. Climate change will play its inexorable part, affecting the movements of animal vectors;

human populations will migrate. And global capitalism continues to fiddle while Rome burns.

What is needed is an early warning radar for identifying emerging diseases and potential new viral threats. This needs to be an international system, where new research can be shared instantly. As Sir Jeremy Farrar put it, 'everything starts with smarter surveillance'.[580] The speed with which scientists across the globe shared the genetic sequence of SARS-Cov-2, and cooperated on producing vaccines, is perhaps a hopeful sign. Similarly, the establishment of COVAX (the COVID-19 Vaccines Global Access programme) in April 2020 to facilitate the equal distribution of COVID vaccines to countries around the world is another step in the right direction. Bodies like the WHO need more funding, and need to be able to work independently of governments. A new global network will also help combat challenges from existing diseases: SARS, MERS, and avian influenza remain major threats; future outbreaks of diseases like Ebola and Nipah could easily become far worse. More research is needed on the interactions between animals and humans. SARS, MERS, avian influenza, Ebola, and Nipah all came from animals; as did, in all probability, COVID-19.

The world needs to be prepared for the next pandemic, whatever it turns out to be. Because there will be another pandemic. Of that we can be sure. When COVID struck, the West was complacent. Not so China. After initially mishandling the crisis, Beijing acted swiftly by initiating lockdowns in Wuhan and other cities. Part of the success in the Chinese reaction can be attributed to the fact that the Chinese government had invested in healthcare infrastructure after the SARS pandemic of 2002–3. The Chinese, in other words, had had recent experience of a pandemic, and were much better placed to deal with a new threat like COVID. Although SARS spread to 29 countries, western governments did not regard it as a sufficient threat; the uncoordinated international response to the coronavirus pandemic during 2020 is the highly visible result of such complacency.

As of early 2022, the ten highest COVID-19 death tolls in the world have been suffered by the United States, Brazil, India, Russia, Mexico,

Peru, the UK, Indonesia, Italy, and Iran. How the pandemic will affect their governments – or the politicians in power when the pandemic struck – remains to be seen. There has been an interesting development in Brazil: in October 2021, the Brazilian senate discussed bringing murder charges against president Jair Bolsonaro. Although it is unlikely that Bolsonaro will end up in court, the fact that such measures are even being discussed is a measure of how far some politicians have rightly earned the opprobrium and contempt of their electorates.

Trying political leaders for murder or manslaughter may certainly make future presidents and prime ministers aware of the dangers of complacency. But changes will need to be made elsewhere, too. Capitalism remains the biggest challenge. Industrial-scale farming not only causes problems for the environment – witness the deforestation of the Amazon – but there are also strong links between Big Farming and disease.[581] Neoliberal economics were also a primary factor in why the West was unprepared for the pandemic in 2020: scientific research budgets had been slashed over the preceding decade, a result of the 2008 financial crisis. Governments fixated on protecting banks, not people. Austerity had weakened the world. To this we can add the related phenomenon of isolationism and toxic nationalism, as exemplified by former US National Security Advisor, John Bolton who, in 2019, abolished the role of White House director for global health security and biothreats, meaning that there was no one in the Trump administration to monitor emerging pandemic threats.[582] This is exactly the opposite of what needs to happen.

We need new ways of thinking about societies, and a rediscovery of the fact that there are non-monetary forms of value. We need investment in people and communities, a 'reweaving [of] the social fabric', as former Bank of England economist Andy Haldane put it in his article on the importance of social capital after the pandemic.[583] What life will be like is very much up to us; everyone may need to become an activist of one kind or another. Perhaps the notion of activism itself needs to be deepened and broadened to include those who would normally balk at defining themselves as such. Perhaps well-informed daily living that acknowledges the need to care for others, and to maintain communities that are healthy in mind as well as body will be a new form of activism. COVID-19 may never go away; it could well become endemic, adding further weight to the need for change. 'We cannot go on the way we have till now,' Slavoj Žižek has written, 'a radical change is needed,'[584] while also reminding us that we need 'to reflect on the sad fact that we need a catastrophe to be able to rethink the very basic features of the society in which we live.'[585]

And thus we stand on the threshold of Arundhati Roy's portal:

> We can choose to walk through it, dragging the carcasses of our prejudice and hatred, our avarice, our data banks and dead ideas, our dead rivers and smoky skies behind us. Or we can walk through lightly, with little luggage, ready to imagine another world. And ready to fight for it.[586]

Envoi

At the beginning of this book, we looked at disease origin myths. Many attribute the origins of disease to the actions of an Eve or a Pandora. While these remain some of the most well-known stories, their patriarchal and sexist attitudes are part of the world that COVID-19 has challenged. With political, economic, and healthcare systems strained almost to breaking point, and the climate crisis poised over all not so much like the Sword of Damocles but the scythe of the Grim Reaper, never has it seemed more evident that all the demons remain out of Pandora's Box, running amok, with little hope of ever coaxing them back in again.

But there is one myth of disease origin that offers not just hope (the only thing to remain in Pandora's Box), but suggests a practical approach for the way out of our current dire predicament. The story is from the Cherokee. In the old days, they say, animals and humans lived in harmony. But as time went by, humans began to multiply and spread out across the earth. The animals suddenly found themselves pushed for space. Not only that, but the ever-increasing numbers of humans invented weapons – bows and arrows, knives, spears – and killed the animals for their meat and skins. The animals got together to decide what to do.

The Bears met first. They decided to declare war on humans, and made a bow and arrow. One of the bears stepped up to test the new weapon. His claws caught on the string, but he fluffed the shot. It was pointed out that if he had his claws trimmed, that might help. So they trimmed his claws, and he tried again. This time, the arrow found its target. However, the chief of the bears, Old White Bear, pointed out that if they all trimmed their claws, they would no longer be able to climb trees. They decided it would be better to trust the teeth and claws that nature had given them, rather than to adopt the weapons that humans used. So the meeting ended.

The Deer were the next to meet, under their leader, Little Deer. They decided to give rheumatism to every hunter who killed one of their number, unless the hunter asked the deer's pardon before taking its life. If Little Deer heard the pardon, then all would be well; if not, the hunter would become a cripple for the rest of their days.

The Fishes and Reptiles decided to send humans bad dreams. In the nightmares, snakes would coil around a person's body, blowing foul breath into their faces; they would dream they were eating raw flesh, or carrion. Revolted by the dead flesh, the human would lose their appetite, sicken and die.

Finally the Birds, Insects, and smaller animals got together, presided over by the humble Grubworm. They decided to vote on humanity's guilt: seven votes would be enough to condemn the human race. They each stepped up and spoke of the cruelty of humans, of how they continually killed, displaced, or mocked all the denizens of the animal kingdom. The vote was carried. Taking their cue from the Deer, Fishes and Reptiles, the animals began to devise more new diseases for humans. They got so carried away that, had they not run out of ideas, it is said that not one human being would have remained alive.

The Plants heard about this, and vowed to intervene on humanity's behalf. Each tree, shrub and herb, even down to grasses, mosses and weeds, agreed to provide a cure for the diseases the animals had devised. When doctors didn't know what medicine to use, the spirits of the plants would tell them.

Thus, disease appeared in the world, but at the same time, also the power to combat it.

To my mind, this remains the best of the disease origin myths. Not only because of its beauty as a story, but also because it reveals a profound awareness of zoonotic disease, and the role of the natural world in maintaining the balance that humanity, with its demon children – war, capitalism, greed, ignorance – threatens to destroy. Adopting the holistic worldview suggested by the Cherokee story is a crucial paradigm shift, in that it allows us to see ourselves not as having the Biblical dominion over the birds of the air and the fishes of the sea and over every living thing, but as part of an infinite fabric. Disease, and pandemics especially, remind us to work with nature, not against it; to re-learn our place in the world.

Notes

1 Keith Weller Taylor, *The Birth of Vietnam* (Berkeley, 1983), 183.
2 *Oxford English Dictionary*, 2nd ed. (Oxford: OUP, 1989), vol. IV, 763.
3 Robert P Hudson, 'Concepts of Disease in the West', in *The Cambridge World History of Human Disease* (hereafter *CWHHD),* 45.
4 Robert P Hudson, 'Concepts of Disease in the West', in *CWHHD*, 45.
5 David Leeming, *The Oxford Companion to World Mythology*, (Oxford, New York: OUP, 2005), 307.
6 43 Vendidad Far II, 3–41, from SGF Brandon, *Creation Legends of the Ancient Near East* (London: Hodder & Stoughton, 1963), 48.
7 Richard Heinberg, *Memories and Visions of Paradise* (Wellingborough: Aquarian Press, 1990), 43.
8 Dorothy H Crawford, *The Invisible Enemy: A Natural History of Viruses* (Oxford: Oxford University Press, 2000), 8.
9 Dorothy H Crawford, *The Invisible Enemy*, 18.
10 Dorothy H Crawford, *Deadly Companions: How Microbes Shaped Our History* (Oxford University Press, 2007), 15.
11 Mary Ellen Snodgrass, *World Epidemics: A Cultural Chronology of Disease from Prehistory to the Era of SARS* (Jefferson, NC; McFarland and Company, 2003), 9.
12 See Tony Waldron, *Paleopathology* (Cambridge: Cambridge University Press, 2009).
13 Charlotte Roberts & Keith Manchester, *The Archaeology of Disease* (1983) (Stroud: The History Press. Third edition, 2010), 13.

14 Charlotte Roberts & Keith Manchester, *The Archaeology of Disease*, 13.
15 Charlotte Roberts & Keith Manchester, *The Archaeology of Disease*, 14.
16 Arno Karlen, *Plague's Progress: A Social History of Man and Disease* (London: Cassell, 1996), 32.
17 Mary Ellen Snodgrass, *World Epidemics: A Cultural Chronology of Disease from Prehistory to the Era of SARS* (Jefferson, NC; McFarland and Company, 2003), 9.
18 Dorothy H Crawford, *Deadly Companions: How Microbes Shaped Our History* (Oxford: Oxford University Press, 2007), 48.
19 Arno Karlen, *Plague's Progress*, 19.
20 Dorothy H Crawford, *Deadly Companions*, 31.
21 Arno Karlen, *Plague's Progress,* 31.
22 Paul S Martin, *Twilight of the Mammoths: Ice Age Extinctions and the Rewilding of America* (Berkeley and Los Angeles: University of California Press, 2005), 1–3.
23 Arno Karlen, *Plague's Progress,* 20.
24 Arno Karlen, *Plague's Progress*, 20.
25 Arno Karlen, *Plague's Progress*, 27–28.
26 Historian Yuval Noah Harari has argued that the agricultural revolution brought more woes than just disease: 'Rather than heralding a new era of easy living, the Agricultural Revolution left farmers with lives generally more difficult and less satisfying than those of foragers. Hunter-gatherers spent their time in more stimulating and varied ways, and were less in danger of starvation and disease. The Agricultural Revolution certainly enlarged the sum total of food at the disposal of humankind, but the extra food did not translate into a better diet or more leisure. Rather, it translated into population explosions and pampered elites. The average farmer worked harder than the average forager, and got a worse diet in return. The Agricultural Revolution was history's biggest fraud.' Yuval Noah Harari, *Sapiens: A Brief History of Humankind* (London: Harvill Secker, 2014), 79.

27 Hershkovitz et al (2008), 'Detection and Molecular Characterization of 9000-Year-Old *Mycobacterium tuberculosis* from a Neolithic Settlement in the Eastern Mediterranean'. http://journals.plos.org/plosone/article?id=10.1371/journal.pone.0003426
28 Helen Bynum, *Spitting Blood: The History of Tuberculosis* (Oxford: Oxford University Press, 2012), 7–8. Dates for the first settlement of the Americas vary, and these are approximate.
29 See Roberts & Manchester, *The Archaeology of Disease*, Ch 19.
30 Theya Molleson and Peter Andrews, 'The Human Remains'. Çatalhöyük 1997 Archive Report. http://www.catalhoyuk.com/archive_reports/1997/ar97_12.html
31 David Quammen, *Ebola: The Natural and Human History* (London: The Bodley Head, 2014), 85.
32 Alfred W Crosby, 'Smallpox', in *CWHHD*, 1009.
33 Naomi Hamilton, 'Burials and Grave Goods', Çatalhöyük 1998 Archive Report. http://www.catalhoyuk.com/archive_reports/1998/ar98_15.html
34 Roy Porter, *The Greatest Benefit to Mankind: A Medical History of Humanity from Antiquity to the Present* (London: HarperCollins, 1997), 35.
35 Roy Porter, *The Greatest Benefit to Mankind: A Medical History of Humanity from Antiquity to the Present* (London: HarperCollins, 1997), 36.
36 The writer Bruce Chatwin had a theory that settlement brought with it more than just disease: 'Gradually the idea for a book began to take shape. It was to be a wildly ambitious and intolerant work, a kind of "Anatomy of Restlessness" that would enlarge on Pascal's dictum about the man sitting quietly in a room. The argument, roughly, was as follows: that in becoming human, man had acquired, together with his straight legs and striding walk, a migratory 'drive' or instinct to walk long distances through the seasons; that this 'drive' was inseparable from his central nervous system; and,

that, when warped in conditions of settlement, it found outlets in violence, greed, status-seeking or a mania for the new. This would explain why mobile societies such as the gypsies were egalitarian, thing-free and resistant to change; also why, to re-establish the harmony of the First State, all the great teachers – Buddha, Lao-tse, St Francis – had set the perpetual pilgrimage at the heart of their message and told their disciples, literally, to follow The Way.' Bruce Chatwin, *The Anatomy of Restlessness*, 12–13.

37 http://www.telegraph.co.uk/science/science-news/7530678/Biblical-plagues-really-happened-say-scientists.html. Accessed 27 February 2014. See also Siro Trevisanato, *The Plagues of Egypt*. Barbara J Sivertsen, in *The Parting of the Sea*, argues that the account of the plagues in Exodus conflates different events several centuries apart.

38 http://www.nbcnews.com/id/43979556/ns/technology_and_science-science/#.Tji4qqjgW5M. Accessed 26 August 2014.

39 Snodgrass, *World Epidemics: A Cultural Chronology of Disease from Prehistory to the Era of Sars* (Jefferson, NC: McFarland & Co, 2003), 10.

40 http://www.sacred-texts.com/hin/sbe42/. Accessed 27 August 2014.

41 William McNeill, *Plagues and Peoples*, 49–50.

42 Possible motives – and much more – discussed in John Byron, *Cain and Abel in Text and Tradition: Jewish and Christian Interpretations of the First Sibling Rivalry* (Leiden: Brill, 2011).

43 Hesiod, *Works and Days*, in *Hesiod and Theognis*, trans. Dorothea Wender (Harmondsworth: Penguin, 1973), 62.

44 John F Nunn, *Ancient Egyptian Medicine*, 103.

45 Nunn, 104.

46 Reuven Yaron, *Eshnunna Code*, 79.

47 Ernest S Tierkel, 'Canine Rabies', in *The Natural History of Rabies*, Vol II, 123.

48 Owsei Temkin, *The Falling Sickness: A History of Epilepsy from the Greeks to Modern Neurology* (Baltimore: Johns Hopkins University Press, 2nd ed., 1971), 3–4.

49 John F Nunn, *Ancient Egyptian Medicine*, 24.
50 John F Nunn, *Ancient Egyptian Medicine*, 26.
51 Nunn, 32.
52 Nunn, 105.
53 Nunn, 68.
54 Nunn, 69.
55 Nunn, 69.
56 Nunn, 89.
57 Nunn, 33.
58 Nunn, 33.
59 Nunn, 61.
60 A number of other papyri contain gynaecological material, such as the Kahun Papyrus; Carlsberg VIII, which is mainly gynaecological and obstetrical; and Ramesseum papyri III, IV and V. These contain information on the eyes, gynaecology and the diseases of children. It's the best preserved, and possibly earliest, medical pap. See Nunn, 39–40.
61 Nunn, 33.
62 Nunn, 33.
63 Nunn, 64.
64 Nunn, 81.
65 Nunn, 81.
66 Nunn, 75.
67 Roy Porter, *The Greatest Benefit to Mankind*, 121
68 Andrew Nikiforuk, *The Fourth Horseman*, 29.
69 Nunn, 83.
70 These, and many more examples, can be found at http://archive.org/stream/incubationorcur00hamigoog/incubationorcur00hamigoog_djvu.txt. Accessed 24.09.14.
71 Roy Porter, *The Greatest Benefit to Mankind*, 53.
72 Roy Porter, *The Greatest Benefit to Mankind*, 53–4.
73 For more on the diseases thought to be represented in Hippocratic writings, see Pappas et al (2007) 'Infectious disease in the age of Hippocrates',

http://www.sciencedirect.com/science/article/pii/S1201971207002123. Accessed 17.09.14.

74 Angela Ki Che Leung, 'Diseases of the Pre-Modern Period in China', *CWHHD*, 354.

75 Angela Ki Che Leung, 'Diseases of the Pre-Modern Period in China', *CWHHD*, 346.

76 Leung, *CWHHD*, 354.

77 William McNeill, *Plagues and Peoples*, 269–72.

78 Walter Scheidel, 'Disease and Death', in Paul Erdkamp (ed.), *The Cambridge Companion to Ancient Rome*, 51.

79 Scheidel, 51.

80 Scheidel, 52.

81 Susan Mattern (2013), *The Prince of Medicine: Galen in the Roman Empire*, 126.

82 For more on Rome's population, see Erdkamp, *The Cambridge Companion to Ancient Rome*, Ch 2.

83 Walter Scheidel, 'Disease and Death', 45–59, in *The Cambridge Companion to Ancient Rome*, 53.

84 Mattern (2013), *The Prince of Medicine: Galen in the Roman Empire*, 118.

85 Mattern (2013), *The Prince of Medicine: Galen in the Roman Empire*, 119.

86 Mattern (2013), *The Prince of Medicine: Galen in the Roman Empire*, 119.

87 A Ascenzi et al (1996), 'The Roman Mummy of Grottarossa', in *Human Mummies: A Global Survey of their Status and the Techniques of Conservation*, ed. K Spindler et al, 205–218. Vienna: Springer.

88 Suetonius, *The Twelve Caesars*, trans. Robert Graves, rev. James B Rives (Penguin, 2007), 278.

89 Suetonius, *The Twelve Caesars*, trans. Robert Graves, rev. James B Rives (Penguin, 2007), 277.

90 Scheidel, 54.

91 Pliny the Elder, *The Natural History*. Trans. John Bostock and HT Riley. London: Taylor and Francis, 1855.

92 Pliny the Elder, *The Natural History*. Trans. John Bostock and HT Riley. London: Taylor and Francis, 1855.

93 Galen, *Methodus medendi* 5.12, quoted in RJ Littman and ML

Littman, 'Galen and the Antonine Plague', *The American Journal of Philology,* Vol. 94, No. 3 (Autumn, 1973), 243–255, 246.

94 Littman and Littman, 250.

95 Scheidel, 52.

96 David E Stannard, 'Disease, Human Migration and History', *CWHHD*, 37.

97 Pontius the Deacon, *The Life and Passion of Cyprian, Bishop and Martyr* (*c.* 260), from http://www.ccel.org/ccel/schaff/anf05.iv.iii.html. Accessed 11 October 2014.

98 William H McNeill, *Plagues and Peoples*, 113.

99 Mark 9:17–27; Matthew 17:14–8; Luke 9:38–43.

100 Porter, *Greatest Benefit to Mankind*, 84.

101 EM Forster, review of Revd. Father J Faivre's *Canopus, Menouthis, Aboukir. Egyptian Mail*, 29 December 1918. Quoted in Dominic Montserrat, 'Carrying on the Work of the Earlier Firm: Doctors, Medicine and Christianity in the Thaumata of Sophronius of Jerusalem', in *Health in Antiquity*, ed. Helen King, 230.

102 The forerunners of hospitals were ancient Egyptian temples, where people sought the help of the gods in recovering their health. Perhaps the earliest recorded hospitals were those built in Sri Lanka in the fourth century BC at Mihintale. Hospitals also existed in northern India by the first or second centuries AD, and the Buddhist monk and traveller Fa Xian (337 – *c.* 422) wrote of visiting them in the fourth century AD.

103 David M Wagner, Jennifer Klunk, Michaela Harbeck, et al, '*Yersinia pestis* and the Plague of Justinian 541–543 AD: A Genomic Analysis', *The Lancet Infectious Diseases*, Volume 14, Issue 4, April 2014, 319–326. http://www.thelancet.com/journals/laninf/article/PIIS1473-3099(13)70323-2/abstract. Accessed 14 October 2014.

104 Lester K Little, 'Life and Afterlife of the First Plague Pandemic', in *Plague and the End of Antiquity: The Pandemic of 541–750*, ed. Lester K Little (Cambridge University Press, 2007), 9.

105 Paul Slack, *Plague: A Very Short Introduction* (Oxford University Press, 2012), 18.

106 Quoted in Little, *Plague and the End of Antiquity*, 7.
107 Quoted in Little, *Plague and the End of Antiquity*, 7.
108 Amir Harrak, ed. and trans., *The Chronicle of Zuqnin, Parts III and IV, AD 488–775* (Toronto: Pontifical Institute of Mediaeval Studies, 1999), 30.
109 Paul Slack, *Plague: A Very Short Introduction*, 56.
110 Paul the Deacon, *Historia Langobardorum* 2.4, p. 74. Quoted in John Maddicott, 'Plague in Seventh-Century England', in Little, *Plague and the End of Antiquity*, 197–8.
111 Jean Durliat's influential essay, 'La Peste du Vle siecle: Pour un nouvel examen des sources byzantines', (1989) questioned reliance on literary sources. Peter Sarris, 'Bubonic Plague in Byzantium: The Evidence of Non-Literary Sources', in Little (ed.), *Plague and the End of Antiquity*, 125.
112 Hugh N Kennedy, 'Justinianic Plague in Syria and the Archaeological Evidence', in Little (ed.), *Plague and the End of Antiquity*, 95.
113 Sarris, in Little (ed.), *Plague and the End of Antiquity*, 127.
114 McNeill, *Plagues and Peoples*, 123.
115 *The Chronicle of Zuqnin, Parts III and IV, AD 488–775*, ed. and trans. Amir Harrak (Toronto: Pontifical Institute of Mediaeval Studies, 1999), 170–171.
116 *The Chronicle of Zuqnin*, ed. and trans. Harrak, 171.
117 *The Chronicle of Zuqnin*, ed. and trans. Harrak, 172.
118 *The Chronicle of Zuqnin*, ed. and trans. Harrak, 172.
119 Arno Karlen, *Plague's Progress*, 78.
120 Karlen, 79.
121 ML Cameron, *Anglo-Saxon Medicine*, 5.
122 Bede, *Ecclesiastical History of the English People*, II.15, ed. Colgrave and Mynors, 182–5. Quoted in Cameron, 5–6.
123 ML Cameron, *Anglo-Saxon Medicine*, 6
124 ML Cameron, *Anglo-Saxon Medicine*, 10.
125 ML Cameron, *Anglo-Saxon Medicine*, 11.
126 ML Cameron, *Anglo-Saxon Medicine*, 12.
127 ML Cameron, *Anglo-Saxon Medicine*, 15.

128 ML Cameron, *Anglo-Saxon Medicine*, 24.
129 ML Cameron, *Anglo-Saxon Medicine*, 38.
130 ML Cameron, *Anglo-Saxon Medicine*, 47.
131 Stephen Pollington, *Leechcraft: Early English Charms, Plant-lore and Healing* (Hockwold-cum-Wilton: Anglo-Saxon Books, 2000), 454.
132 Bede, *Ecclesiastical History of the English People*, ed. Bertram Colgrave and RAB Mynors (Oxford: Clarendon Press, 1991), 461.
133 McNeill, 123.
134 John Maddicott, 'Plague in Seventh-Century England,' in Little (ed.), *Plague and the End of Antiquity*, 171.
135 Bede, *Historical Works* Vol I, 485.
136 Charles Creighton, *A History of Epidemics in Britain*, Vol. I, 15.
137 Frederick Cartwright and Michael Biddiss, *Disease and History*, 3.
138 McNeill, *Plagues and Peoples*, 124.
139 John C Snyder, 'The Typhus Fevers', in *Viral and Rickettsial Infections of Man*, ed. Thomas M Rivers, (Philadelphia, London and Montreal: JB Lippincott, 1948), 463.
140 Snyder, 'The Typhus Fevers', 464.
141 Quoted in Zinsser, *Rats, Lice and History* (London: Penguin, 2000), 242. Snyder (1948) cites the 1083 outbreak with caution, stating that the 'first medical record which is sufficiently clear to identify typhus fever' is the 1546 description by Fracastorius. Snyder (1948), 462.
142 Creighton, Vol. I, 9.
143 Creighton, Vol. I, 9.
144 Creighton, Vol. I, 9.
145 Creighton, Vol. I, 11.
146 Later in the Middle Ages, another St Anthony also became identified with the disease, St Anthony of Padua (1195–1231), who had a reputation as a healer.
147 LSD can be extracted from the basic ergot alkaloid.
148 Ergot poisoning has been suggested as the cause of the witch craze in Salem, Massachusetts, in 1692. See Kiple, 'Ergotism',

in Kiple (ed.), *Plague, Pox & Pestilence*, 34–5. Given the prevalence of religious mania in the seventeenth century, one wonders if America could have been founded by religious extremists tripping out of their minds on infected rye, hallucinating the apocalypse. Surely it couldn't still be going on, could it?

149 Kenneth F Kiple, 'Ergotism', in Kiple (ed.), *Plague, Pox and Pestilence*, 32.

150 John S Haller, 'Ergotism', *CWHHD*, 719.

151 Carole Rawcliffe, *Leprosy in Medieval England*, 1.

152 Carole Rawcliffe, *Leprosy in Medieval England*, 1.

153 Margaret Cox and Charlotte Roberts, *Health and Disease in Britain*, 267.

154 Nikiforuk, *The Fourth Horseman*, 31.

155 Cox and Roberts, 269. Methods of attempted treatment were equally well-intentioned, strange and futile.

156 Nikiforuk, 35.

157 Cox and Roberts, 267

158 Cox and Roberts, 270.

159 Nikiforuk, *The Fourth Horseman*, 31.

160 Saul Nathaniel Brody, *The Disease of the Soul*, 93.

161 For more on the varieties of *separatio leprosarum*, see Brody, 64–9.

162 Nikiforuk, *Fourth Horseman*, 28.

163 Brody, *The Disease of the Soul*, 89.

164 Brody, 91. Fastoul appears to have been successful in getting into the leprosarium after Bodel's death.

165 See Keith Manchester, 'Tuberculosis and Leprosy: Evidence for Interaction of Disease', in DJ Ortner and AC Aufderheide, eds., *Human Paleopathology: Current Syntheses and Future Options* (Washington DC: Smithsonian Institution Press, 1991).

166 Rawcliffe, *Leprosy in Medieval England*, 228–229.

167 Cox and Roberts, 271.

168 Cox and Roberts, 272. The authors elaborate on the liminality of the leprosaria: 'In fact, some sites of leprosy houses are still called 'no man's land' on modern maps.' Some, such as St Mary

Magdalene, Winchester, became extra-parochial areas somewhat like the mediaeval liberties, which were exempt from paying tax to the crown and which could be subject to different laws. 'The Winchester site [St Mary Magdalene] seems to have persisted in the landscape as a place of "infection" becoming an isolation hospital in the C19 and the "sanitising" unit for a suite of First World War barracks in the C20. The history of this site would suggest an unusual and evidently powerful form of continuity of the concept of the contagion of the landscape.' Cox and Roberts, 272.

169 Roy Porter, *Greatest Benefit*, 122.

170 Carole Rawcliffe, *Leprosy in Medieval England*, 6.

171 Rawcliffe, *Leprosy in Medieval England,* 59.

172 Rawcliffe, *Leprosy in Medieval England*, 52.

173 Rawcliffe, *Leprosy in Medieval England*, 4.

174 Beroul, *The Romance of Tristan*, trans. Alan S. Fedrick (Penguin, 1970), 73–74.

175 Seán Martin, *The Black Death* (Harpenden: Oldcastle Books, 2007), 27.

176 See Michael W Dols, *The Black Death in the Middle East* (Princeton: Princeton University Press, 1977), 92–95.

177 Dols, 58.

178 Dols, 65.

179 See Graham Twigg, *The Black Death: A Biological Reappraisal* (London: Batsford, 1984) and *Bubonic Plague: A Much Misunderstood Disease* (Ascot: Derwent Press, 2013).

180 David Herlihy, *The Black Death and the Transformation of the West* (Harvard University Press, 1997), 2.

181 Columbus, entry for 14 October 1492. *The Four Voyages of Christopher Columbus* (Penguin, 1969), 59.

182 Rape of an indigenous woman, *The Four Voyages of Christopher Columbus*, 139. This incident is from the voyage of 1493–6. The rape was carried out by one of Columbus's lieutenants.

183 Quoted in Donald R Hopkins, *The Greatest Killer*, 204.

184 Snodgrass, *World Epidemics*, 55.

185 Snodgrass, *World Epidemics*, 13.

186 Frank Fenner, et al, *Smallpox and its Eradication* (Geneva: World Health Organization, 1988), 96.

187 Gareth Williams, *The Angel of Death*, 16.

188 Alfred W Crosby, 'Smallpox', in *CWHHD*, 1009.

189 Alfred W Crosby, 'Smallpox', in *CWHHD*, 1009–1010.

190 Hopkins, *The Greatest Killer*, 205.

191 EA Foster, *Motolinia's History of the Indians of New Spain* (Berkeley: Cortes Society, 1950), 38.

192 GS D'Ardois 'La Viruela en la Nueva España' (*Gaceta Médica de México* 91, 1961), 1016.

193 Hopkins, *The Greatest Killer*, 207.

194 Karlen, *Plague's Progress*, 99.

195 McNeill, *Plagues and Peoples*, 186.

196 McNeill, *Plagues and Peoples*, 304.

197 Karlen, *Plague's Progress*, 100. For more on pre-Columbian malaria, see Robert Desowitz, *Tropical Diseases: From 50,000 BC to 2500 AD* (London: HarperCollins, 1997), 74–82.

198 Marvin J Allion, 'Chagas' Disease', *CWHHD*, 637.

199 Quoted in Kevin Brown, *The Pox: The Life and Near Death of a Very Social Disease* (Stroud: Sutton Publishing, 2006), 2.

200 Quoted in Brown, *The Pox: The Life and Near Death of a Very Social Disease*, 2.

201 Jon Arrizabalaga, 'Syphilis', in *CWHHD*, 1025.

202 http://www.britannica.com/EBchecked/topic/560509/spirochete: Accessed 25.11.14.

203 Nikiforuk, *The Fourth Horseman*, 88.

204 Nikiforuk, *The Fourth Horseman*, 92.

205 Brown, *The Pox: The Life and Near Death of a Very Social Disease*, 3.

206 Brown, *The Pox: The Life and Near Death of a Very Social Disease*, 3.

207 Quoted in Nikiforuk, *The Fourth Horseman*, 90/91.

208 Brown, *The Pox: The Life and Near Death of a Very Social Disease*, 4.

209 Brown, *The Pox*, 9.

210 Brown, *The Pox*, 9.

211 S dei Conti da Foligno, *Le Storie de suoi Tempi* (1883), vol 2, 272; quoted in Brown, 9.
212 S dei Conti da Foligno, *Le Storie de suoi Tempi* (1883), vol 2, 273; quoted in Brown, 9.
213 Brown, *The Pox,* 11.
214 Brown, *The Pox,* 12. See also: Claude Quétel, *History of Syphilis*, 34.
215 See Ira K Schwartz, Felicia Guest, 'Promiscuity and the Abuse of Stigma', http://www.thelancet.com/journals/lancet/article/PIIS0140-6736(05)72404-1/fulltext#back-bib4. Accessed 04.12.14.
216 The story that the Magdalene was a repentant prostitute, one of the Church's most successful smear campaigns, originated in the C6 with Pope Gregory the Great.
217 RS Morton, *Venereal Diseases* (Harmondsworth: Penguin, 1972), 25.
218 Nikiforuk, *The Fourth Horseman*, 91.
219 Claude Quétel, *History of Syphilis*, 35.
220 Robert Desowitz, *Tropical Diseases*, 56.
221 Claude Quétel, *History of Syphilis* (Cambridge: Polity Press, 1990), 38.
222 RS Morton, *Venereal Diseases,* (Harmondsworth: Penguin, 1972), 28.
223 For a recent defence of the Columbian theory, see KN Harper, MK Zuckerman, ML Harper, JD Kingston, and GJ Armelagos, (2011), 'The Origin and Antiquity of Syphilis Revisited: An Appraisal of Old World pre-Columbian evidence for treponemal infection.' *American Journal of Physical Anthropology*, 146: 99–133. doi: 10.1002/ajpa.21613.
224 See Cox and Roberts, 272–273. Also CA Roberts, (1994) 'Treponematosis in Gloucester, England: a theoretical and practical approach to the pre-Columbian theory', in Olivier Dutour, et al, *L'origine de la syphilis en Europe: avant ou après 1493?: actes du colloque international de Toulon, 25–28 Novembre 1993*. Toulon, France: Centre Archeologique du Var; Editions Errance, 101–108.

225 G Cole, and T Waldron, (2011), 'Apple Down 152: A putative case of syphilis from sixth century AD Anglo-Saxon England.' *American Journal of Physical Anthropology*, 144: 72–79. doi: 10.1002/ajpa.21371.
226 Ann G Carmichael, 'Diseases of the Renaissance and Early Modern Europe,' in *CWHHD*, 283.
227 Ann G Carmichael, 'Sweating Sickness,' in *CWHHD*, 1024.
228 Ann G Carmichael, 'Sweating Sickness,' in *CWHHD*, 1023.
229 Ann G Carmichael, 'Sweating Sickness,' in *CWHHD*, 1023.
230 Neil Harding McAlister, 'The Dancing Pilgrims at Muelebeek', *Journal of the History of Medicine and Allied Sciences* 32 (1977): 315–19.
231 Hecker's book on dancing mania can be read on Project Gutenberg: gutenberg.org/files/1739/1739–h/1739–h.htm. Heck also details the bizarre episode of the 'Paris convulsionaires' of 1727, where an outbreak of dancing mania was also accompanied by an apparent resistance to pain and torture. See Michael Talbot, *The Holographic Universe*, (London: 1991), 128–132.
232 John Waller, *A Time to Dance, A Time to Die* (Thriplow: Icon Books, 2008).
233 Roger K French, 'Scurvy', in *CWHHD*, 1001.
234 Roger K French, 'Scurvy', in *CWHHD*, 1002.
235 Roger K French, 'Scurvy', in *CWHHD*, 1002.
236 Elizabeth W Etheridge, 'Pellagra', in *CWHHD*, 920. The eventual elimination of pellagra from much of Europe and North America in the twentieth century was achieved through a virtual reverse of this policy – governments encouraged better farming practices, which saw the planting of a wider variety of crops, and which ultimately led to better diets.
237 Elizabeth W Etheridge, 'Pellagra', in *CWHHD*, 923.
238 Porter, *Greatest Benefit*, 497.
239 Paul Chambers, *Bedlam: London's Hospital for the Mad*, 26.
240 Ned Ward, *The London Spy*, ed. Hyland, 55.
241 Chambers, *Bedlam*, 13.

242 William Willis Moseley, *Eleven Chapters on Nervous or Mental Complaints* (1838), in *The Faber Book of Madness*, Porter (ed.), 38–39.
243 Porter, *Greatest Benefit*, 495.
244 Chambers, *Bedlam*, 201.
245 Dols, *Majnun: The Madman in Medieval Islamic Society*, 173.
246 Dols, *Majnun*, 173.
247 Dols, *Majnun,* 120. See also *The Travels of Ibn Jubayr*, trans. RJC Broadhurst (London, 1952), 44, 296.
248 Dols, *Majnun,* 127.
249 Dols, *Majnun,* FN: 129. Powys Mathers trans. (London, 1986), IV: 55.
250 Sir Thomas More, *The Apologie of Syr T More, Knyght* (1533), in Porter (ed.), *The Faber Book of Madness*, 98.
251 Chambers, *Bedlam*, 13.
252 Chambers, *Bedlam*, 13.
253 Chambers, *Bedlam*, 23.
254 Kiple, *PPP*, 41.
255 Stephen V Beck, 'Epilepsy', in Kiple (ed.), *Plague, Pox and Pestilence*, 40.
256 Temkin, *The Falling Sickness*, 9.
257 *Arthur Mervyn*, Ch 18: http://www.gutenberg.org/files/18508/18508-h/18508–h.htm.
258 Diego López de Cogolludo, *Historia de Yucathan*, quoted in Pierce & Writer, *Yellow Jack*, 12. They are quoting HR Carter, LA Carter & WH Frost (eds.), *Yellow Fever: An Epidemiological and Historical Study of its Place of Origin*, Baltimore: Williams & Wilkins, 1931, 147–9.
259 Diego López de Cogolludo, *Historia de Yucathan*, quoted in Pierce & Writer, *Yellow Jack*, Ch 12.
260 Cogolludo, quoted in Pierce & Writer, *Yellow Jack,* 13, again quoting Carter et al 1931, 147–9.
261 Pierce & Writer, *Yellow Jack,* 11.
262 Pierce & Writer, *Yellow Jack,* 14.
263 Mark Harrison, *Contagion: How Commerce has Spread Disease*, 19.
264 Pierce & Writer, *Yellow Jack,* 14.

265 Kiple, *PPP*, 89.
266 Mary J Dobson, *Disease*, 149.
267 Kiple, *PPP*, 91.
268 DF Stickle, 'Death and Class in Baltimore: The Yellow Fever Epidemic of 1800', *Maryland History Magazine*, vol. 74 no. 3, 1979, 293. Quoted in Pierce and Writer, *Yellow Jack*, 21.
269 Dobson, *Disease*, 128.
270 Joseph Needham, *Science & Civilization in China VI, Biology & Biological Technology, Pt. 6, Medicine*, 154.
271 Needham, *Science & Civilization in China*, 134.
272 Lady Mary Wortley Montagu, *The Turkish Embassy Letters* (Virago, 1994), 81.
273 Isobel Grundy, *Lady Mary Wortley Montagu: Comet of the Enlightenment* (OUP, 1999), 101.
274 Lady Mary Wortley Montagu, *The Turkish Embassy Letters*, 81.
275 Snodgrass, *World Epidemics*, 106.
276 Dorothy H Crawford, *Deadly Companions*, 159.
277 William D Johnston, 'Tuberculosis', *CWHHD*, 1063.
278 Dorothy H Crawford, *Deadly Companions*, 158.
279 Kiple, *PPP*, 44.
280 Kenneth Kiple, 'Scrofula', in Kiple (ed.), *Plague, Pox and Pestilence*, 45.
281 https://mercuriuspoliticus.wordpress.com/2008/07/28/john-taylor-charles-i-and-the-royal-touch/. Accessed 18.2.15.
282 Peter Martin, *Samuel Johnson: A Biography* (London: Weidenfeld and Nicolson, 2008), 20.
283 August Hirsch, *Handbuch der historisch-geographischen Pathologie* (2 vols, 1860/64). Charles Creighton, whom we met in Chapter 3, translated the second edition into English as the *Handbook of Geographical and Historical Pathology* (3 vols, 1883–6). As the *Cambridge World History of Human Disease* noted, 'The *Handbook* represented a Herculean effort to detail the distribution of diseases of historical and geographic interest in time and in place.' *CWHHD*, 1.

284 Kiple, *PPP*, 44.
285 Charles Dickens, *Nicholas Nickleby* (1838–9), Ch 55.
286 Charles Dickens, *Nicholas Nickleby* (1838–9), Ch 58.
287 Helen Bynum, *Spitting Blood*, 19.
288 Helen Bynum, *Spitting Blood*, 20.
289 Helen Bynum, *Spitting Blood*, 19.
290 Helen Bynum, *Spitting Blood*, 19.
291 J Blondiaux, et al. 'Epidemiology of Tuberculosis: A 4th–12th *c.* AD picture in a 2498–skeleton series from northern France', in *Tuberculosis Past and Present,* G Pálfi, O Dutour, J Deák, I Hutás, (eds). Golden Book Publishers TB Foundation: Budapest (1999): 521–530.
292 Bynum, 26.
293 Crawford, *Deadly Companions*, 158.
294 See Helen D Donoghue, et al, 'Co–infection of Mycobacterium tuberculosis and Mycobacterium leprae in human archaeological samples: a possible explanation for the historical decline of leprosy'. DOI: 10.1098/rspb.2004.2966 Published 22 February 2005
295 Chopin wrote the letter on 3 December 1838. *Chopin's Letters*, EL Voynich & Henryk Opienski (eds.) (New York: Dover, 1988), 186.
296 August Hirsch, quoted by Kiple, 104.
297 Snodgrass, 114.
298 JN Hays, *Epidemics and Pandemics*, 239.
299 Hays, 242.
300 Frank Neal, *Black '47: Britain and the famine Irish*, 131.
301 John Belchem, *Irish, Catholic and Scouse: The History of the Liverpool Irish, 1800–1939* (Liverpool University Press, 2007), 60.
302 This quote is from an 1866 article in the *Quarterly Journal of Science*, quoted in Belchem, 61.
303 Belchem, 61.
304 Neal, *Black '47*, 153.
305 Quoted in Belchem, *Irish, Catholic and Scouse*, 60.
306 Charles W LeBaron and David W Taylor, 'Typhoid Fever', in *CWHHD*, 1075.

307 Margaret Humphreys, 'Typhoid and its Carriers', in Kiple, *PPP*, 16.
308 Dobson, *Disease*, 54.
309 Dobson, *Disease*, 54.
310 Hays, *Epidemics and Pandemics*, 213.
311 There seem to have been sporadic cases of what may have been cholera in Sunderland as early as August 1831. See Norman Longmate, *King Cholera: A Biography* (London: Hamish Hamilton, 1966), 24–5.
312 Norman Longmate, *King Cholera: A Biography* (London: Hamish Hamilton, 1966), 31
313 Longmate, *King Cholera,* 31–2.
314 Longmate, *King Cholera,* 33.
315 Longmate, *King Cholera*, 86.
316 Hays, 197.
317 Hays, 193.
318 Christopher Hamlin, *Cholera: The Biography*, 82.
319 Heinrich Heine, *French Affairs: Letters from Paris, Vol. I*, in *The Works of Heinrich Heine, Vol. VII*, trans. Charles Godfrey Leland (London: William Heinemann, 1893), 166–7.
320 Literally, 'To the lamppost!' The French revolutionary equivalent of 'String them up!' 'Them' in that context usually meant the aristocracy or their supporters, who were often hanged on Parisian lampposts.
321 A right wing, pro-Bourbon faction, active mainly in Spain.
322 Heinrich Heine, *French Affairs: Letters from Paris, Vol. I,* in *The Works of Heinrich Heine, Vol. VII*, trans. Charles Godfrey Leland (London: William Heinemann, 1893), 170–2.
323 Heinrich Heine, *French Affairs: Letters from Paris, Vol. I*, in *The Works of Heinrich Heine, Vol. VII*, trans. Charles Godfrey Leland (London, 1893), 165–6.
324 Hamlin, 63.
325 Cartwright and Biddiss, Ch 6.
326 There is some debate about the dating of the second and third pandemics. Most scholars agree that the second started in 1829,

with an end date usually given as either 1835 or 1851. The dates for the third can vary between early – 1839 to 1856 – and late – 1852–60.

327 Reinhard S Speck, 'Cholera', in *CWHHD*, 647.

328 Snow's findings can be read online at http://www.ph.ucla.edu/EPI/snow/cholerasouthlondon.html

329 Cartwright & Biddiss, *Disease and History*, Ch 6.

330 Mark Harrison, *Contagion*, 139.

331 John Waller, *The Discovery of the Germ*, 146.

332 Waller, *The Discovery of the Germ*, 148.

333 Waller, *The Discovery of the Germ*, 156.

334 Waller, *The Discovery of the Germ*, 158.

335 Waller, *The Discovery of the Germ*, 124.

336 K Codell Carter, 'Puerperal Fever', in *CWHHD*, 956.

337 Richard W Wertz & Dorothy C Wertz, *Lying-in: A History of Childbirth in America* (New Haven, CT: Yale University Press, 1989), 122.

338 Erysipelas also has links to the gangrenous form of ergotism, for which it was often mistaken.

339 Quoted in Waller, *The Discovery of the Germ*, 140.

340 Waller, *The Discovery of the Germ*, 138.

341 Waller, *The Discovery of the Germ*, 140.

342 William Winwood Reade, *The Martyrdom of Man* (1872), quoted in Myron Echenberg, *Plague Ports* (New York University Press, 2007), 1.

343 Karlen, *Plague's Progress*, 110.

344 Mark Harrison, *Contagion*, x.

345 Porter, *Greatest Benefit*, 466.

346 Porter, *Greatest Benefit*, 462–3.

347 Sonia Shah, *The Fever: How Malaria has Ruled Humankind for 500,000 Years*, 152.

348 Shah, 152.

349 Shah, 155.

350 ML Cameron, *Anglo-Saxon Medicine*, 10.

351 Shah, 175.

352 Shah, *The Fever*, 176; Packard, *The Making of a Tropical Disease*, 99–101.

353 Ian Cameron, *The Impossible Dream: The Building of the Panama Canal* (London: Hodder & Stoughton, 1971), 18.

354 Cameron, *The Impossible Dream*, 136.

355 Packard, *The Making of a Tropical Disease*, 121.

356 Cameron, *The Impossible Dream*, 134.

357 Mike Davis, *Late Victorian Holocausts*, 127.

358 Quoted in Davis, *Late Victorian Holocausts,* 131.

359 Quoted in Davis, *Late Victorian Holocausts,* 131.

360 Richard Pankhurst, *The History of Famine and Epidemics in Ethiopia Prior to the Twentieth Century* (Addis Ababa, 1986), 59 and 91–2. Quoted in Davis, *Late Victorian Holocausts,* 128.

361 Porter, *Greatest Benefit*, 465–6.

362 Davis, *Late Victorian Holocausts*, 139. The David Landes quotation is from his *The Unbound Prometheus: Technological Change and Industrial Development in Western Europe from 1750 to the Present* (Cambridge: Cambridge University Press, 1969), 231.

363 Davis, *Late Victorian Holocausts*, 140.

364 Waller, *The Discovery of the Germ*, 186.

365 http://sussexhistoryforum.co.uk/index.php?topic=7811.0;wap2 Accessed 2 March 2015.

366 Kenneth F Kiple and Kriemhild Coneè Ornelas, 'Typhus, Ships and Soldiers', in Kiple, *PPP*, 108.

367 http://www.influenzaarchive.org/cities/city-newyork.html# Accessed 4 March 2015.

368 Katherine Anne Porter's *Pale Horse, Pale Rider* (1939) is one of the few works of fiction about the pandemic.

369 Quoted in Dobson, *Disease*, 176.

370 Mark Honigsbaum, *Living with Enza* (London: Macmillan, 2009), xiii. *The Times*, 18 December 1918.

371 Honigsbaum, 41.

372 Honigsbaum, 22.

373 Honigsbaum, 46.

374 Honigsbaum, 47.
375 Honigsbaum, 50.
376 Niall Johnson, *Britain and the 1918–19 Influenza Pandemic: A Dark Epilogue* (London: Routledge, 2006), 192.
377 ID Mills, 'The 1918–1919 Influenza Pandemic – The Indian Experience'. *Indian Economic and Social History Review* 23:1–40, 1986, 35–6. Quoted in Hays, 387.
378 Johnson, 206.
379 Nikiforuk, *The Fourth Horseman*, 152.
380 Nikiforuk, 152.
381 Crawford, *Deadly Companions*, 204.
382 Dobson, *Disease*, 172.
383 Dobson, *Disease*, 174.
384 Thomas Randolph writing to Sir William Cecil, November 1562. Quoted in Charles Creighton, *A History of Epidemics in Britain, Volume II*, 308.
385 Alfred Crosby, 'Influenza: In the Grip of Grippe', Kiple, *PPP*, 149.
386 Alfred Crosby, 'Influenza: In the Grip of Grippe', Kiple, *PPP*, 149.
387 FB Smith, 'The Russian Influenza in the United Kingdom, 1889–1894', *Social History of Medicine*, 8 (1): 55–73, 64. Quoted in Johnson, 137.
388 Honigsbaum, 9.
389 John M Barry, *The Great Influenza: The Story of the Deadliest Pandemic in History*, 396–397.
390 See Gina Kolata, *Flu*, Ch 10.
391 See Honigsbaum, 17–32.
392 Nikiforuk, *The Fourth Horseman*, 154.
393 Honigsbaum, xiv.
394 Quoted in Joanne Reilly, *Belsen: The Liberation of a Concentration Camp* (London: Routledge, 1998), 24.
395 Reilly, 46.
396 Arthur Allen, *The Fantastic Laboratory of Dr. Weigl* (New York: WW Norton, 2014), 14.
397 Kenneth F Kiple and Kriemhild Coneè Ornelas, 'Typhus, Ships

and Soldiers', in Kiple, *PPP*, 109.

398 K David Patterson, 'Typhus and its Control in Russia, 1870–1940', *Medical History*, 1993, 37: 361–381, 361.

399 Hans Zinsser, *Rats, Lice and History*, 301.

400 Kenneth F Kiple and Kriemhild Coneè Ornelas, 'Typhus, Ships and Soldiers', in Kiple, *PPP*, 109.

401 Garrett, *The Coming Plague*, 30.

402 Garrett, 32.

403 Garrett, 30.

404 Garrett, 36.

405 JG Farrell, *The Lung* (London: Corgi, 1968), 56.

406 Alastair Cooke, *Letter from America*, 18 April 1955. Quoted in Gareth Williams, *Paralysed with Fear: The Story of Polio*, 209.

407 Garrett, 30.

408 World Health Organization, Resolution WHA33.3, 8 May 1980.

409 Randy Shilts, *And the Band Played On: Politics, People, and the AIDS Epidemic*, 48.

410 Shilts, 48.

411 Shilts, 48.

412 Dobson, *Disease*, 192. Also quoted in Shilts, 40.

413 Crawford, *Virus Hunt*, 4.

414 Peter Piot, 121.

415 Crawford, *Virus Hunt*, 35–36.

416 Piot, 122.

417 Piot, 131.

418 Piot et al (1984), 'Acquired immunodeficiency syndrome in a heterosexual population in Zaire', *The Lancet* ii: 65–69. The same issue also included another paper – Van de Perre et al (1984) – on AIDS in Rwanda.

419 Crawford, *Virus Hunt*, 38.

420 Crawford, *Virus Hunt*, 38.

421 Even that wasn't his real name, which was Arne Vidar Røed; 'Arvid Noe' was an anagram derived from this.

422 1984 figures, Dobson, *Disease*, 197. Crawford (2013:7) puts the

1984 US figures at 6993 with 3342 deaths.

423 Crawford, *Virus Hunt*, 8.

424 Dobson, *Disease*, 193.

425 http://espn.go.com/classic/biography/s/Ashe_Arthur.html Accessed 10 March 2015.

426 Ed Hooper, *Slim: A Reporter's Own Story of AIDS in East Africa* (London: The Bodley Head, 1990), 20.

427 Ed Hooper, *Slim*, 20–21.

428 Ed Hooper, *Slim*, 26.

429 See Crawford, *Virus Hunt*, 202–204.

430 See Crawford, *Virus Hunt*, 133–149, for an account of the OPV theory and its demise. The original article, by Tom Curtis, appeared in *Rolling Stone* in 1992, issue 626, 54–60. Another early proponent of the theory was Ed Hooper, in his follow-up to *Slim*, *The River: A Journey back to the Source of HIV and AIDS* (Little, Brown, 1999).

431 Crawford, *Virus Hunt*, 165.

432 Crawford, *Virus Hunt*, 166.

433 http://www.bbc.co.uk/news/health-29442642 Accessed 3 October 2014. The paper the BBC article reports is Oliver G Pybus, Philippe Lemey, et al, 'The Early Spread and Epidemic Ignition of HIV-1 in Human Populations', *Science* 3 October 2014: Vol. 346 no. 6205, pp. 56–61. DOI: 10.1126/science.1256739.

434 Dobson, *Disease*, 200–201.

435 John Iliffe, *The African AIDS Epidemic: A History* (Oxford: James Currey Ltd, 2006), 159.

436 Quoted in Iliffe, *The African AIDS Epidemic*, 25.

437 Garrett, *The Coming Plague*, 33.

438 Dobson, *Disease*, 243.

439 Dobson, *Disease*, 247.

440 Dobson, *Disease*, 234.

441 Joel D Howell, 'Concepts of Heart-Related Diseases', in *CWHHD*, 92.

442 Dobson, *Disease*, 240.
443 Dobson, *Disease*, 240.
444 Dobson, *Disease*, 240.
445 Dobson, *Disease*, 239.
446 Joel D Howell, 'Concepts of Heart-Related Diseases', in *CWHHD*, 92.
447 Joel D Howell, 'Concepts of Heart-Related Diseases', in *CWHHD*, 94.
448 Joel D Howell, 'Concepts of Heart-Related Diseases', in *CWHHD*, 94.
449 Tattersall, *Diabetes: The Biography*, 9.
450 Tattersall, *Diabetes: The Biography*, 9.
451 Tattersall, *Diabetes: The Biography*, 12.
452 Tattersall, *Diabetes: The Biography*, 14.
453 Tattersall, *Diabetes: The Biography*, 14.
454 Tattersall, *Diabetes: The Biography*, 18.
455 The full text can be read online at https://archive.org/details/ondiabetesandit00campgoog
456 Tattersall, *Diabetes: The Biography*, 179.
457 EP Joslin, LI Dublin and HH Marks, 'Studies in Diabetes mellitus: III. Interpretation of the variations in diabetes incidence', *American Journal of the Medical Sciences*, 189 (1935), 163–93. Quoted in Tattersall, 179.
458 E Bulmer, 'The Menace of Obesity', *British Medical Journal* 1 (1932), 1024–26. Quoted in Tattersall, 180.
459 Robert Saundby, 'Diabetes mellitus', *Medical Annual* (Bristol, 1897), 675. Quoted in Tattersall, 178.
460 CL Bose, 'Discussion on Diabetes in the Tropics', British Medical Journal 2 (1907), 1051–64, quoted in Tattersall, 179.
461 CL Bose, quoted in Tattersall, 179.
462 Sander L Gilman, *Obesity: The Biography* (OUP, 2010), ix.
463 Sander L Gilman, *Obesity: The Biography* (OUP, 2010), ix.
464 Umberto Eco, *Faith in Fakes* (Vintage, 1998), 257.
465 Gilman, *Obesity: The Biography*, xv.

466 In John Wycliffe's translation of the Bible, we read 'But eschew thou unholy and vain speeches, for why those profit much to unfaithfulness, and the word of them creepeth as a canker'. (2 Timothy 2:16–17)

467 See, among others, Francis Barrett, *The Magus*, Book II (London: 1801); H Stanley Redgrove, *Alchemy Ancient and Modern* (London: 1922).

468 See Siddhartha Mukherjee, *The Emperor of All Maladies: A Biography of Cancer*, 92.

469 See Rock Brynner and Trent Stephens, *Dark Remedy: The Impact of Thalidomide and its Revival as a Vital Medicine* (New York: Basic Books, 2001).

470 See Valerie Steele, *The Corset: A Cultural History* (New Haven and London: Yale University Press, 2001), Ch 3, 'Dressed to Kill: The Medical Consequences of Corsetry.'

471 Clive Bates and Andy Rowell, *Tobacco Explained: The Truth about the Tobacco Industry… in its own words*, available from the World Health Organization: https://www.researchgate.net/publication/46438695_Tobacco_Explained_The_truth_about_the_tobacco_industry_in_its_own_words.

472 Laurie Garrett, *Coming Plague: Newly Emerging Diseases in a World out of Balance*, (Penguin: 1994), 53.

473 Laurie Garrett, *The Coming Plague*, 55.

474 Garrett, *The Coming Plague*, 75–76.

475 Garrett, *The Coming Plague*, 78.

476 Garrett, *The Coming Plague*, 82.

477 Garrett, *The Coming Plague*, 82.

478 Garrett, *The Coming Plague*, 83.

479 Garrett, *The Coming Plague*, 103–104.

480 Garrett, *The Coming Plague*, 111.

481 Garrett, *The Coming Plague*, 124.

482 David Quammen, *Ebola: The Natural and Human History* (London: The Bodley Head, 2014), 24.

483 Quammen, *Ebola*, 24.

484 Quammen, *Ebola*, 32.
485 See, for instance, J Michael Fay's study of gorillas detailed in Quammen, *Ebola*, Ch 1.
486 For more on the 1976 Sudan outbreak, see http://www.ncbi.nlm.nih.gov/pmc/articles/PMC2395561/
487 Quammen, *Ebola*, 27.
488 Quammen, *Ebola*, 41.
489 Quammen, *Ebola*, 42.
490 Quammen, *Ebola*, 111.
491 See the World Health Organization's *Ebola Situation Report* of 11 March 2015.
492 Quammen, *Ebola*, 107.
493 Quammen, *Ebola*, 41.
494 Karlen, *Plague's Progress*, 6.
495 Dobson, *Disease*, 221.
496 Nathan Wolfe, *The Viral Storm: The Dawn of a New Pandemic Age* (Penguin, 2013), 82.
497 Thomas Abraham, *Twenty-First Century Plague: The Story of SARS* (Baltimore: Johns Hopkins University Press, 2005), 2.
498 Andrew Nikiforuk, *Pandemonium: Bird Flu, Mad Cow Disease, and Other Biological Plagues of the 21st Century* (Toronto: Viking Canada, 2006), 5.
499 Nikiforuk, *Pandemonium*, 6.
500 William McNeill, *Plagues and Peoples*, 13–21.
501 Karlen, *Plague's Progress*, 6. The list is selective.
502 Sally Davies, *The Drugs Don't Work* (Penguin, 2013), 45. Davies notes that over one million people died of TB in 2010.
503 Michael Shnayerson and Mark Plotkin, *The Killer Within*, 165.
504 Hugh Pennington, 'Don't Pick Your Nose', in *London Review of Books*, Vol. 27 No. 24, 15 December 2005, 29–31.
505 Nikiforuk, *Pandemonium*, 235.
506 Hugh Pennington, 'Don't Pick Your Nose', in *London Review of Books*, Vol. 27 No. 24, 15 December 2005, 29–31.
507 Davies, *The Drugs Don't Work*, xii.

508 See Martin J Blaser, *Missing Microbes: How the Overuse of Antibiotics is Fueling our Modern Plagues* (New York: Henry Holt/London: Oneworld Publications, 2014).

509 James Le Fanu, *The Rise and Fall of Modern Medicine* (London: Abacus, 2011), 465–466.

510 Davies, *The Drugs Don't Work*, x.

511 See, amongst others, Steven Salzberg, 'Anti-Vaccine Movement Causes Worst Measles Epidemic In 20 Years', *Forbes*, 1 February 2015.

512 Dr Jolyon M Medlock and Steve A Leach, PhD, 'Effect of climate change on vector-borne disease risk in the UK'. *The Lancet*, published Online: 23 March 2015. DOI: http://dx.doi.org/10.1016/S1473–3099(15)70091–5

513 Dr Jolyon M Medlock and Steve A Leach, PhD, 'Effect of climate change on vector-borne disease risk in the UK'. *The Lancet*, published Online: 23 March 2015. DOI: http://dx.doi.org/10.1016/S1473–3099(15)70091–5

514 Roxanne Khamsi, 'Were "cursed" rams the first biological weapons?', *New Scientist*, 26 November 2007.

515 See David Willman, *The Mirage Man: Bruce Ivins, the Anthrax Attacks, and America's Rush to War* (Bantam, 2011).

516 Thomas Abraham, *Twenty-first Century Plague: The Story of SARS*, 143.

517 Thomas Abraham, *Twenty-first Century Plague: The Story of SARS*, 143.

518 Andrew Nikiforuk, *Pandemonium*, 267.

519 Nikiforuk, *Pandemonium*, 268.

520 Davies, *The Drugs Don't Work*, 46–50.

521 AncientBiotics: 'A medieval remedy for modern day superbugs?' https://www.nottingham.ac.uk/life-sciences/news/a-medieval-remedy-for-modren-day-superbugs.aspx (sic). Accessed 8 April 2015.

522 Of course, it's wrong to think of myths as happening 'back then'. They are timeless and ongoing. As Sallust said, 'These things never

happened, but are, always.'
523 Farrar & Ahuja, 12.
524 Farrar & Ahuja, 14.
525 Farrar & Ahuja, 18.
526 Farrar & Ahuja, 36
527 https://www.reuters.com/article/us-china-health-who-idUSKBN1ZM1G9. Accessed 16 December 2021.
528 Wang, Horby, et al, 'A novel coronavirus outbreak of global health concern', *The Lancet (London, England)* vol. 395, 10223 (2020): 470–473; Huang, Wang, Li, et al, 'Clinical features of patients infected with 2019 novel coronavirus in Wuhan, China, *The Lancet (London, England)* vol. 395, 10223 (2020): 497–506.
529 Farrar & Ahuja, 81.
530 Huang, Wang, Li, et al.
531 Wang, Horby, et al.
532 https://www.who.int/director-general/speeches/detail/who-director-general-s-remarks-at-the-media-briefing-on-2019-ncov-on-11-february-2020. Accessed 16 December 2021.
533 https://www.who.int/news/item/30-01-2020-statement-on-the-second-meeting-of-the-international-health-regulations-(2005)-emergency-committee-regarding-the-outbreak-of-novel-coronavirus-(2019-ncov). Accessed 16 December 2021.
534 For a detailed account of the creation of the Oxford AstraZeneca vaccine, see Professor Sarah Gilbert's and Dr Catherine Green's *Vaxxers* (Hodder, 2021).
535 Horton, 16–17.
536 Horton, 17.
537 Andres Schipani, Henry Foy, Jude Webber, and Max Seddon, 'The "Ostrich Alliance": the leaders denying the coronavirus threat.' *Financial Times*, 17 April 2020.
538 Africanews/AFP, 'Magufuli died from Covid, says Tanzania opposition leader Tundu Lissu'. https://www.africanews.com/2021/03/18/magufuli-died-from-covid-says-tanzania-opposition-leader-tundu-lissu/. Accessed 17 January 2022.

539 Horton, 53.
540 Lily Kuo, 'Trump sparks anger by calling coronavirus the "Chinese virus"', *The Guardian*, 17 March 2020.
541 Horton, 70.
542 Jon Henley, 'World's media ask how it went so wrong for "Plague Island" Britain'. https://www.theguardian.com/world/2020/dec/22/worlds-media-ask-how-it-went-so-wrong-for-plague-island-britain-covid. Accessed 23 December 2021.
543 UK chief medical adviser, Professor Dame Sally Davies, quoted in Calvert and Arbuthnott, 88.
544 Interview on ITV's *This Morning*, 5 March 2020.
545 Calvert & Arbuthnott, 153.
546 Although the UK government did not know it at the time, the first UK death from COVID-19 occurred on 30 January 2020, when Peter Attwood, an 84-year-old man from Chatham in Kent, succumbed to the disease. Mr Attwood had fallen ill on 28 December 2019, suggesting that the virus may have entered the UK much earlier than previously thought. See Calvert & Arbuthnott, 51–2, 55.
547 Heather Stewart and Ian Sample, 'Coronavirus: enforcing UK lockdown one week earlier "could have saved 20,000 lives"', *The Guardian*, 11 June 2020. https://www.theguardian.com/world/2020/jun/10/uk-coronavirus-lockdown-20000-lives-boris-johnson-neil-ferguson. Accessed 27 December 2021.
548 Nick Triggle, 'Covid-19: NHS Test and Trace "no clear impact" despite £37bn budget.' *BBC News*, 10 March 2021. https://www.bbc.co.uk/news/health-56340831. Accessed 24 December 2021.
549 Claire Press, 'Coronavirus: The NHS workers wearing bin bags as protection.' *BBC News*, 5 April 2020. https://www.bbc.co.uk/news/health-52145140. Accessed 24 December 2021.
550 Horton, 133–5.
551 Daniel Martin, Emine Sinmaz, and Martin Robinson, 'Fury over

£18 billion PPE scandal.' *Daily Mail*, 18 November 2020. https://www.dailymail.co.uk/news/article-8961343/Fury-18bn-PPE-scandal.html. Gareth Iacobucci,'Covid-19: Government has spent billions on contracts with little transparency, watchdog says.' *British Medical Journal*, 18 November 2020. https://www.bmj.com/content/371/bmj.m4474. Accessed 24 December 2021.

552 See, for instance: Sophie Hill, 'The Tories' "chumocracy" over Covid contracts is destroying public trust.' *The Guardian*, 21 November 2020. https://www.theguardian.com/commentisfree/2020/nov/21/tories-covid-contracts-public-trust-government. Accessed 28 December 2021. T. J. Coles, 'How the Tories normalised corruption: In the past, corruption brought down politicians. But today, it's a business model.' *The London Economic*, 14 October 2020. https://www.thelondoneconomic.com/politics/how-the-tories-normalised-corruption-report-205523/. Accessed 28 December 2021. David Collins, Andrew Gregory, Gabriel Pogrund and Tom Calver, 'Tory backers net £180m PPE deals.' *The Sunday Times*, 9 August 2020. https://www.thetimes.co.uk/article/tory-backers-net-180m-ppe-deals-xwd5kmnqr. Accessed 28 December 2021. Laura Webster, '£1bn of government contracts given to Tory "friends and donors" during crisis.' *The National*, 22 October 2020. https://www.thenational.scot/news/18813681.1bn-government-contracts-given-tory-friends-donors-crisis/. Accessed 28 December 2021. Justin Parkinson, 'Government acted unlawfully over firm's £560,000 Covid contract.' *BBC News*, 9 June 2021. https://www.bbc.co.uk/news/uk-politics-57413115. Accessed 28 December 2021. Sam Bright, 'Government Awards £122 million PPE contract to one-month-old firm.' *Byline Times*, 14 September 2020. https://bylinetimes.com/2020/09/21/government-ppe-deals-conservatives-364-million/. Accessed 28 December 2021. Bethany Reilly, 'Government has spent nearly £2 billion on 'crony contracts' to Tory donors during pandemic.' *The Morning Star*, 7 February 2021.
https://morningstaronline.co.uk/article/b/government-has-

spent-nearly-2-billion-on-crony-contracts-tory-donors-during-pandemic. Accessed 28 December 2021. Craig Murray, 'Banana republic corruption.' 8 July 2020.
https://www.craigmurray.org.uk/archives/2020/07/banana-republic-corruption/. Accessed 28 December 2021.
Craig Murray, 'Stinking Tory corruption.' 6 August 2020. https://www.craigmurray.org.uk/archives/2020/08/stinking-tory-corruption/. Accessed 28 December 2021. Emma Youle, 'Revealed: Who Profited From The Government's Coronavirus Spending Boom: Firms with no history of supplying the products they were paid for, a business linked to Brexit lobbyists, and a dormant company were among the beneficiaries.' *Huffington Post*, 19 August 2020. https://www.huffingtonpost.co.uk/entry/who-profits-coronavirus-government-spending-boom_uk_5f0890c0c5b63a72c3413817. Accessed 28 December 2021. Danyal Hussain and David Wilcock, 'New Tory sleaze row over PPE deals as ex-Conservative chairman Lord Feldman and shamed former health Secretary Matt Hancock are revealed among those who helped total of 47 firms win "VIP" contracts worth more than £1.5billion at the height of the Covid pandemic.' *The Daily Mail*, 16 November 2021.
https://www.dailymail.co.uk/news/article-10207949/Matt-Hancock-Lord-Feldman-Tories-helped-47-firms-win-Covid-contracts-worth-millions.html. Accessed 28 December 2021.

553 'Covid: Government's PPE "VIP lane" unlawful, court rules'. *BBC News*, 13 January 2022. https://www.bbc.co.uk/news/uk-59968037. Accessed 17 January 2022.

554 Calvert & Arbuthnott, 273.

555 'How many Covid lockdown parties were held in Downing Street?' *BBC News*, 14 January 2022.
https://www.bbc.co.uk/news/uk-politics-59952395. Accessed 17 January 2022.

556 Calvert & Arbuthnott, 345.

557 Farrar & Ahuja, 183.

558 See Calvert & Arbuthnott, 354–60; Farrar & Ahuja, 172–84.
559 Calvert & Arbuthnott, 360–1.
560 Calvert & Arbuthnott, 368.
561 Simon Walters, 'Boris Johnson: "Let the bodies pile high in their thousands". PM's incendiary remark during fight over lockdowns is latest claim in No. 10 drama – amid spectacular row with Cummings.' *Daily Mail*, 25 April 2021. The claim that Johnson uttered these words was later confirmed by both Dominic Cummings, and political journalist Robert Peston.
562 Sam Lister, 'Boris Johnson battles experts to save Christmas with 40 mass vaccination centres.' *Daily Express*, 20 November 2020. https://www.express.co.uk/news/uk/1362343/boris-johnson-coronavirus-save-christmas-vaccination-centres-latest. Accessed 4 October 2021.
563 Niamh McIntyre, Pamela Duncan and Caelainn Barr, 'January's daily UK Covid death toll averages more than 1,000, figures show.' *The Guardian*, 30 January 2021. https://www.theguardian.com/world/2021/jan/30/januarys-daily-uk-covid-death-toll-averages-more-than-1000-figures-show. Accessed 28 December 2021.
564 T. J. Coles, 'The Tories have taken credit for the vaccine rollout—here's who is really behind the remarkable success: Team Johnson benefitted politically from the hard work of scientists, frontline workers, the Armed Forces and, of course, the NHS.' *The London Economic*, 2 June 2021. https://www.thelondoneconomic.com/news/the-tories-have-taken-credit-for-the-vaccine-rollout-heres-who-is-really-behind-the-remarkable-success-272920/. Accessed 28 December 2021.
565 Nick Triggle, 'Covid: UK's early response worst public health failure ever, MPs say.' *BBC News*, 12 October 2021. https://www.bbc.co.uk/news/health-58876089. Accessed 28 December 2021.
566 The House of Commons report, *Coronavirus: lessons learned to date*, is available here: https://committees.parliament.uk/publications/7496/documents/78687/default/.
567 Peter Walker, 'Damning Commons Covid report should be seen

only as a start.' *The Guardian*, 12 October 2021. https://www.theguardian.com/world/2021/oct/12/damning-commons-covid-report-should-be-seen-only-as-a-start. Accessed 28 December 2021.

568 Farrar & Ahuja, 226.

569 Farrar & Ahuja, 226.

570 Arundhati Roy, 'The pandemic is a portal'. *Financial Times*, 3 April 2020.

571 Žižek (2020), 3.

572 See Peter Baldwin, *Fighting the First Wave: Why the Coronavirus was Tackled So Differently Across the Globe.*

573 Richard Horton, 'COVID-19 is not a pandemic', *The Lancet*, 2020; 396: 874. https://www.thelancet.com/journals/lancet/article/PIIS0140-6736(20)32218-2/fulltext. Accessed 6 January 2022. Giovanni Di Guardo, 'CoViD-19 a "syndemic" rather than a "pandemic" disease', *British Medical Journal*, 14 December 2020, https://www.bmj.com/content/370/bmj.m3702/rapid-responses. Accessed 6 January 2022.

574 Emily Mendenhall, 'The COVID-19 syndemic is not global: context matters', *The Lancet*, 22 October 2020. https://www.thelancet.com/journals/lancet/article/PIIS0140-6736(20)32218-2/fulltext. Accessed 6 January 2022.

575 Jake Horton, 'Covid: Are some states lifting restrictions too soon?' *BBC News*, 12 March 2021. https://www.bbc.co.uk/news/world-us-canada-56297329. Accessed 1 February 2022.

576 Dartunorro Clark, 'San Francisco had the 1918 flu under control. And then it lifted the restrictions. A cautionary tale about the dangers of reopening too soon.' *NBC News*, 25 April, 2020. https://www.nbcnews.com/politics/politics-news/san-francisco-had-1918-flu-under-control-then-it-lifted-n1191141. Accessed 1 February 2022.

577 Farrar & Ahuja, 44.

578 Horton, 183.

579 Horton, 184.

580 Farrar & Ahuja, 214.

581 See, for instance, Rob Wallace's *Big Farms Make Big Flu: Dispatches on Influenza, Agribusiness and the Nature of Science*, and Mike Davis's *The Monster Enters: COVID-19, Avian Flu and the Plagues of Capitalism*.

582 Horton, 79.

583 Andy Haldane, 'Reweaving the social fabric after the crisis.' *Financial Times*, 24 April 2020.

584 Žižek (2020),41.

585 Žižek (2020), 41.

586 Arundhati Roy, 'The pandemic is a portal'. *Financial Times*, 3 April 2020.

Glossary of Diseases

An A-Z of the major diseases mentioned in the book

AIDS: Acquired Immunodeficiency Syndrome, first identified 1981. Thought to have originated in chimpanzees in West Africa, it causes the immune system to collapse, making the body vulnerable to diseases not usually fatal. Initially portrayed in the media as a 'gay plague', it became apparent that the disease could be transmitted via heterosexual intercourse, blood transfusions and from mother to baby.

Amebiasis: Deadly parasitic disease causing dysentery and diarrhoea, often transmitted by the faecal-oral route.

Anthrax: Affects primarily cattle, sheep and goats. Humans can become infected through contact with animals or animal products, although can't spread it from person to person. Robert Koch's and Louis Pasteur's work on anthrax played a crucial part in the development of germ theory. The Biblical plagues of Egypt might have included anthrax; Virgil describes the disease in *The Georgics.* During World War Two and the Cold War, anthrax was considered for use as a biological weapon.

Arthritis: One of the oldest known diseases, causing pain and stiffness in the joints. Traces have been found in human bones dating from 3500 BC (in its rheumatoid form). We have fifth century BC descriptions from Hippocrates for the more common form, osteoarthritis. The ancient Greeks believed the disease to have been divine retribution for the destruction of the Temple of Ashkelon by the Scythians in the seventh century BC.

Asclepia: Temples built in ancient Greece dedicated to the god of medicine, Asclepius. Rituals at Asclepia involved incubation, or temple sleep. The patient would sleep before an image of the god, and hope they would either be made well during the night by Asclepius, or be given the cure in a dream. People came to Asclepia seeking cures from blindness, paralysis, edema, tapeworms, abdominal abscesses, lice, headaches, wounds sustained in battle, infertility, gout, even baldness.

Avian influenza: Bird flu (H5N1) broke out in China in 1996, causing the culling of over a million birds. Influenza is notorious for being able to mutate. H5N1 is linked to the Spanish Flu of 1918, the deadliest pandemic of all time, and the next pandemic is expected to be a form of bird flu.

Bats: Bats are vectors (or the carriers) of many diseases – including **Ebola**, it is suspected, and **Marburg virus**. Other bat diseases include Hendra virus, **SARS**, **Nipah**, **Rabies,** Duvenhage and Kyasanur Forest virus.

Beriberi: Caused by a deficiency of thiamine, or vitamin B1, it produces swelling of the legs, arms, and face. The nerves and cardiovascular system may also be affected. Known since antiquity in China and Japan, where it is described in some of the world's oldest medical texts. The name derives from the Sinhalese word for weakness.

Bronchitis: Known since antiquity, where the Chinese text *Yueh Ling* (*Monthly Ordinances*) refers to it as a disease particularly prevalent in summer months.

BSE: Bovine spongiform encephalopathy, otherwise known as mad cow disease, first appeared in the UK in 1984. BSE is a neurodegenerative condition that is thought to have been caused by feeding cows the brains and spinal cords of sheep. Dubbed 'high-tech cannibalism', its human form is **variant CJD**. Both human and bovine forms cause the rapid onset of dementia and death, and are incurable.

Cancer: 'Canker' first appeared in the English language in the fourteenth century, although records of tumours that 'eat' date back to the second millennium BC in Egyptian papyri. Cancer saw a rise in the twentieth century, although this could be the result of improvements in methods of detection. It is now one of the world's major killers.

Carrión's disease: Discovered by conquistadores in the sixteenth century, Carrión's disease is a New World disease with a very old provenance: it seems to have been represented on pieces of pre-Columbian Peruvian pottery known as *huacos*. Originating in the Andes, it is a parasitic condition that can cause fever and anaemia and can lead to unsightly boils known as 'Peruvian warts'.

Cattle plague (rinderpest): Although it does not affect humans, cattle plague has a long history of causing devastation in human communities, causing loss of livelihood, famine and the diseases that follow in its wake, such as **typhus**.

Chagas' disease: Like **Carrión's disease**, Chagas' disease was unknown in the Old World. Similar to sleeping sickness, it seems to have originated in northeastern Brazil and evolved independently. It is at least two thousand years old: mummies from the Tarapaca Valley in northern Chile have revealed Chagas' signature digestive tract problems, and it remains endemic in parts of Chile to this day.

Chicken pox: Common childhood disease in many parts of the world, chickenpox is caused by a virus that remains latent within the body and can reappear in later life as shingles.

Cholera: Probably endemic in India since time immemorial. The nineteenth century saw a succession of cholera pandemics that killed millions. The first outbreak in the UK in 1832 was heralded by an official day of national penance and prayer in an attempt to try and stop the disease from reaching British shores. It is caused by a bacterium, and John Snow discovered it was transmitted by dirty water. Cholera was eradicated in Britain with the invention of Victorian sewerage systems.

COVID-19: Contagious respiratory disease caused by the coronavirus SARS-CoV-2. Symptoms include fever, headache, loss of taste and smell, aches, vomiting, fatigue, and difficulty breathing, although some cases can be asymptomatic. Complications include pneumonia, respiratory failure, pulmonary fibrosis, kidney failure, and long COVID. The original reservoir is thought to be bats, although research is ongoing. The disease emerged in China in the autumn of 2019, with the first cases being reported in December.. The ensuing pandemic was the most serious global health emergency since the Spanish Flu a hundred years earlier.

Crimean-Congo haemorrhagic fever: Tick-borne virus first identified in the Crimea in 1944, later in the Congo (1969), although an account from twelfth century Tajikistan may be the same disease. Symptoms include fever, back, joint and stomach pain, red spots on the palate, vomiting and bleeding and bruising, mood swings and changes in sensory perception. Fatality rates can be anywhere from 9 to 50 per cent.

Dengue fever: Known as breakbone fever due to the intense pains it causes in bones and joints, dengue is a mosquito-borne viral disease that also causes a measles-like rash. Has seen a huge increase in cases since the 1960s, and is now endemic in more than 100 countries.

Diabetes: Known since antiquity as a disease that causes 'honey-tasting' urine – people were employed as professional tasters – it was known in the seventeenth century as the 'Pissing Evil'. Caused by irregularities in the pancreas, diabetes has seen an upsurge in the twentieth century, largely due to an increase in obesity. In British India, it was seen as one of the 'penalties of an advanced civilisation'.

Diphtheria: A 'throat distemper' that causes a hide-like membrane on the tonsils and a 'bullneck'. Frequently a disease of the poor in the nineteenth century, the first recorded epidemics were in the seventeenth century. The Spanish outbreak of 1613 was known as The Year of Strangulations, a reference to the severe sore throat and breathing difficulties that diphtheria produces.

Dracunculiasis: Old Testament references to a 'fiery serpent' are, it has been suggested, references to the guinea worm, which causes dracunculiasis, a parasitic infection caused by drinking infected water. Egyptian mummies from *c.* 1450–1500 BC also show evidence of worm infestation, and the Indian Rig Veda offers magical charms against the worm. The female worms move through the person's subcutaneous tissue, causing intense pain, and eventually emerge through the skin, usually at the feet, producing blisters and ulcers, accompanied by fever, nausea, and vomiting.

Dropsy: An abnormal accumulation of fluid in the interstitium, between the skin and in the cavities of the body. Galen noted that it was a common condition in ancient Rome. Its principal causes are congestive heart failure, liver failure, kidney failure, and malnutrition.

Dysentery: A major killer of children in ancient Rome, dysentery (bloody diarrhoea) also saw King John and Henry V of England and Louis IX of France to their graves.

Ebola: One of the deadliest diseases known, Ebola is an acute viral haemorrhagic fever that first broke out in South Sudan and northern Democratic Republic of Congo in 1976. In the latter case, the mortality rate was 88 per cent. Its animal reservoir is unknown, although bats are strongly suspected. The 2014 outbreak in West Africa was the first time Ebola had reached epidemic proportions, with over 10,000 deaths.

Elephantiasis: Caused by a parasitic worm, elephantiasis can cause thickening of the skin and horrific swellings of the lower body.

Encephalitis: A viral swelling of the brain, encephalitis comes in a variety of forms. Many can be fatal. Some survivors can develop parkinsonism.

English Sweate: A mysterious sweating sickness that first affected England in 1485 after the Battle of Bosworth. Dutch mercenaries fighting for Henry VII were immune. It could kill within 24 hours. German medical historian Justus Hecker attributed the disease to the

English weather and habits of the aristocracy – gluttony and heavy drinking in particular. The English Sweate disappeared after 1551, although the equally mysterious Picardy sweat, noted in the C18 and C19, could be a descendant.

Epilepsy: A neurological disease of ancient pedigree. Ancient Babylonians attributed epilepsy to the touch of a god, or the influence of the star Marduk (Jupiter). Hippocrates believed the disease had a natural explanation, although was not able to identify a cause. The ancient Romans believed fresh human blood could cure epilepsy, and sufferers were allowed into the arena to drink from gladiators' wounds. In the early modern period, epileptics were frequently confined in mental asylums.

Ergotism (St Anthony's Fire): A fungal disease that can cause convulsions and, in its gangrenous form, rashes and hallucinations. An outbreak in 922 of the gangrenous type was said to have killed 40,000 people, while another killed 14,000 in Paris in 1128–9. Ergotism has been proposed as the disease behind the Salem witch trials in 1692, as the accused girls all showed signs of ergot poisoning, including eating bread that was coloured red – a classic indicator of ergot-infested rye.

Erysipelas: Long confused with ergotism, which also produces rashes on the skin, erysipelas was identified as a separate disease in the nineteenth century. It was noted that erysipelas often happened in conjunction with puerperal or childbed fever, one of the main causes of deaths in childbirth. Puerperal fever was eventually found to be caused by the doctors attending women in labour not washing their hands.

Fatal familial insomnia: A very rare neurological disease caused by prions, fatal familial insomnia produces progressively worsening insomnia, leading to hallucinations, delirium, and confusional states like that of dementia. It is usually fatal within 18 months of onset.

Gerstmann–Sträussler–Scheinker syndrome: A very rare neurodegenerative disease caused by prions. Initial symptoms include difficulty speaking and unsteadiness, followed by worsening dementia.

Gout: A disease that causes the joints, particularly the knee and ankles, to swell due to the formation of crystals as a result of higher levels of uric acid in the blood. 90 per cent of the sufferers are male. Long associated with fine living and overindulgence, its nickname 'the Disease of Kings' reflects the fact that the well-to-do were often its victims. The poor had to make do with **pellagra**.

Haemorrhagic fevers: Viral diseases characterised by a high fever, bleeding from all orifices, shock and high mortality rates. Yellow fever is one of the oldest known, characterised by jaundice and the production of black vomit, while **Ebola** is the most well-known of the newer haemorrhagic fevers. The group also includes **Marburg virus**, **Lassa fever**, and **Crimean-Congo haemorrhagic fever**, which all originated in Africa and Asia. A South American group includes Argentine, Bolivian, Brazilian and Venezuelan haemorrhagic fevers.

Halfdead disease: A condition known to the Anglo-Saxons, who referred to it as *seo healfdeade adl*, which was probably hemiplegia, a form of partial paralysis often caused by a stroke.

Heart disease: The heart attack is a particularly twentieth century phenomenon. Although demographer John Graunt (1620–74) recorded people dying 'suddenly', which could be heart-related, the term was not coined until 1912. Like diabetes, heart disease has seen a rise of cases in the twentieth century, and is now the biggest killer.

Hepatitis: Producing inflammation of the liver, often leading to jaundice, hepatitis exists in a number of different forms. It can be caused by excess consumption of alcohol or drugs, autoimmune deficiencies, and can be sexually transmitted.

HIV: Human immunodeficiency virus, the virus that causes **AIDS**. HIV has been one of the worst pandemics in history, infecting around

65 million people and killing around 25 million. Half of all HIV deaths have occurred in Africa.

Huntington's chorea: Neurodegenerative disorder than can lead to erratic movements and mental impairment. It has been suggested as a cause of dancing mania and **St Vitus Dance**.

Influenza: Also known as flu, influenza is a disease of humans, pigs, horses, and several other species of mammal and birds. In humans it is a very contagious respiratory disease characterised by sudden onset and symptoms of sore throat, cough, runny nose, fever, chills, headache, weakness, muscle and joint pain. The first recorded epidemics were in the sixteenth century, and an eighteenth century epidemic gave the disease its name, from the Italian for 'influence' (meaning the influence of the stars, which were thought to be responsible for so apparently universal an affliction.) A particularly virulent strain was responsible for the **Spanish Flu** pandemic in 1918–19.

Kuru: A degenerative neurological disease endemic among the Fore people of Papua New Guinea. It is similar to **variant CJD**. In the case of the Fore, it is usually caused by their practice of funerary cannibalism.

Lassa fever: An acute viral haemorrhagic fever first reported in Nigeria in 1969. Symptoms include high fever, lethargy, muscle and joint pains, sore throat, back pain, nausea, liver failure, and bleeding. Lassa can simulate the appearance of other endemic African diseases such as malaria, yellow fever and typhoid. Lassa is a Risk Group 4 pathogen, meaning it's one of the deadliest diseases known.

Legionnaires' disease: First breaking out at a convention of the American Legion in a Philadelphia hotel in 1976, Legionnaires' is a sudden form of pneumonia caused by a previously unknown bacterium, *legionella*. An airborne infection, the disease is frequently spread by air conditioning, cooling towers and condensers.

Leprosy: Along with plague, leprosy is perhaps the most feared disease in history. There are numerous references to leprosy in the Bible, although these could be any number of skin conditions. Leprosy reached epidemic proportions in Europe in the late Dark Ages through to the High Middle Ages. It declined after the fourteenth century, possibly being replaced by **tuberculosis**. Frequently seen in the Middle Ages as a disease caused by sin, lust in particular. Lepers were given bells and clappers to warn of their approach. The medical cause of the disease was finally identified in 1880 and it is now known as Hansen's Disease.

***Lupus vulgaris*:** A form of **tuberculosis** that attacks the skin, mainly around the face and neck. The name means 'common wolf'.

Lyme disease: First reported in Lyme, Connecticut, in 1975, Lyme is a tick-borne disease that can cause fever, headache, fatigue, and a distinctive skin rash called *erythema migrans*. If left untreated, infection can spread to the joints, the heart, and the nervous system.

Malaria: One of the oldest known diseases, malaria has probably killed more human beings than any other. Caused by the bacteria *Plasmodium falciparum*, it is transmitted to humans by the bite of the female *Anopheles* mosquito.

Marburg fever: Lethal viral haemorrhagic fever first reported in 1967, when it affected laboratory workers in Marburg and Frankfurt, Germany, and Belgrade, Yugoslavia. The outbreak was traced to monkeys from Uganda. It can have a fatality rate of 90 per cent, and is one of the World Health Organization's Risk Group 4 pathogens, meaning it's one of the deadliest diseases known.

Measles: Now one of the diseases of childhood, measles is a viral disease that causes a distinctive red rash. Measles is what is known as a crowd disease, meaning it needs a certain number of susceptibles to remain active. In prehistory, communities were not thought to be of sufficient size to sustain measles. The disease was initially far more virulent, and has been proposed as the cause of the Antonine Plague of AD 165–190, and the Plague of Cyprian, 251–70.

Meningitis: An acute inflammation of the meninges, the membranes that cover the brain and spinal cord. Usually the result of bacterial infection, but can also be caused by fungi and viruses.

MERS: Middle East Respiratory Syndrome was first identified in Saudi Arabia in 2012. MERS is a coronavirus, caused by the virus MERS-CoV, and produces fever, cough and shortness of breath. (Gastrointestinal symptoms have also been reported in some cases.) Infection with MERS can lead to pneumonia and death. Dromedary camels have been identified as a reservoir for MERS, with bats as the possible original reservoir. Since 2012, MERS has also been reported in the UK (2013), the Philippines (2014), the Netherlands (2014), South Korea (2015) and Saudi Arabia again in 2018. The fatality rate of MERS is in the region of 35%, making it a much more deadly disease than either SARS or COVID-19. There is no known vaccine.

MRSA: Known as a 'superbug' for its resistance to antibiotics, methicillin resistant *Staphylococcus aureus* first broke out in an English hospital in 1963, but became headline news in the 1990s as a disease increasingly prevalent in hospitals and other healthcare facilities. MRSA is a bacterium that can live on any surface, including the nostrils and skin, and can cause life-threatening infections such as blood poisoning, heart problems, pneumonia, urinary tract infection, septic arthritis, osteomyelitis and septic bursitis. MRSA can also cause **toxic shock syndrome.**

Mosquitoes: Along with **bats** and ticks, perhaps the most common disease vector. The most significant mosquito-borne disease is **malaria.** Others include **yellow fever, dengue fever** and **West Nile virus**.

Nipah: A zoonosis that sprang to bats to humans via pigs. The first outbreak occurred in Malaysian piggeries in 1999. Initially causing fever, vomiting and flu-like symptoms, Nipah then attacks the nervous system, and can cause brain damage and hallucinations before death occurs. It caused 100 human fatalities, and the culling of over one million pigs.

Obesity: A condition of the body, rather than a disease, obesity has nevertheless been linked to growing incidences of heart disease and diabetes. Increasingly sedentary western lifestyles, together with processed food, are largely responsible.

Omsk haemorrhagic fever: A highly contagious viral disease discovered in Western Siberia, it is transmitted to humans via contaminated water, an infected tick or rat, or by drinking the milk of an infected sheep or goat.

Pellagra: Dubbed 'land scurvy' for its similarities to the disease that afflicted sailors, pellagra is caused most often by a deficiency of vitamin B3. Characteristic symptoms include the 'Three Ds': diarrhoea, dementia and dermatitis.

Phthisis: One of the old Greek names for **tuberculosis.**

Pinta: a skin disease endemic to Central and South America caused by the spirochete, *Treponema pallidum carateum*, which is highly similar to the organism that causes **syphilis.**

Plague: Arguably the most notorious disease in history. Caused by the bacterium *Yersinia pestis*, plague is a rodent disease endemic in many parts of the world that is spread to humans by the rodent's fleas, or by eating infected rodent meat. There are three principal forms: bubonic, which settles in the lymphatic system and produces the black tumours or 'buboes' that give the disease its name; pneumonic, which attacks the lungs, and causes respiratory problems and the vomiting of blood; and septicaemic, which poisons the blood stream. Bubonic, although the most famous form, is the least lethal, with mortality rates anywhere between 30 to 60 per cent. Untreated pneumonic and septicaemic plague have death rates of almost 100 per cent. There have been three pandemics: the Plague of Justinian (542–*c.*750), the second (*c.*1330–1771), whose most notorious phase (*c.*1330–*c.*1350) was known as the Black Death, and a third pandemic that began in China in 1855, reached its apogee in the 1890s, when a vaccine for plague was developed, and was considered over by 1959. The Black Death is the most devastating pandemic in history, killing approximately one in three people across Asia, Europe, North Africa and the Middle East in less than twenty years. It did most of its work in Europe, the Middle East and North Africa in less than three (1347–50).

Pneumonia: An acute inflammatory condition of the lung tissue caused by numerous infectious agents and toxins. The name derives from the Greek for 'condition of the lung'. Symptoms include fever, cough, chest pain, and difficulty in breathing. Untreated, it can have a mortality rate of up to 30 per cent. Pneumonia can also be the result of another disease, such as AIDS, plague or Legionnaires' disease.

Polio: An acute disease caused by inflammation and destruction of motor neurons after infection by a poliovirus. Frequently asymptomatic, only a small number of those infected go on to develop full-blown polio. Symptoms can include fever, infection of the central nervous system, meningitis, paresis or paralysis. When the muscles of respiration are affected, death can occur. Although possibly known to the ancient Egyptians, polio suddenly became an epidemic disease in the nineteenth and twentieth centuries.

Pott's disease: A form of **tuberculosis** that attacks the spine, causing deformity. Thought to be depicted in funerary stelae from ancient Egypt.

Psoriasis: A disease of the skin that can cause rashes, scabs and irritation. Its cause is still not fully understood. It may have been taken for a form of **leprosy** in the past.

Puerperal fever: Also known as childbed fever, this was a major cause of mothers dying in childbirth, until it was suggested in the mid nineteenth century that mortality could be reduced by the doctor or midwife washing their hands. Doctors who had performed autopsies immediately prior to working in the delivery room were found to be inadvertently transmitting bacteria to the mother-to-be.

Pyorrhea: A dental disease that causes gradual loss of the alveolar bone around the teeth, and if left untreated, can lead to the loosening and subsequent loss of teeth.

Rabies: First recorded in a Babylonian legal tablet from *c.* 2300 BC, rabies is one of the oldest known diseases, and also one of the deadliest. Usually transmitted to humans via the bite of a rabid dog, it is impossible to survive without urgent treatment. A vaccine was developed by Louis Pasteur in 1885.

Relapsing fever: The endemic form of relapsing fever is transmitted to humans by ticks and rodents; the epidemic form by a spirochete, transmitted by human head and body lice. Often confused with **malaria** and **typhus**, due to the similarity of its symptoms.

Rickets: Mainly caused by a lack of vitamin D, rickets can cause various abnormalities of the bone, muscle weakness and dental problems.

Rinderpest (cattle plague): Although it does not affect humans, cattle plague has a long history of creating devastation in human communities, causing loss of livelihood, famine and the diseases that follow in its wake, such as **typhus**.

Ringworm: Skin condition caused by a fungal infection.

Risk Group 4 pathogens: The World Health Organization's highest hazard level classification for diseases. Group 4 pathogens are the deadliest diseases known to humanity, and include Ebola, Marburg, Lassa, Kyasanur Forest Virus, Machupo, Crimean Congo haemorrhagic fever and Nipah virus.

Salmonella: Infection with salmonella, known as salmonellosis, can cause diarrhoea, fever, and abdominal pain. Usually lasts up to a week, and most individuals recover without treatment. In rare cases, the infection can spread to the bloodstream, which can prove fatal unless treated.

SARS: Sudden Acute Respiratory Syndrome was the first pandemic of the twenty first century. Breaking out in China in November 2002, it spread to 32 countries over the coming months, with 8,000 cases and 900 deaths. It is thought to have originated in bats, and spread to humans via meat sold in Chinese markets.

Scabies: From the Latin word 'to scratch', scabies is a contagious skin disease caused by the mite *Sarcoptes scabiei*. The mite burrows under the skin and can cause intense itching.

Scarlet fever (scarlatina): A disease usually associated with childhood, scarlet fever causes a sore throat with difficulty swallowing, chills, vomiting and pain in the abdomen. After a couple of days, a distinctive red rash appears, giving the disease its name.

Schistosomiasis: Also known as bilharzia, schistosomiasis is a disease caused by the eggs of parasitic worms. The disease is transmitted by contact with freshwater, in which the snails that carry the worms live. Symptoms include a rash, itchy skin, fever, chills, cough, and muscle aches. Repeated infection can cause anaemia, malnutrition, and learning difficulties.

Scrofula: Also known as the King's Evil, scrofula is a form of tuberculosis that attacks the lymph nodes, where it causes swellings in the neck. In mediaeval and early modern France and England, the disease was thought to be curable by being touched by the monarch.

Scurvy: Caused by a deficiency of vitamin C, scurvy was one of the hazards of life on board ship. Symptoms include lethargy, spots on the skin (especially the legs), a softness of the gums that can lead to loss of teeth, jaundice and death. Early attempts at prevention included growing fruit and vegetables on board ship, a technique developed by the Dutch. The Royal Navy experimented with cider before settling on lime juice, earning Britons the nickname 'limeys' in the process.

Septicaemia: Blood poisoning usually caused by bacteria entering the bloodstream.

Sheep liver fluke: A zoonotic parasitic disease that affects the livers of sheep and cattle, but can also affect humans. Symptoms include vomiting, weight loss and liver problems.

Shigellosis: Caused by a bacteria closely related to **salmonella**, symptoms can range from abdominal discomfort to serious dysentery and seizures. Commonly transmitted by the faecal-oral route (contaminated water or unsanitary preparation of food).

Sickle cell anaemia: The most common form of sickle cell disease, it produces sickle-shaped red blood cells that can cause severe pain and strokes. Mainly found in sub-Saharan Africa, sickle cell disease can confer a certain degree of resistance to **malaria**.

SIV: Simian immunodeficiency virus is the monkey equivalent of HIV. It is thought that HIV made the species jump to humans from sooty mangabeys and chimpanzees sometime in the late nineteenth or early twentieth century.

Smallpox: A viral disease caused by two viruses, *Variola major* and *Variola minor*. Symptoms include the body being covered by rashes of pustules that can leave permanent scarring. *V. major*, the more serious form, can be fatal. The history of smallpox remains debated. The Egyptian pharaoh Ramses V (d. 1145 BC) may have suffered from smallpox, and it has been suggested as being the cause of the Antonine Plague (AD 165–190). Gregory of Tours was the first writer to use the term 'variola' in 580. Possibly due to a mutation, the disease became much more virulent during the Renaissance and early modern period, when it became known as 'smallpox' to differentiate it from the 'great pox' – syphilis. The World Health Organization launched a campaign to eradicate smallpox in 1967, and the disease was officially declared extinct in 1980. Samples, however, remain in high security storage facilities.

Spanish Flu: A pandemic of unusually virulent influenza, Spanish Flu broke out in the spring of 1918. Due to war broadcasting restrictions, the first reports came from Spain (a neutral country), and it became known as the Spanish Flu. It is now thought to have killed at least 50 million people in the space of 12 months, more than died in the First World War. It is the deadliest pandemic in history.

Sydenham's chorea: A neurological disease caused by bacteria that can produce spasmodic movements, loss of motor control and impaired cognitive function. It has been suspected as being the disease behind **St Vitus Dance**.

Syphilis: The most infamous sexually transmitted disease prior to AIDS, syphilis is thought to have been brought back to Europe by Christopher Columbus's expeditions to the Americas. Due to the horrific disfigurement it causes, syphilis spread fear and revulsion across Europe. It became less virulent over time. Effective treatments against it were not developed until the early twentieth century.

Taterapox: Posited as one of the diseases **smallpox** could have evolved from, it affects mainly rodents.

Tetanus: A bacterial disease that, due to the severe spasms it can cause, has long been known as lockjaw. It is transmitted to humans via wounds, and can be fatal in up to 50 per cent of untreated cases.

Toxic shock syndrome: A bacterial disease first reported in 1978. Symptoms can include high fever, accompanied by low blood pressure, malaise and confusion, which can worsen to stupor, coma, and multiple organ failure. Also produces a sunburn-like rash. It can be fatal if untreated.

Trench fever and trench foot: Diseases that affected soldiers in the First World War. Trench fever is a relapsing fever caused by the human body louse (see **typhus**), while trench foot was a gangrenous condition of the feet caused by prolonged exposure to the cold, dirty water of the trenches. Although most associated with the First World War, it was first noted on Napoleon's 1812 campaign in Russia.

Tuberculosis: A bacterial disease that can affect almost any organ of the body, tuberculosis most frequently settles in the lungs (pulmonary TB). The remains dating from around 7000 BC of a mother and child found in the submerged village of Atlit Yam off the coast of Israel both showed signs of tuberculosis, making it one of the oldest definitely identifiable diseases.

Tularemia: A bacterial disease that can affect aquatic rodents, but is especially virulent in rabbits and humans. Clinical signs in humans include fever, lethargy, skin lesions, loss of appetite, signs of sepsis, and possibly death. The face and eyes redden, becoming inflamed. If inflammation spreads to the lymph nodes, they can enlarge and suppurate (resembling bubonic plague).

Typhoid: The name, meaning 'like typhus', was coined in the 1830s when it became clear it was a separate disease. One of the great nineteenth century diseases of urban filth, typhoid is caused by the bacterium *salmonella typhi*, and thrives in areas with poor sanitation, transmitted via faecal-oral contamination. Symptoms include abdominal pain, intense headache, high fever and a distinctive 'rose rash' on the chest and abdomen. Untreated it can be fatal in 10 to 20 per cent of cases.

Typhus: Transmitted by the human body louse, typhus routinely follows armies and famines. (It defeated Napoleon's huge army in 1812 when he attempted to take Moscow.) It was also prevalent in prisons, where it was known as jail fever, and caused the Black Assizes – courtroom epidemics – of the early modern period. Symptoms include fever, headache, delirium, high temperature and, after a few days, a rash. The name derives from the Greek word for 'smoky' or 'hazy', a reference to the delirious state many typhus patients suffer.

St Vitus Dance: Notable outbreaks of dancing mania occurred in 1374 at Aachen and in 1518 at Strasbourg. These have been attributed to convulsive **ergotism** (St Anthony's Fire), **Huntington's chorea**, **Sydenham's chorea** or the effects of stress. Tarantism, thought to be caused by the bite of a tarantula, was long thought to be the same phenomenon.

West Nile virus: Tropical mosquito borne disease discovered in 1937 that was not thought to be a serious threat until it reached Romania in 1996, and New York City in 1999. In severe cases can lead to neurological damage.

Whooping cough (pertussis): A highly contagious respiratory tract infection. With initial cold-like symptoms, whooping cough can become more serious, especially in infants. The distinctive cough can be so hard that it can cause fainting, vomiting, broken ribs, hernias and incontinence.

Yaws: An ancient skin disease related to syphilis, although is not sexually transmitted. Bone evidence suggests humans were susceptible to yaws 1.5 million years ago.

Yellow fever: First recorded in Barbados in 1647, yellow fever causes severe jaundice and death. Its other colourful characteristic, black vomit, earned it the nickname *el vomito negro.*

Zika: First identified in Uganda in 1947, Zika is a virus usually transmitted by the bite of a female *Aedes* mosquito. Zika can also be transmitted through sexual intercourse, and blood transfusions. Symptoms of Zika include fever, rash, conjunctivitis, and muscle and joint pain. Infection during pregnancy can lead to birth defects such as microcephaly, and can cause premature birth and miscarriage. Zika can also lead to neurologic complications including Guillain-Barré syndrome, neuropathy, and myelitis. An epidemic of Zika occurred in Brazil in 2015-6, spreading throughout the Americas and the Caribbean.

Bibliography

Aberth, John, *The Black Death: The Great Mortality of 1348–1350: A Brief History with Documents*. Boston: Bedford/St Martin's, 2005.

Abraham, Thomas, *Twenty-first Century Plague: The Story of SARS*. Baltimore: Johns Hopkins University Press, 2005.

Alcabes, Philip, *Dread: How Fear and Fantasy Have Fueled Epidemics from the Black Death to Avian Flu*. New York: Public Affairs Books, 2009.

Allen, Terence and Cowling, Graham, *The Cell: A Very Short Introduction*. Oxford: Oxford University Press, 2011.

Alexander, John T, *Bubonic Plague in Early Modern Russia: Public Health and Urban Disaster*. Oxford: Oxford University Press, 2003.

Allen, Arthur, *Vaccine: The Controversial Story of Medicine's Greatest Lifesaver*. New York, London: WW Norton, 2007.

______, *The Fantastic Laboratory of Dr. Weigl: How Two Brave Scientists Battled Typhus and Sabotaged the Nazis*. New York: WW Norton & Company, 2014.

Amyes, Sebastian, *Bacteria: A Very Short Introduction*. Oxford: Oxford University Press, 2013.

Andrews, Jonathan, Briggs, Asa, Porter, Roy, Tucker, Penny & Waddington, Keir, *The History of Bethlem*. London: Routledge, 1997.

Andrews, Jonathan and Scull, Andrew T, *Undertaker of the Mind: John Monro and Mad-Doctoring in Eighteenth-Century England*. Berkeley, London: University of California Press, 2001.

______, *Customers and Patrons of the Mad-trade: The Management of Lunacy in Eighteenth-century London: With the Complete Text of John Monro's 1766*

Case Book. Berkeley, London: University of California Press, 2003.
Arrizabalaga, Jon, Henderson, John and French, Roger, *The Great Pox: The French Disease in Renaissance Europe*. New Haven; London: Yale University Press, 1997.
Aufderheide, Arthur C & Rodrígues-Martín, Conrado, *The Cambridge Encyclopedia of Human Paleopathology*. Cambridge: Cambridge University Press, 1998.
Baer, George M (ed.), *The Natural History of Rabies* (2 vols). New York, San Francisco, London: Academic Press, 1975.
Baldwin, Peter, *Fighting the First Wave: Why the Coronavirus was Tackled So Differently Across the Globe*. Cambridge: Cambridge University Press, 2021.
Barnes, David S, *The Great Stink of Paris and the Nineteenth-century Struggle against Filth and Germs*. Baltimore: Johns Hopkins University Press, 2006.
Barrett, Francis, *The Magus*. London: Lackington, Allen & Co, 1801.
Barry, John M, *The Great Influenza: The Story of the Deadliest Pandemic in History*. New York: Penguin Books, 2009.
Bartosiewicz, László, *Shuffling Nags, Lame Ducks: The Archaeology of Animal Disease*. Oxford : Oxbow Books; Oakville, CT: David Brown Book Company, 2013.
Bassett, Steve (editor), *Death in Towns: Urban Responses to the Dying and the Dead, 100–1600*. Leicester, London, New York: Leicester University Press, 1992.
Bates, Clive and Rowell, Andy, *Tobacco Explained: The Truth about the Tobacco Industry… in its own words*. ASH/World Health Organization, n.d.
Bede, *Historical Works*, trans. JE King (2 vols). Loeb Classical Library. London: Heinemann/Cambridge, MA: Harvard University Press, 1962.
Belchem, John, *Irish, Catholic and Scouse: The History of the Liverpool-Irish, 1800–1939*. Liverpool: Liverpool University Press, 2007.
Benedict, Carol, *Bubonic Plague in Nineteenth-century China*. Stanford: Stanford University Press, 1996.

BIBLIOGRAPHY

Benedictow, Ole J, *The Black Death, 1346–1353: The Complete History*. Woodbridge: Boydell Press, 2004.

Beroul, *The Romance of Tristan*. Trans. Alan S Fedrick. Harmondsworth: Penguin, 1970.

Berman, Jonathan M., *Anti-Vaxxers: How to Challenge a Misinformed Movement*. Cambridge, MA: MIT Press, 2020.

Bibby, Geoffrey, *Looking for Dilmun*. London: Collins, 1970. Penguin, 1984.

Blaser, Martin J, *Missing Microbes: How Killing Bacteria Creates Modern Plagues*. New York: Henry Holt; London: Oneworld Publications, 2014.

Bonser, Wilfrid, *The Medical Background of Anglo-Saxon England: A Study in History, Psychology, and Folklore*. London: The Wellcome Historical Medical Library,1963.

Borsch, Stuart J, *The Black Death in Egypt and England: A Comparative Study*. Austin: University of Texas Press, 2005.

Bowker, John, *Is God a Virus?: Genes, Culture and Religion: The Gresham Lectures, 1992–3*. London: SPCK, 1995.

Brandon, SGF, *Creation Legends of the Ancient Near East*. London: Hodder & Stoughton, 1963.

Brands, Hal, and Gavin, Francis J. (eds.), *COVID-19 and World Order: The Future of Conflict, Competition and Cooperation*. Baltimore: Johns Hopkins University Press, 2020.

Brockden Brown, Charles, *Arthur Mervyn; Or, Memoirs Of The Year 1793*. Philadelphia: David McKay, 1889.

Brody, Saul Nathaniel, *The Disease of the Soul: Leprosy in Medieval Literature*. Ithaca and London: Cornell University Press, 1974.

Brown, Kevin, *Penicillin Man: Alexander Fleming and the Antibiotic Revolution*. Stroud: Sutton, 2005.

______, *The Pox: The Life and Near Death of a Very Social Disease*. Stroud: Sutton, 2006.

______, *Poxed and Scurvied: The Story of Sickness & Health at Sea*. Barnsley: Seaforth Publishing, 2011.

Brunton, Deborah (ed.), *Health, Disease and Society in Europe, 1800–1930:*

A Source Book. Manchester: Manchester University Press, 2004.

Burnet, Sir Macfarlane, *Natural History of Infectious Disease*. Cambridge: Cambridge University Press, 1972.

Bynum, Helen, *Spitting Blood: The History of Tuberculosis*. Oxford: Oxford University Press, 2012.

Bynum, WF et al., *The Western Medical Tradition: 1800 to 2000*. New York: Cambridge University Press, 2006.

Bynum, William, *The History of Medicine: A Very Short Introduction*. Oxford: Oxford University Press, 2008.

Byrne, Joseph P, *Daily Life During the Black Death*. Westport, CT: Greenwood Press, 2006.

Byron, John, *Cain and Abel in Text and Tradition: Jewish and Christian Interpretations of the First Sibling Rivalry*. Leiden: Brill, 2011.

Calvert, Jonathan, & Arbuthnott, George. *Failures of State: The Inside Story of Britain's Battle with Coronavirus*. London: HarperCollins, 2021.

Cameron, Ian, *The Impossible Dream: The Building of the Panama Canal*. London: Hodder and Stoughton, 1971.

Cameron, ML, *Anglo-Saxon Medicine*. Cambridge, Cambridge University Press, 1993.

Campbell, Bruce MS (ed.), *Before the Black Death: Studies in the 'Crisis' of the Early Fourteenth Century*. Manchester: Manchester University Press, 1991.

Camplin, John M, *On Diabetes and its Successful Treatment*. New York: SS and W Wood, 1861.

Carter, HR, Carter, LA & Frost WH (eds.), *Yellow Fever: An Epidemiological and Historical Study of its Place of Origin*, Baltimore: Williams & Wilkins, 1931.

Cartwright, Frederick F & Biddiss, Michael, *Disease & History*. London, 1972. 3rd Ed: London: Thistle Publishing, 2014.

Chamberlin, ER (ed.), *The Black Death: A Collection of Contemporary Material*. London: Jonathan Cape, 1968.

Chambers, Paul, *Bedlam: London's Hospital for the Mad*. Hersham: Ian Allan Publishing, 2009.

Chan, Alina, and Ridley, Matt. *Viral: The Search for the Origin of COVID-19*.

London: Fourth Estate, 2021.
Chatwin, Bruce, *The Anatomy of Restlessness: Uncollected Writings*. London: Picador, 1997.
Clark, Linda and Rawcliffe, Carole (eds.), *The Fifteenth Century: Society in an Age of Plague*. Woodbridge: The Boydell Press, 2013.
Close, William T, *Ebola*. New York: Ivy Books, 1995. London: Arrow, 1995.
______, *Ebola: Through the Eyes of the People*. New York: Meadowlark Springs, 2002.
Cockburn, Aidan, Cockburn, Eve and Reyman, Theodore A (eds.), *Mummies, Disease and Ancient Cultures*. Cambridge: Cambridge University Press, 2nd ed. 1998.
Cohen, JM (ed. and trans.), *The Four Voyages of Christopher Columbus*. Harmondsworth: Penguin Books, 1969.
Cole, G and Waldron, T, 'Apple Down 152: A putative case of syphilis from sixth century AD Anglo-Saxon England.' *American Journal of Physical Anthropology*, 144, 2011.
Collier, Richard, *The Plague of the Spanish Lady: The Influenza Pandemic of 1918–1919*. London: Allison & Busby, 1974.
Conrad, Lawrence I, Neve, Michael, Nutton, Vivian, Porter, Roy & Wear, Andrew, *The Western Medical Tradition, 800 BC to AD 1800*. Cambridge: Cambridge University Press, 1995.
Conrad, Lawrence I and Wujastyk, Dominik (eds.), *Contagion: Perspectives from Pre-modern Societies*. Aldershot: Ashgate, 2000.
Conti da Foligno, S Dei, *Le Storie de suoi Tempi*, vol 2. Rome, 1883.
Crawford, Dorothy H, *The Invisible Enemy: A Natural History of Viruses*. Oxford: Oxford University Press, 2000.
______, *Deadly Companions: How Microbes Shaped Our History*. Oxford: Oxford University Press, 2007.
______, *Viruses: A Very Short Introduction*. Oxford: Oxford University Press, 2011.
______, *Virus Hunt: The Search for the Origin of HIV*. Oxford: Oxford University Press, 2013.
Creighton, Charles, *A History of Epidemics in Britain: from A.D. 664 to*

the Extinction of the Plague. Cambridge: Cambridge University Press, 1891.

______, *A History of Epidemics in Britain: from the Extinction of Plague to the Present Time*. Cambridge: Cambridge University Press, 1894.

Crosby, Alfred W, *America's Forgotten Pandemic: The Influenza of 1918*. Cambridge: Cambridge University Press, 1989.

Curtin, Philip D, *Death by Migration: Europe's Encounter with the Tropical World in the Nineteenth Century*. Cambridge: Cambridge University Press, 1989.

D'Ardois, GS, 'La Viruela en la Nueva España'. *Gaceta Médica de México* 91, 1961.

Davies, Professor Dame Sally C, Grant, Dr Jonathan and Catchpole, Professor Mike, *The Drugs Don't Work: A Global Threat*. London: Penguin, 2013.

Davis, Mike, *Late Victorian Holocausts: El Niño, Famines and the Making of the Third World*. London; New York: Verso, 2001.

______, *The Monster at our Door: The Global Threat of Avian Flu*. New York, London: The New Press, 2005.

______, *The Monster Enters: COVID-19, Avian Flu and the Plagues of Capitalism*. New York-London: OR Books, 2020.

Graaf, John de, Wann, David & Naylor, Thomas H, *Affluenza: How Overconsumption is Killing Us – and How We Can Fight Back*. San Francisco: Berrett-Koehler Publishers, Inc., 2014.

Delaporte, François, trans. Arthur Goldhammer, *Disease and Civilization: The Cholera in Paris, 1832*. Cambridge, MA: MIT Press, 1986.

Demaitre, Luke, *Leprosy in Premodern Medicine: A Malady of the Whole Body*. Baltimore: Johns Hopkins University Press, 2007.

Desowitz, Robert, *The Malaria Capers: Tales of Parasites and People*. New York: WW Norton, 1993.

______, *Tropical Diseases: From 50,000 BC to 2500 AD*. London: Flamingo, 1997.

Dickens, Charles, *Nicholas Nickleby*. London: 1838–9.

Dobson, Mary J, *Contours of Death and Disease in Early Modern England*. Cambridge: Cambridge University Press, 1997.

______, *Disease: The Extraordinary Stories Behind History's Deadliest Killers.* London: Quercus, 2007

Dodds, Ben and Britnell, Richard (eds.), *Agriculture and Rural Society after the Black Death: Common Themes and Regional Variations.* Hatfield: University of Hertfordshire Press, 2008.

Dols, Michael W, *The Black Death in the Middle East*. Princeton: Princeton University Press, 1977.

Dols, Michael W, edited by Diana E Immisch, *Majnūn: The Madman in Medieval Islamic Society.* Oxford: Clarendon Press, 1992.

Donoghue, Helen D, Marcsik, Antónia, Matheson, Carney, Vernon, Kim, Nuorala, Emilia, Molto, Joseph E, Greenblatt, Charles L & Spigelman, Mark, 'Co–infection of Mycobacterium tuberculosis and Mycobacterium leprae in human archaeological samples: a possible explanation for the historical decline of leprosy'. DOI: 10.1098/rspb.2004.2966. Published 22 February 2005.

Dubos, René and Dubos, Jean, *The White Plague: Tuberculosis, Man, and Society.* New Brunswick, NJ: Rutgers University Press, 1987.

Dunn, Oliver and Kelley, James E (editors and translators), *The Diario of Christopher Columbus's First Voyage to America 1492–1493*, Norman, Oklahoma, and London: University of Oklahoma Press, 1989.

Dutour, Olivier et al, *L'origine de la syphilis en Europe: avant ou après 1493?: actes du colloque international de Toulon, 25–28 novembre 1993*. Toulon: Centre Archéologique du Var, 1994.

Dutton, Diana B with contributions by Thomas A Preston & Nancy E Pfund, *Worse than the Disease: Pitfalls of Medical Progress.* Cambridge: Cambridge University Press, 1988.

Echenberg, Myron, *Black Death, White Medicine: Bubonic Plague and the Politics of Public Health in Colonial Senegal, 1914–1945*. Oxford: James Currey, Ltd, 2002.

______, *Plague Ports: The Global Urban Impact of Bubonic Plague, 1894–1901.* New York University Press, 2007.

______, *Africa in the Time of Cholera: A History of Pandemics from 1817 to the Present*. New York: Cambridge University Press, 2011.

Eco, Umberto, *Faith in Fakes*. London: Vintage, 1998.

Edmond, Rod, *Leprosy and Empire: A Medical and Cultural History*. Cambridge: Cambridge University Press, 2006.

Elmer, Peter, *The Miraculous Conformist: Valentine Greatrakes, the Body Politic, and the Politics of Healing in Restoration Britain*. Oxford: Oxford University Press, 2013.

Elmer, Peter (editor), *The Healing Arts: Health, Disease and Society in Europe, 1500–1800*. Manchester: Manchester University Press, 2004.

Elmer, Peter & Grell, Ole Peter (eds.), *Health, Disease and Society in Europe, 1500–1800: A Source Book*. Manchester: Manchester University Press, 2004.

Erdkamp, Paul (ed.), *The Cambridge Companion to Ancient Rome*. Cambridge: Cambridge University Press, 2013.

Ewald, Paul W, *Evolution of Infectious Disease*. Oxford: Oxford University Press, 1996.

Farrar, Jeremy, with Ahuja, Anjana. *Spike: The Virus vs. the People – The Inside Story*. London: Profile Books, 2021.

Farrell, JG, *The Lung*. London: Corgi, 1968.

Fenner, Frank, Henderson, Donald A, Arita, Isao, Ježek, Zdeněk & Ladnyi, Ivan D, *Smallpox and its Eradication*. Geneva: World Health Organization, 1988.

Fiennes, Richard, *Man, Nature and Disease*. London: Weidenfeld & Nicolson, 1964.

Finkel, Irving L and Geller, Markham J (eds.), *Disease in Babylonia*. Leiden: Brill, 2013.

Fletcher, Angus, *Allegory: The Theory of a Symbolic Mode*. Ithaca, London: Cornell University Press, 1970 (orig. 1964)

Foster, EA, *Motolinia's History of the Indians of New Spain*. Berkeley: Cortes Society, 1950.

Garrett, Laurie, *Betrayal of Trust: The Collapse of Global Public Health*. Oxford: Oxford University Press, 2002.

______, *The Coming Plague: Newly Emerging Diseases in a World out of Balance*. Penguin: 1994.

Gatacre, WF, *Report on the Bubonic Plague in Bombay: 1896–97*. Bombay: Times of India, 1897.

Gilbert, Sarah, and Green, Catherine, with Crewe, Deborah. *Vaxxers: The Inside Story of the Oxford AstraZeneca Vaccine and the Race Against the Virus*. London: Hodder & Stoughton, 2021.

Gilman, Sander L, *Obesity: The Biography*. Oxford: Oxford University Press, 2010.

Goldacre, Ben, *Bad Pharma: How Medicine is Broken, and How we can Fix It*. London: Fourth Estate, 2013.

Goldsmith, Connie, *Understanding Coronaviruses: SARS, MERS, and the COVID-19 Pandemic*. Minneapolis, MN: Twenty-First Century Books, 2022.

Gould, Tony, *Don't Fence Me In: Leprosy in Modern Times*. London: Bloomsbury, 2005.

Grainger, Ian et al., *The Black Death Cemetery, East Smithfield, London*. London: Museum of London Archaeology Services, 2008.

Green, Monica H, *Women's Healthcare in the Medieval West: Texts and Contexts*. Aldershot: Ashgate, 2000.

Greenfield, Karl Taro. *China Syndrome: The True Story of the 21st Century's First Great Epidemic*. London: Penguin, 2006.

Grmek, Mirko D, *Diseases in the Ancient Greek World*. trans. Mireille Muellner and Leonard Muellner. Baltimore, MD: The Johns Hopkins University Press, 1989.

Gross, Charles G, *Brain, Vision, Memory: Tales in the History of Neuroscience*. Cambridge, MA; London: MIT Press, 1998.

______, *A Hole in the Head: More Tales in the History of Neuroscience*. Cambridge, MA; London: MIT Press, 2009.

Grove, David I, *Tapeworms, Lice and Prions: A Compendium of Unpleasant Infections*. Oxford: Oxford University Press, 2013.

Grundy, Isobel, *Lady Mary Wortley Montagu*. Oxford: Oxford University Press, 1999.

Guillemin, Jeanne, *Anthrax: The Investigation of a Deadly Outbreak*. Berkeley; London: University of California Press, 1999.

Gummer, Benedict, *The Scourging Angel: The Black Death in the British Isles*. London: The Bodley Head, 2009.

Halliday, Stephen, *The Great Stink of London: Sir Joseph Bazalgette and the*

Cleansing of the Victorian Capital. Stroud: Sutton, 1999.

Hamilton, Mary *The Cure Of Disease in Pagan Temples and Christian Churches*. St Andrews: W. C. Henderson & Son; London: Simpkin, Marshall, Hamilton, Kent & Co, 1906.

Hamilton, Naomi, 'Burials and Grave Goods', Çatalhöyük 1998 Archive Report.

Hamlin, Christopher, *Cholera: The Biography*. Oxford: Oxford University Press, 2009.

_____, *More than Hot: A Short History of Fever*. Baltimore, MD: Johns Hopkins University Press, 2014.

Harari, Yuval Noah, *Sapiens: A Brief History of Humankind*. London: Harvill Secker, 2014.

Harper, KN et al, 'The Origin and Antiquity of Syphilis Revisited: An Appraisal of Old World pre-Columbian evidence for treponemal infection', *American Journal of Physical Anthropology*, 146, 2011.

Harrak, Amir (trans. and ed.), *The Chronicle of Zuqnin, parts III and IV: AD 488–775*. Toronto: Pontifical Institute of Mediaeval Studies, 1999.

Harrison, Mark, *Disease and the Modern World: 1500 to the Present Day*. Cambridge: Polity Press, 2004.

_____, *Contagion: How Commerce has Spread Disease*. New Haven, London: Yale University Press, 2012.

Hart, Gerald D, *Asclepius: The God of Medicine*. London: Royal Society of Medicine Press, 2000.

Hatcher, John, *Plague, Population and the English Economy, 1348–1530*. London: Macmillan, 1977.

_____, *The Black Death: An Intimate History*. London: Weidenfeld & Nicolson, 2008.

Häusler, Thomas, *Viruses Vs. Superbugs: A Solution to the Antibiotics Crisis?* Basingstoke: Palgrave Macmillan, 2006.

Hayden, Deborah, *Pox: Genius, Madness, and the Mysteries of Syphilis*. New York: Basic Books, 2003.

Hays, JN, *Epidemics and Pandemics: Their Impacts on Human History*. Santa Barbara, CA: ABC-CLIO, 2005.

Hecker, Justus (trans. BG Babington), *The Black Death and The Dancing*

Mania. London: Cassell, 1888.

Heinberg, Richard, *Memories and Visions of Paradise: Exploring the Universal Myth of a Lost Golden Age*. London: Aquarian Press, 1990.

Heine, Heinrich, *French Affairs: Letters from Paris, Vol. I*, in *The Works of Heinrich Heine, Vol. VII*, trans. Charles Godfrey Leland. London: William Heinemann, 1893.

Hempel, Sandra, *The Medical Detective: John Snow, Cholera and the Mystery of the Broad Street Pump*. London: Granta, 2007.

Herlihy, David, *The Black Death and the Transformation of the West*. New Haven and London: Harvard University Press, 1997.

Hershkovitz, Israel et al, 'Detection and Molecular Characterization of 9000-Year-Old *Mycobacterium tuberculosis* from a Neolithic Settlement in the Eastern Mediterranean', 2008.

Hesiod, *Works and Days*, in *Hesiod and Theognis*, trans. Dorothea Wender. Harmondsworth: Penguin, 1973.

Hirsch, August, *Handbook of Geographical and Historical Pathology*, trans. Charles Creighton, 3 vols, London: 1883–6.

Honigsbaum, Mark, *Living with Enza: The Forgotten Story of Britain and the Great Flu Pandemic of 1918*. London: New York: Macmillan, 2009.

______, *The Pandemic Century: A History of Global Contagion from the Spanish Flu to COVID-19*. London: Penguin, 2020.

Hopkins, Donald R, *The Greatest Killer: Smallpox in History*. Chicago/London: University of Chicago Press, 2002. Originally published as *Princes and Peasants: Smallpox in History*, 1983.

Hooper, Ed, *Slim: A Reporter's Own Story of AIDS in East Africa*. London: The Bodley Head, 1990.

______, *The River: A Journey Back to the Source of HIV and AIDS*. London: Allen Lane, 1999.

Hope, Tony, *Medical Ethics: A Very Short Introduction*. Oxford: Oxford University Press, 2004.

Horrox, Rosemary (ed.), *The Black Death*. Manchester Medieval Sources Series. Manchester; New York: Manchester University Press, 1994.

Horton, Richard. *The COVID-19 Catastrophe: What's Gone Wrong and How to Stop it Happening Again*. 2nd edition. London, Polity Press. 2021.

Huet, Marie Hélène, *The Culture of Disaster*. Chicago, IL; London: University of Chicago Press, 2012.

Iliffe, John, *The African AIDS Epidemic: A History*. Oxford: James Currey Ltd, 2006.

Jackson, Mark, *Allergy: The History of a Modern Malady*. London: Reaktion, 2006.

______, *Asthma: The Biography*. Oxford: Oxford University Press, 2009.

James, Oliver, *Affluenza: How to be Successful and Stay Sane*. London: Vermilion, 2007.

______, *The Selfish Capitalist: Origins of Affluenza*. London: Vermilion, 2008.

Jannetta, Ann Bowman, *Epidemics and Mortality in Early Modern Japan*. Princeton, NJ: Princeton University Press, 2014.

Jillings, Karen, *Scotland's Black Death: The Foul Death of the English*. Stroud: Tempus, 2002.

Johnson, Niall, *Britain and the 1918–19 Influenza Pandemic: A Dark Epilogue*. Abingdon: Routledge, 2006.

Johnson, Steven, *The Ghost Map: A Street, an Epidemic and the Hidden Power of Urban Networks*. London: Penguin Books, 2008.

Jones, Susan D, *Death in a Small Package: A Short History of Anthrax*. Baltimore, MD.: Johns Hopkins University Press, 2010.

Karlen, Arno, *Plague's Progress: A Social History of Man and Disease*. London: Indigo, 1996.

Kaufmann, Stefan (trans. by Michael Capone), *The New Plagues: Pandemics and Poverty in a Globalized World*. London: Haus Publishing, 2009.

Kelly, John, *The Great Mortality: An Intimate History of the Black Death*. London: Harper Perennial, 2006.

Khamsi, Roxanne, 'Were "cursed" rams the first biological weapons?', *New Scientist*, 26 November 2007.

King, Helen, *Greek and Roman Medicine*. London: Bristol Classical Press, 2001.

______, *The Disease of Virgins: Green Sickness, Chlorosis and the Problems of Puberty*. London: Routledge, 2004.

______ (ed.), *Health in Antiquity*. London: Routledge, 2005.

Kiple, Kenneth F (ed.), *The Cambridge World History of Human Disease.* Cambridge: Cambridge University Press, 1993.

______ (ed.), *Plague, Pox and Pestilence: Disease in History.* London: Weidenfeld & Nicolson, 1997. Phoenix Illustrated: 1999.

______, *The Cambridge Historical Dictionary of Disease.* Cambridge: Cambridge University Press, 2003.

Koch, Tom, *Disease Maps: Epidemics on the Ground.* Chicago, London: University of Chicago Press, 2011.

______, *Cartographies of Disease: Maps, Mapping, and Medicine.* 2005.

Kohn, George C (ed.), *The Wordsworth Encyclopedia of Plague and Pestilence.* Ware: Wordsworth Reference, 1998.

Kolata, Gina, *Flu: The Story of the Great Influenza Pandemic of 1918 and the Search for the Virus that Caused It.* London: Pan, 2001.

Landes, David S, *The Unbound Prometheus: Technological Change and Industrial Development in Western Europe from 1750 to the Present.* London: Cambridge University Press, 1969.

Lane, Joan, *A Social History of Medicine: Health, Healing and Disease in England, 1750–1950.* London: Routledge, 2001.

Lax, Eric, *The Mould in Dr Florey's Coat: The Remarkable True Story of the Penicillin Miracle.* London: Abacus, 2005.

Lee, Richard B and Daly, Richard (eds.), *The Cambridge Encyclopedia of Hunters and Gatherers.* Cambridge: Cambridge University Press, 2004.

Le Fanu, James, *The Rise and Fall of Modern Medicine.* London: Abacus, 2011.

Leeming, David, *The Oxford Companion to World Mythology.* Oxford, New York: Oxford University Press, 2005.

Little, Lester K (ed.), *Plague and the End of Antiquity: The Pandemic of 541–750.* New York: Cambridge University Press in association with The American Academy in Rome, 2007.

Littman, RJ and Littman, ML, 'Galen and the Antonine Plague', *The American Journal of Philology,* Vol. 94, No. 3, Autumn, 1973.

Lloyd, GER (ed.), *Hippocratic Writings.* Trans, Chadwick, et al. 2nd edition, 1978. Harmondsworth: Penguin Classics, 1983.

Longmate, Norman, *King Cholera: The Biography of a Disease.* London: Hamish Hamilton, 1966.

Lord, Evelyn, *The Great Plague: A People's History.* New Haven and London: Yale University Press, 2014.

MacGowan, AT, *Malaria, the Common Cause of Cholera.* London: 1866.

Major, Ralph Hermon, *Classic Descriptions of Disease.* Springfield, IL: CC Thomas, 1932. London, 1948.

Marcombe, David, *Leper Knights.* Woodbridge: Boydell Press, 2003.

Marsh, Henry, *Do No Harm: Stories of Life, Death and Brain Surgery.* London: Weidenfeld & Nicolson, 2014.

Martin, Paul S, *Twilight of the Mammoths: Ice Age Extinctions and the Rewilding of America.* Berkeley, CA; London: University of California Press, 2005.

Martin, Peter, *Samuel Johnson: A Biography.* London: Weidenfeld and Nicolson, 2008.

Martin, Seán, *The Black Death.* Harpenden: Oldcastle Books, 2007.

Matossian, Mary Kilbourne, *Poisons of the Past: Molds, Epidemics, and History.* New Haven: Yale University Press, 1991.

Mattern, Susan P, *Galen and the Rhetoric of Healing.* Baltimore, MD: The Johns Hopkins University Press, 2008.

______, *The Prince of Medicine: Galen in the Roman Empire.* Oxford: Oxford University Press, 2013.

McAlister, Neil Harding, 'The Dancing Pilgrims at Muelebeek', *Journal of the History of Medicine and Allied Sciences* 32, 1977.

McCormick, Joseph B, Fisher-Hoch, Susan with Horvitz, Leslie Alan, *The Virus Hunters: Dispatches from the Frontline.* London: Bloomsbury, 1997.

______, *Level 4 Virus Hunters of the CDC.* New York: Barnes and Noble, 1999.

McKenna, Maryn, *Superbug: The Fatal Menace of MRSA.* New York: Free Press, 2010.

McKeown, Thomas, *The Origins of Human Disease.* Oxford: Basil Blackwell, 1988.

McNeill, William H, *Plagues and Peoples.* Garden City, NY; Anchor

Press, 1976. London: Penguin, 1994.

Medlock, Dr Jolyon M and Leach, Steve A, 'Effect of climate change on vector-borne disease risk in the UK'. *The Lancet*, published online: 23 March 2015. DOI: http://dx.doi.org/10.1016/S1473–3099(15)70091–5.

Miller, Timothy S, Nesbitt, John W, *Walking Corpses: Leprosy in Byzantium and the Medieval West*. Ithaca, NY and London: Cornell University Press, 2014.

Mills, ID, 'The 1918–1919 Influenza Pandemic – The Indian Experience', *Indian Economic and Social History Review* 23, 1986.

Mitchell-Boyask, Robin, *Plague and the Athenian Imagination: Drama, History and the Cult of Asclepius*. Cambridge: Cambridge University Press, 2008.

Mithen, Steven, *After the Ice: A Global Human History, 20,000–5000 BC*. London: Weidenfeld & Nicolson, 2003.

Molleson, Theya and Andrews, Peter, 'The Human Remains'. Çatalhöyük 1997 Archive Report.

Money, Nicholas P, *Microbiology: A Very Short Introduction*. Oxford: Oxford University Press, 2014.

_____, *The Amoeba in the Room: Lives of the Microbes*. Oxford: Oxford University Press, 2014.

Montagu, Lady Mary Wortley, with an introduction by Anita Desai; text edited and annotated by Malcolm Jack, *The Turkish Embassy Letters*. London: Virago Press, 1984.

Mooney, James. *Myths of the Cherokee: Extract from the Nineteenth Annual Report of the Bureau of American Ethnology*. Washington DC, Government Printing Office, 1902.

More, Sir Thomas, *The Apologie of Syr T More, Knyght*.

Morton, RS, *Venereal Diseases*. Harmondsworth: Penguin, 1972.

Moseley, William Willis, *Eleven Chapters on Nervous or Mental Complaints*. London: Simpkin, Marshall, 1838.

Mukherjee, Siddhartha, *The Emperor of all Maladies: A Biography of Cancer*. London: Fourth Estate, 2011.

Muntner, Suessman (ed.), *The Medical Writings of Moses Maimonides*.

Philadelphia: JB Lippincott Company, 1963.
Naphy, William and Spicer, Andrew, *The Black Death: A History of Plagues, 1345–1730*. Stroud: Tempus, 2001.
Neal, Frank, *Black '47: Britain and the famine Irish*. Basingstoke: Macmillan, 1997.
Needham, Joseph, with the collaboration of Lu Gwei-Djen; edited and with an introduction by Nathan Sivin, *Science and Civilisation in China, Vol. 6, Pt. 6: Medicine*. Cambridge: Cambridge University Press, 2000.
Nikiforuk, Andrew, *The Fourth Horseman: A Short History of Epidemics, Plagues and Other Scourges*. London: Fourth Estate, 1991.
______, *Pandemonium: Bird Flu, Mad Cow Disease and Other Biological Plagues of the 21st Century*. Toronto: Viking Canada, 2006.
Nohl, Johannes, *The Black Death: A Chronicle of the Plague*. Translated by CH Clarke. London, 1926.
Nunn, John F, *Ancient Egyptian Medicine*. London: British Museum Press, 1996.
Nutton, Vivian, *Ancient Medicine*. London: Routledge, 2004. 2nd edition: London: Routledge, 2013.
Oberhelman, Steven M (ed.), *Dreams, Healing, and Medicine in Greece: From Antiquity to the Present*. Farnham: Ashgate, 2013.
Oldstone, Michael BA, *Viruses, Plagues & History: Past, Present and Future*. New York: Oxford University Press, 2010.
Ortner, DJ and Aufderheide, AC (eds.), *Human Paleopathology: Current Syntheses and Future Options*. Washington DC: Smithsonian Institution Press, 1991.
Oshinsky, David M, *Polio: An American Story*. Oxford: Oxford University Press, 2006.
Packard, Randall M, *The Making of a Tropical Disease: A Short History of Malaria*. Baltimore, MD: Johns Hopkins University Press, 2007.
Pálfi, G, Dutour, O, Deák J and Hutás, I (eds.), *Tuberculosis Past and Present*. Golden Book Publishers TB Foundation: Budapest, 1999.
Pankhurst, Richard, *The History of Famine and Epidemics in Ethiopia Prior to the Twentieth Century*. Addis Ababa, 1986.

Pappas, Georgios et al, 'Insights into Infectious Disease in the Era of Hippocrates', *International Journal of Infectious Diseases*, vol. 12 issue 4, July 2008.

Patterson, K David, 'Typhus and its Control in Russia, 1870–1940', *Medical History* 37, 1993.

Paul the Deacon, *Historia Langobardorum*.

Pennington, Hugh, 'Don't Pick Your Nose', in *London Review of Books*, Vol. 27 No. 24, 15 December 2005, 29–31.

Pierce, John R and Writer, Jim, *Yellow Jack: How Yellow Fever Ravaged America and Walter Reed Discovered its Deadly Secrets.* Hoboken, NJ: Wiley, 2005.

Piot, Peter et al, 'Acquired Immunodeficiency Syndrome in a Heterosexual Population in Zaire', *The Lancet* ii, 1984.

Piot, Peter with Marshall, Ruth, *No time to Lose: A Life in Pursuit of Deadly Viruses.* New York: WW Norton, 2012.

Pliny the Elder, *The Natural History.* Trans. John Bostock and HT Riley. London: Taylor and Francis, 1855.

Pollington, Stephen, *Leechcraft: Early English Charms, Plant Lore, and Healing*. Hockwold-cum-Wilton: Anglo-Saxon Books, 2000.

Pontius the Deacon, *The Life and Passion of Cyprian, Bishop and Martyr.* Online e-text.

Porter, Katherine Anne, *Pale Horse, Pale Rider.* London, Penguin: 2011.

Porter, Roy, *The Medical History of Waters and Spas.* London: Wellcome Institute for the History of Medicine, 1990.

______, (ed.), *The Faber Book of Madness.* London: Faber and Faber, 1991.

______, *The Greatest Benefit to Mankind: A Medical History of Humanity from Antiquity to the Present.* London: Fontana Press, 1997.

______, *Quacks: Fakers and Charlatans in English Medicine.* Stroud: Tempus, 2000.

______, *Bodies Politic: Disease, Death and Doctors in Britain, 1650–1900.* London: Reaktion, 2001

______, *The Cambridge Illustrated History of Medicine.* Cambridge: Cambridge University Press, 2001.

______, *Blood & Guts: A Short History of Medicine.* London: Penguin, 2003.

Porter, Roy and Rousseau, GS, *Gout: The Patrician Malady*. New Haven, CT; London: Yale University Press London, 1998.

Preston, Richard, *The Hot Zone: The Chilling True Story of an Ebola Outbreak*. London: Arrow, 1994.

Pybus, Oliver G, Lemey, Philippe et al, 'The Early Spread and Epidemic Ignition of HIV-1 in Human Populations', *Science*, 3 October 2014.

Quammen, David, *Spillover: Animal Infections and the Next Human Pandemic*. London: Vintage Books, 2013.

______, *Ebola: The Natural and Human History*. London: The Bodley Head, 2014.

Quétel, Claude, *History of Syphilis*. Translated by Judith Braddock and Brian Pike. Cambridge: Polity Press, 1990.

Quinn, Tom, *Flu: A Social History of Influenza*. London: New Holland, 2008.

Ranger, Terence and Slack, Paul (eds.), *Epidemics and Ideas: Essays on the Historical Perception of Pestilence*. Cambridge: Cambridge University Press, 1992.

Rawcliffe, Carole, *Medicine for the Soul: The Life, Death and Resurrection of an English Medieval Hospital, St Giles's, Norwich, c.1249–1550*. Stroud: Sutton, 1999.

______, *Medicine & Society in Later Medieval England*. Stroud: Sutton, 1997.

______, *Leprosy in Medieval England*. Woodbridge: Boydell, 2009.

______, *Urban Bodies: Communal Health in Late Medieval English Towns and Cities*. Woodbridge: The Boydell Press, 2013.

Reader, John, *Cities*. London: Vintage, 2005.

Redgrove, H Stanley, *Alchemy Ancient and Modern*. London: Rider, 1922.

Reilly, Joanne, *Belsen: The Liberation of a Concentration Camp*. London: Routledge, 1997.

Rhodes, John, *The End of Plagues: The Global Battle Against Infectious Disease*. New York: Palgrave Macmillan, 2013.

Richards, Peter, *The Medieval Leper and his Northern Heirs*. Cambridge: DS Brewer, 2000.

Rivers, Thomas M (ed.), *Viral and Rickettsial Infections of Man*.

Philadelphia: JB Lippincott Company, 1948.
Roberts, Charlotte and Manchester, Keith, *The Archaeology of Disease.* 1983. 3rd ed. Stroud: History Press, 2010.
Roberts, Charlotte & Cox, Margaret, *Health & Disease in Britain: From Prehistory to the Present Day.* Stroud: Sutton Publishing, 2003.
Roberts, Charlotte A, Lewis, Mary E and Manchester, Keith (eds.), *The Past and Present of Leprosy: Archaeological, Historical, Palaeopathological and Clinical Approaches.* Oxford: Archaeopress, 2002.
Rocco, Fiammetta, *The Miraculous Fever-tree: Malaria, Medicine and the Cure that Changed the World.* London: HarperCollins, 2003
Rosebury, Theodor, *Microbes and Morals: The Strange Story of Venereal Disease.* New York: Viking, 1971.
Salzberg, Steven, 'Anti-Vaccine Movement Causes Worst Measles Epidemic In 20 Years', *Forbes*, 1 February 2015.
Saracci, Rodolfo, *Epidemiology: A Very Short Introduction.* Oxford: Oxford University Press, 2010.
Sargent, Carolyn F and Johnson, Thomas M (eds.), *Medical Anthropology: Contemporary Theory and Method.* Westport, CT: Praeger, 1996.
Scull, Andrew, *Hysteria: The Biography.* Oxford: Oxford University Press, 2009.
______, *Madness: A Very Short Introduction.* Oxford: Oxford University Press, 2011.
Shah, Sonia, *The Fever: How Malaria has Ruled Humankind for 500,000 Years.* Crows Nest, NSW: Allen & Unwin, 2010.
Shilts, Randy, *And the Band Played On: Politics, People, and the AIDS Epidemic.* New York: St Martin's Press, 1987. London: Souvenir Press, 2011.
Shnayerson, Michael and Mark Plotkin, *The Killers Within: The Deadly Rise of Drug Resistant Bacteria.* London: Time Warner Books, 2003.
Shrewsbury, JFD, *A History of Bubonic Plague in the British Isles.* Cambridge: Cambridge University Press, 1970.
Shuttleton, David E, *Smallpox and the Literary Imagination, 1660–1820.* Cambridge: Cambridge University Press, 2012.
Singer, PN (ed.), with Daniel Davies and Vivian Nutton, *Galen:*

Psychological Writings. New York: Cambridge University Press, 2013.

Sipress, Alan, *The Fatal Strain: On the Trail of Avian Flu and the Coming Pandemic*. London: Penguin, 2010.

Sivertsen, Barbara J, *The Parting of the Sea: How Volcanoes, Earthquakes and Plagues Shaped the Story of Exodus*. Princeton, NJ: Princeton University Press, 2009.

Slack, Paul, *Plague: A Very Short Introduction*. Oxford: Oxford University Press, 2012.

Smallman-Raynor, Matthew and Cliff, Andrew, *War Epidemics: An Historical Geography of Infectious Diseases in Military Conflict and Civil Strife, 1850–2000*. Oxford: Oxford University Press, 2004.

______, *Atlas of Epidemic Britain: A Twentieth Century Picture*. Oxford: Oxford University Press, 2012.

Smallman-Raynor, Matthew, Cliff, Andrew and Haggett, Peter, *World Atlas of Epidemic Diseases*. Boca Raton, FL: CRC Press, 2004.

Smith, Christopher, *Late Stone Age Hunters of the British Isles*. London: Routledge, 1992.

Smith, FB, 'The Russian Influenza in the United Kingdom, 1889–1894', *Social History of Medicine*, 8 (1), 1995.

Snodgrass, Mary Ellen, *World Epidemics: A Cultural Chronology of Disease from Prehistory to the Era of SARS*. Jefferson, NC: McFarland & Company, 2003.

Sontag, Susan, *Illness as Metaphor*. New York: Farrar, Strauss, Giroux, 1978.

______, *AIDS and its Metaphors*. London: Allen Lane, 1989.

Speck, Reinhard S, *Bubonic Plague in San Francisco*. San Francisco: Book Club of California, 1977.

Spinage, CA, *Cattle Plague: A History*. New York: Kluwer Academic/ Plenum Publishers, 2003.

Spindler, K et al (eds.), *Human Mummies: A Global Survey of their Status and the Techniques of Conservation*. Vienna; New York: Springer, 2006.

Steele, Valerie, *The Corset: A Cultural History*. New Haven, CT ; London: Yale University Press, 2001.

Stephens, Trent and Brynner, Rock, *Dark Remedy: The Impact of*

Thalidomide and its Revival as a Vital Medicine. New York: Basic Books, 2001.

Stol, Marten, *Epilepsy in Babylonia*. Groningen: Styx Publications, 1993.

Suetonius, *The Twelve Caesars*, trans. Robert Graves, rev. James B Rives. London: Penguin, 2007.

Talbot, Michael, *The Holographic Universe*. London: Grafton, 1991.

Tattersall, Robert, *Diabetes: The Biography*. Oxford: Oxford University Press, 2009.

Taylor, Keith Weller, *The Birth of Vietnam*. Berkeley, London: University of California Press, 1983.

Temkin, Owsei, *The Falling Sickness: A History of Epilepsy from the Greeks to the Beginnings of Modern Neurology*. Baltimore, London: Johns Hopkins University Press, 1971.

Thirsk, Joan, *Alternative Agriculture: A History: From the Black Death to the Present Day*. Oxford: Oxford University Press, 1997.

Totaro, Rebecca, *Suffering in Paradise: The Bubonic Plague in English Literature from More to Milton*. Pittsburgh, Pa.: Duquesne University Press, 2005.

Trevisanato, Siro Igino, *The Plagues of Egypt: Archaeology, History and Science Look at the Bible*. Gorgias Press, 2005.

Twigg, Graham *The Black Death: A Biological Reappraisal*. London: Batsford Academic and Educational, 1984.

______, *Bubonic Plague: A Much Misunderstood Disease*. Ascot: Derwent Press, 2013.

Van Arsdall, Anne, *Medieval Herbal Remedies: The Old English Herbarium and Anglo-Saxon Medicine*. New York, London: Routledge, 2002.

Van der Eijk, Philip J, *Medicine and Philosophy in Classical Antiquity: Doctors and Philosophers on Nature, Soul, Health and Disease*. Cambridge: Cambridge University Press, 2005.

Voynich, EL & Opienski, Henryk (eds.), *Chopin's Letters*. New York: Dover, 1988.

Wagner, David M, Klunk, Jennifer, Harbeck, Michaela et al, '*Yersinia pestis* and the Plague of Justinian 541–543 AD: A Genomic Analysis', *The Lancet Infectious Diseases*, Volume 14, Issue 4, April 2014.

Waldron, Tony, *Palaeopathology*. New York, Cambridge: Cambridge University Press, 2009.

Wallace, Rob. *Big Farms Make Big Flu: Dispatches on Influenza, Agribusiness and the Nature of Science*. New York: Monthly Review Press, 2016.

Waller, John, *The Discovery of the Germ*. Duxford: Icon Books, 2002.

______, *A Time to Dance, A Time to Die: The Extraordinary Story of the Dancing Plague of 1518*. Thriplow: Icon Books, 2008.

Wallis, Faith (ed.), *Medieval Medicine: A Reader*. Toronto: University of Toronto Press, 2010.

Ward, Ned, *The London Spy* (1709). Paul Hyland, ed. East Lansing, MI: Colleagues Press, 1993.

Wasik, Bill and Murphy, Monica, *Rabid: A Cultural History of the World's Most Diabolical Virus*. New York: Penguin, 2013.

Watts, Sheldon, *Epidemics and History: Disease, Power, and Imperialism*. New Haven; London: Yale University Press, 1997.

Weatherall, David, *Thalassaemia: The Biography*. Oxford: Oxford University Press, 2010.

Webster, Charles (ed.), *Health, Medicine and Mortality in the Sixteenth Century*. Cambridge: Cambridge University Press, 1979.

Weindling, Paul Julian, *Epidemics and Genocide in Eastern Europe, 1890–1945*. Oxford: Oxford University Press, 2000.

Wertz, Richard W & Wertz, Dorothy C, *Lying-in: A History of Childbirth in America*. Yale University Press, 1989.

Williams, Gareth, *The Angel of Death: The Story of Smallpox*. London: Palgrave Macmillan, 2010.

______, *Paralysed with Fear: The Story of Polio*. Basingstoke: Palgrave Macmillan, 2013.

Willman, David, *The Mirage Man: Bruce Ivins, the Anthrax Attacks, and America's Rush to War*. London: Bantam, 2011.

Wills, Christopher, *Plagues: Their Origin, History and Future*. London: HarperCollins, 1996.

Wolfe, Nathan D, *The Viral Storm: The Dawn of a New Pandemic Age*. London: Penguin, 2012.

WHO/International Study Team, 'Ebola Haemorrhagic Fever in

Sudan, 1976'. *Bulletin of the World Health Organization*, issue 56, 1978.

Wright, Thomas, *Circulation: William Harvey's Revolutionary Idea*. London: Chatto & Windus, 2012.

Yaron, Reuven, *The Laws of Eshnunna*. Leiden: Brill, 1988.

Ziegler, Philip, *The Black Death*. London: Collins, 1969. Stroud: Sutton, 2003.

Zinsser, Hans, *Rats, Lice and History*. Boston: Little, Brown, 1935. London: Penguin Books, 2000.

Živanović, Srboljub, *Ancient Diseases: The Elements of Palaeopathology*. (Translated by Lovett F Edwards) London: Methuen, 1982.

Žižek, Slavoj, *Pandemic! COVID-19 Shakes the World*. New York-London: OR Books, 2020.

______, *Pandemic! 2: Chronicles of a Time Lost*. New York-London: OR Books, 2021.

Index

About the Author

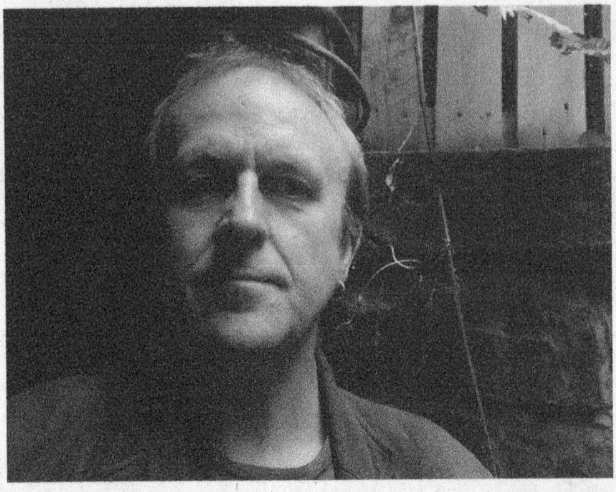

SEÁN MARTIN is the author of *The Knights Templar*, *The Cathars*, *The Gnostics*, *The Black Death*, *Alchemy and Alchemists*, *A Short History of Disease* and, for Kamera Books, *Andrei Tarkovsky* and *New Waves in Cinema*. His own films include *Lanterna Magicka: Bill Douglas & the Secret History of Cinema*, *Folie à Deux*, and a series of documentaries on Tarkovsky: *Tarkovsky's Andrei Rublev: A Journey* and *The Dream in the Mirror*.

oldcastlebooks.co.uk/sean-martin

Also by Seán Martin

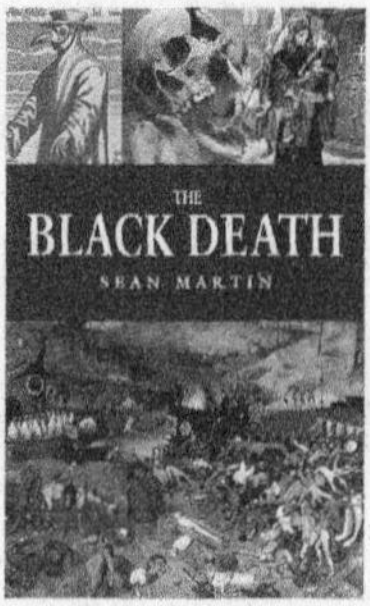

The Black Death is the name most commonly given to the pandemic of bubonic plague that ravaged the medieval world in the late 1340s. From Central Asia the plague swept through Europe, leaving millions of dead in its wake. A vivid and dramatic account of one of the great catastrophes of history, *The Black Death* examines the origins of the disease and traces its terrible march through Europe from the Italian cities to the far-flung corners of Scandinavia.

978-1-84344-604-0 £8.99

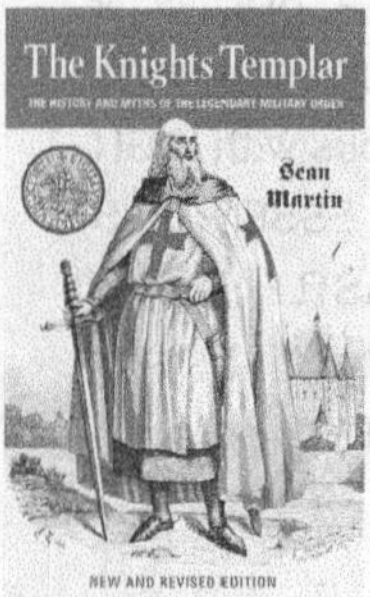

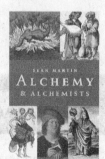

The Knights Templar were the most powerful military religious order of the Middle Ages. Formed to protect pilgrims in the Holy Land, they participated in the Crusades and rapidly gained wealth, lands and influence and were answerable to none save the Pope himself. They were also involved in developments in navigation, architecture, medicine, and engineering, amongst others.

978-1-84243-563-2 £12.99

Often alchemy is seen as an example of medieval gullibility and the alchemists as a collection of eccentrics and superstitious fools. In this Pocket Essential Seán Martin shows that nothing could be further from the truth. Tracing the history of alchemy from ancient times to the 20th century, the book covers a major, if neglected area of Western thought.

978-1-84344-609-5 £12.99